An Introduction to Medical Terminology

A SELF-TEACHING PACKAGE

Andrew Hutton BSc MSc

Lecturer in Life Science
EDINBURGH'S TELFORD COLLEGE, EDINBURGH, UK

SECOND EDITION

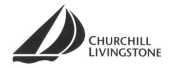

CHURCHILL LIVINGSTONE

EDINBURGH LONDON NEW YORK PHILADELPHIA SAN FRANCISCO SYDNEY AND TORONTO 1998

CHURCHILL LIVINGSTONE
A Division of Harcourt Brace and Company Limited

First edition 1993
Second edition 1998

ISBN 0 443 059659

British Library of Cataloguing in Publication Data
A catalogue record for this book is available from the British
Library.

Library of Congress Cataloging in Publication Data
A catalog record for this book is available from the Library of
Congress.

Note
Medical knowledge is constantly changing. As new information
becomes available, changes in treatment, procedures, equipment
and the use of drugs become necessary. The author and the
publishers have, as far as it is possible, taken care to ensure that
the information given in this text is accurate and up to date.
However, readers are strongly advised to confirm that the
information, especially with regard to drug usage, complies with
latest legislation and standards of practice.

The
publisher's
policy is to use
**paper manufactured
from sustainable forests**

Produced through Longman Malaysia, PP

About this book

This book is designed to introduce medical terms to students who have little prior knowledge of the language of medicine. Included in the text are simple, nontechnical descriptions of pathological conditions, medical instruments and clinical procedures.

The medical terms introduced by the text are based on body systems and each set of exercises provides the student with the opportunity to learn, review and assess new words. Once complete, the exercises will be a valuable reference text.

No prior knowledge of medicine is required to follow the text and, to ensure ease of use, the more complex details of word origins and analysis have been omitted. The book will thus be of great value to anyone who needs to learn medical terms quickly and efficiently.

Edinburgh 1997   Andrew Hutton

Acknowledgements

We are grateful to Aesculap Ltd incorporating Downs Surgical for permission to reproduce Figures 17, 18, 56 and 57. Figure 23 was redrawn from a catalogue supplied by A.C. Cossor & Son (Surgical) Ltd.

How to use this book

Before you begin working through the units, read through the introduction which explains the basic principles of reading, writing and understanding medical terms.

Once you have understood the elementary rules of medical word building, complete Units 1–20 which are based on different medical topics. These units can be studied in sequence or independently.

For ease of use each unit has the same basic plan and is arranged into:

 WORD EXERCISES

 AN ANATOMY EXERCISE

 A WORD CHECK

 A SELF-ASSESSMENT

The different parts of each unit are indicated by icons. For each unit:

1 Complete the word exercises . These are written exercises which can be completed using the exercise guide which lists prefixes and suffixes at the beginning of each unit. The answers to the word exercises are on p 231.

2 Complete the anatomy exercise which accompanies each body system unit.

3 You can now complete the word check , which lists all the relevant prefixes, roots and suffixes, to help you to revise all the word components introduced in the unit.

4 Try the self-assessment at the end of each unit. Aim to complete each test without the aid of your word lists. Check your answer on p 251 and record your score.

Note. A Quick Reference box containing medical word roots relevant to each system is given after the final word exercise of each unit.

Contents

Introduction

Students beginning any kind of medical or paramedical course are faced with a bewildering number of complex medical terms. Surprisingly it is possible to understand many medical terms and build new ones by learning relatively few words that can be combined in a variety of ways. Even the longest medical terms are easy to understand if you know the meaning of each component of the word. For example, you may never have heard of **laryngopharyngitis** but if you learn that **-itis** always means inflammation, **laryng/o** refers to the larynx or voice box and **pharyng/o** refers to the throat or pharynx, its meaning becomes apparent, i.e. inflammation of the pharynx and larynx. Laryngopharyngitis is an inflammation of the upper respiratory tract with symptoms of sore throat and loss of voice.

Most doctors, however, do not use precise medical terminology when conversing with patients. If patients hear a complex medical description of their illness, they may become frightened rather than reassured. Precise medical terms are used when medical records and letters are completed. They are also used when doctors discuss a patient and when medical material is published.

The terms you will use in this book describe common diseases and disorders, instruments, diagnostic techniques and therapies.

The components of medical words

In this introduction you will learn how to split medical terms into their components and deduce their meanings. Skills developed here will enable you to derive the meanings of unfamiliar medical words and improve your ability to understand medical literature.

Let us begin by using a medical word associated with an organ with which you are familiar, the stomach:

GASTROTOMY

First we can split the word and examine its individual components:

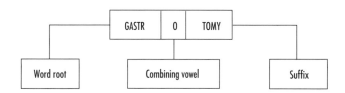

The word root

Roots are the basic medical words. Most are derived from Greek and Roman (Latin) words. Others have their origins in Arabic, Anglo-Saxon and German. Some early Greek words have been retained in their original form whilst others have been latinized. In their migrations throughout Europe and America many words have changed their spelling, meaning and pronunciation.

In our first example we have used the root **gastr** which always means stomach.

The combining vowel

Combining vowels are added to word roots to aid pronunciation and to connect the root to the suffix. In our first example we have used 'o'. All the combining vowels a, e, i, o and u are used but the most commonly used is o.

In our first example we have added the combining vowel **o** to the word root.

The suffix

The suffix follows the word root, i.e. it is found at the end of the word. It also adds to or modifies the meaning of the word root.

In our first example we have used the suffix **-tomy** which always means to form an incision.

We can now fully understand the meaning of our first medical word:

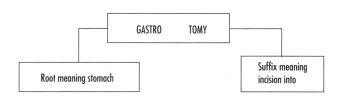

Therefore the meaning of gastrotomy is – incision into the stomach. Gastrotomy is a name used by surgeons to describe an operation in which a cut is made into the wall of the stomach.

The combining form

Notice that in our first example the root gastr is combined with the vowel o to make gastro. This word component is called a combining form of a word root, i.e.

Word root	+	combining vowel	=	combining form
gastr	+	o	=	gastro

Most combining forms end in o.
Now we have learnt the meaning of our first root we can use it again with a new word component:

EPIGASTRIC

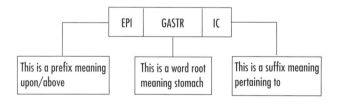

Here we have split the word into its components and we can see that it begins with a prefix.

The prefix

The prefix precedes the word root and changes its meaning. The prefix **epi-** means upon and so it modifies the word to mean upon or above the stomach. Prefixes are also derived from Greek and Latin words.

The suffix -ic meaning pertaining to was also used in our second example so we can now write the full meaning of epigastric:

EPI	GASTR	IC
This is a prefix meaning upon/above	This is a word root meaning stomach	This is a suffix meaning pertaining to

The full meaning of epigastric is – pertaining to above or upon the stomach.

> **Key Point**
> The components of medical words are:
> - prefixes
> - roots
> - suffixes
> - combining vowels
> - combining forms.

The use of prefixes, combining forms and suffixes

There are certain simple 'rules' which need to be applied when building and analysing medical words. To learn these rules we will use some new word components with which you will soon become familiar.

First we will use the combining form gastr/o again.

Rule 1: Adding a combining form to a suffix

If we add the suffixes **-logy**, meaning study of, and **-algia**, meaning condition of pain, to the combining form gastr/o we can make two new words:

gastr/o	+	-logy	=	gastrology	(study of the stomach)
gastr/o	+	-algia	=	gastralgia	(condition of pain in the stomach)

Notice that in gastrology the combining vowel o has been left in place whilst in gastralgia it has been dropped. The o has been dropped in gastralgia because -algia begins with a, a vowel. Gastroalgia is not used and it would be more difficult to pronounce.

> **Key Point**
> When a root combines with a suffix, the combining vowel is left in place if the suffix begins with a letter other than a vowel.

Here are some more examples where the vowel is left in place because the suffix begins with a letter other than a vowel:

gastr/o	+	-tomy	=	gastrotomy (incision into the stomach)
gastr/o	+	-scope	=	gastroscope (instrument to view the stomach)

Here are some examples where the vowel is dropped:

gastr/o	+	-itis	=	gastritis (inflammation of the stomach)
gastr/o	+	-ectomy	=	gastrectomy (removal of the stomach)

Rule 2: Combining two word roots

Some medical words contain two or more roots:

GASTROENTEROLOGY

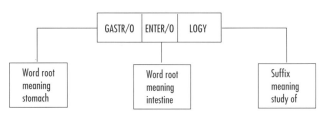

The full meaning of gastroenterology is the study of the intestines and stomach. Notice that the vowel between the two roots is left in place.

> **Key Point**
> When two roots are combined, the combining vowel is kept.

Here are some more examples:

pylor/o + gastr/o + ectomy = pylorogas-
                                       trectomy
duoden/o + enter/o + stomy = duodenoen-
                                       terostomy

We will learn the meaning of these words later.

Rule 3: Adding a prefix to a root

When a prefix that ends in a vowel is added to a root that begins with a vowel or 'h', the vowel of the prefix is dropped.

If we examine our second example, epigastric, again, here the vowel 'i' of epi- was retained because gastric begins with 'g' which is not a vowel.

Consider another example, which may be familiar to you – antacid, a drug used to neutralize stomach acid. This word is made from:

anti   +   acid   =   antacid
Prefix meaning   Root meaning
against   acid

The 'i' is dropped because acid begins with the vowel 'a'.

Here are some more examples, we will learn their meanings later.

Here the vowel is retained:

hemi   +   col/o   +   ectomy   =   hemicolectomy

Here the vowel of the prefix is dropped:

endo   +   arter/i   +   ectomy   =   endarterectomy
anti   +   helminth   +   ic   =   anthelminthic

Note. This is not a strict rule and there are many exceptions to it, e.g. periosteitis.

> **Key Point**
> When a prefix ends in a vowel, the vowel of the prefix is dropped if the root begins with a vowel or 'h'.

Reading and understanding medical words

Now you have learnt the basic principle of building medical words, you should be able to deduce the meaning of an unfamiliar word. To do this:

> **First**
>   Split the word into its components endo-, gastr/o, -itis, etc.
> **Then**
>   Think of or look up the meaning of these components.
> **Finally**
>   Read the meaning of the word *beginning with the suffix and reading backwards*:
>   e.g. gastr/o[3], enter/o[2], -logy[1]
>   1 study of
>   2 the intestines and
>   3 the stomach.

Once you have an understanding of these simple rules you should be able to complete the exercises in Units 1–20. Each unit introduces different medical terms associated with a body system or medical specialty. The units can be completed in an order which complements your studies in anatomy, physiology and health care.

1 Levels of organization

Objectives

Once you have completed Unit 1 you should be able to:

- understand the meaning of medical words relating to levels of organization
- build medical words relating to levels of organization
- understand medical abbreviations relating to cells and tissues.

Exercise Guide

Use this list of word components and their meanings to complete the word exercises in this unit.

Prefixes

micro-   small

Roots/Combining forms

chem/(istry)   chemicals (study of)
chondr/o   cartilage
erythr/o   red
fibr/o   fibre
granul/o   granule
haem/o   blood
hem/o (Am.)   blood
leuc/o   white
leuk/o (Am.)   white
lymph/o   lymph
melan/o   pigment/melanin
oo   egg/ovum
path/o   disease
spermat/o   sperm
tox/o   poisonous

Suffixes

-blast   immature germ cell/cell which forms …
-genesis   formation of
-ic   pertaining to
-ist   specialist
-logist   specialist who studies …
-logy   study of
-lysis   breakdown/disintegration
-pathy   disease of
-scope   instrument to view/examine
-scopist   specialist who uses viewing instrument
-scopy   technique of viewing/examining
-trophic   pertaining to nourishing

Levels of organization

The human body consists of basic units of life known as **cells**. Groups of cells similar in appearance, function and origin join together to form **tissues**. Different tissues then interact with each other to form **organs**. Finally groups of organs interact to form body **systems**. Thus there are four levels of organization in the human body: cells, tissues, organs and systems. Let us begin by examining the first level of organization.

Cells

The cell is the basic unit of life and the bodies of all plants and animals are built up of cells. Your body consists of millions of very small specialized cells. It is interesting to note that all non-infectious disorders and diseases of the human body are really due to the abnormal behaviour of cells.

Body cells are all built on the same basic plan. Figure 1 represents a model cell.

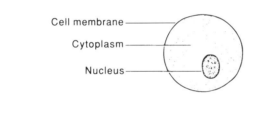

Cell membrane ————

Cytoplasm ————

Nucleus ————

Figure 1   A cell

Most cells have the same basic components as are shown in the model but they are all specialized to carry out particular functions within the body. In your studies you will come across many terms which relate to these different types of cell. Now we will look at our first word root:

Root	**Cyt**
	(From a Greek word **kytos,** *meaning cell.)*
Combining forms	**Cyt/o, -cyte**
	(Remember from our introduction that combining forms are made by adding a combining vowel to the word root.)

Here is a reminder about writing the meaning of medical words. First split the word into its components, then find the meaning of each component. Finally write the meaning of the word beginning with the suffix. Here we have a word which contains the root cyt:

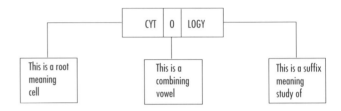

CYT	O	LOGY

This is a root meaning cell

This is a combining vowel

This is a suffix meaning study of

Reading from the suffix back, cytology means the study of cells.

Cytology is a very important topic in medicine as many diseases and disorders can be diagnosed by studying cells. Cells removed from patients are sent for cytological examination to a hospital cytology laboratory where they are examined with a microscope.

The exercises which follow rely on the use of the Exercise Guide which appears at the beginning of this unit; use this to look up the meaning of path/o and -pathy and then try Word Exercise 1.

WORD EXERCISE 1

(a) Name the components of the word and give their meanings:

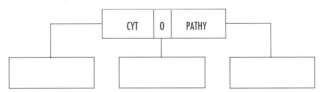

CYT	O	PATHY

(b) Reading from the suffix back, the meaning of cytopathy is:

_____

The root **path** can be used at the beginning and in the middle of a compound word as in the next two examples. Write the meaning of these words:

(c) path/o/logy   _____

(d) cyt/o/path/o/logy   _____

Using the Exercise Guide again find the meaning of -ic, -ist, tox/o, and -lysis and write the meaning of the words below. Remember to read the meaning from the suffix back to the beginning of each word:

(e) cytolysis   _____

(f) cytotoxic   _____

(g) cytologist   _____

In the above examples, **cyt/o** was used at the beginning of words. It can also be used at the end of words in combination with other roots, its meaning remaining the same. Remember, when two roots are joined the combining vowel remains in place.

WORD EXERCISE 2

Here we have an example of two roots joined to make a compound word:

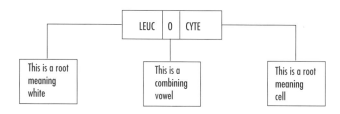

LEUC	O	CYTE

This is a root meaning white

This is a combining vowel

This is a root meaning cell

The meaning of leucocyte is therefore: white cell (actually a type of blood cell) (Am. leukocyte).

(a) Name the components of the following word and give their meaning:

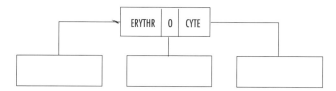

ERYTHR	O	CYTE

(b) The meaning of erythrocyte is: _____

WORD EXERCISE 3

Figure 2 and Figure 3 show two specialized cells, each one carrying out a different function.

(i) This is a cell which is found in the skin. It produces the pigment melanin which gives the dark colour to skin.

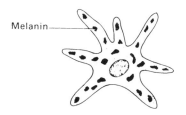

Melanin

Figure 2   A pigment cell

(ii) This is a cell also found in the skin which produces the white collagen fibres that give the skin support.

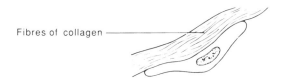

Fibres of collagen

Figure 3   A fibre cell

Use your Exercise Guide to find the combining forms of melanin and fibre to build words which name these cells.

(a) A cell containing melanin _____

(b) A cell that produces fibres _____

(c) Complete the table by looking up the combining forms of the following roots in your Exercise Guide and building words which refer to cell types.

Root	Combining form	Name of cell
oste	osteo	osteocyte (bone cell)
lymph	_____	_____
spermat	_____	_____
oo	_____	_____
granul	_____	_____
chondr	_____	_____

All of the above examples show how the combining vowel is retained when two roots are joined.

Now we will examine another root which also refers to cells:

Root

Blast
(A Greek word meaning bud or germ. It is used to denote an immature stage in cell development or a cell which is forming something.)

Combining forms   **Blast/o, -blast**

WORD EXERCISE 4

Without using your Exercise Guide, write the meaning of:

(a) osteo**blast** _____

(b) fibro**blast** _____

Using your Exercise Guide, write the meaning of:

(c) Haemocyto**blast** _____
(Am. hemocytoblast)

Tissues

As cells become specialized, they form groups of cells known as tissues. A definition of a tissue is a group of cells similar in appearance, function and origin. There are four basic types of tissue: epithelial, muscle, connective and nervous tissue. These form the second level of organization in the body. Figure 4 illustrates how cells form a tissue. Here we can see a cuboidal epithelium from the kidney.

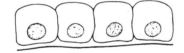

Figure 4   Cuboidal epithelium

The study of tissues is known as histology, the combining form coming from a Greek word *histos* meaning web (web of cells). Histology is an important branch of biology and medicine because it is used to identify diseased tissues. The histology and cytology laboratories are usually sections of the pathology laboratory of a large hospital.

Root   **Hist**
(From a Greek word **histos,** *meaning web. It is used to mean the tissues of the body.)*

Combining forms   **Hist/o, histi/o**

 WORD EXERCISE 5

Using your Exercise Guide, find the meaning of:

(a) **histo**chemistry _____

Without using your Exercise Guide, write the meaning of:

(b) **histo**pathology _____

(c) **histo**logist _____

(d) **histo**lysis _____

Cells and tissues are very small and need to be examined using an instrument known as a microscope.

 WORD EXERCISE 6

Using your Exercise Guide, find the meaning of:

(a) **micro-** _____

(b) **micro**scope _____

(c) **micro**scopy _____

(d) **micro**scop/ist _____

Note carefully the differences between **-scope**, **-scopy** and **-scopist**.

Organs

Groups of different tissues interact to produce larger structures known as organs. These form the third level of organization. A familiar example is the heart (Fig. 5), which consists of muscle tissue, a covering of epithelium, nerve tissue and connective tissue. All these tissues interact so that the heart pumps blood.

Root   **Organ**
(From a Greek word **organon,** *meaning tool. Here we are using it to mean a body organ.)*

Combining forms   **Organ/o**

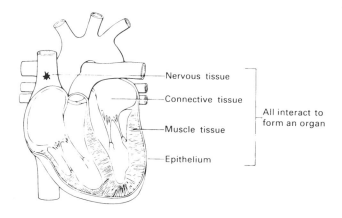

Nervous tissue

Connective tissue

All interact to form an organ

Muscle tissue

Epithelium

 Figure 5   The heart

WORD EXERCISE 7

Using your Exercise Guide, find the meaning of:

(a) **organo**genesis _____
(synonymous with organogeny)

(b) **organo**trophic _____

Body systems

Groups of organs interact to form the fourth level of organization, the system, e.g. the stomach, duodenum, colon, etc. interact to form the digestive system which digests and absorbs food. Units 2–16 introduce medical terms associated with the main body systems.

Quick Reference

Medical roots relating to levels of organization:

Blast/o	immature cell/forming cell
Chondr/o	cartilage
Cyt/o	cell
Granul/o	granule
Hist/i/o	tissue/web
Lymph/o	lymph
Melan/o	pigment/melanin
Oo	egg/ovum
Organ/o	organ
Oste/o	bone
Path/o	disease
Spermat/o	sperm

Abbreviations

You should learn common abbreviations related to cells and tissues. Those listed below have been taken from patients' notes in use in hospitals and general practice. However, some are not standard abbreviations and their meaning may vary from one hospital to another. There is a more extensive list of abbreviations for reference on page 259.

Diff	differential blood count (of cell types)
FBC	full blood count (of cells)
GCSF	granulocyte colony stimulating factor
Histo	histology (lab)
HLA	human lymphocyte antigen
Lymphos	lymphocytes
NK	natural killer (cells)
Pap	Papanicolaou smear test (of cervical cells)
PCV	packed cell volume
RBC	red blood count/red blood cell
RCC	red cell count
WBC	white blood cell/white blood count

 NOW TRY THE WORD CHECK

WORD CHECK

This self-check exercise lists all the word components used in this unit. First write down the meaning of as many word components as you can. Then check your answers using the Exercise Guide and Quick Reference box or the Glossary of Word Components (pp. 269–279).

Prefixes

micro- _____

Combining forms of word roots

blast/o _____

chem/o _____

chondr/o _____

cyt/o _____

erythr/o _____

fibr/o   _____

granul/o   _____

hist/i/o   _____

leuc/o   _____

lymph/o   _____

melan/o   _____

oo-   _____

organ/o   _____

oste/o   _____

path/o   _____

spermat/o   _____

tox/o   _____

Suffixes

-blast   _____

-ic   _____

-ist   _____

-log(ist)   _____

-logy   _____

-lysis   _____

-pathy   _____

-scope   _____

-scop(ist)   _____

-scopy   _____

-tox(ic)   _____

-trophic   _____

> **NOW TRY THE SELF-ASSESSMENT** ◀

SELF-ASSESSMENT

Test 1A

Prefixes, suffixes and combining forms of word roots

Match each word component in Column A with a meaning in Column C by inserting the appropriate number in Column B.

	Column A	Column B		Column C
(a)	chem/o	_____	1.	egg
(b)	cyt/o	_____	2.	bone
(c)	erythr/o	_____	3.	white
(d)	granul/o	_____	4.	study of
(e)	hist/i/o	_____	5.	pigment (black)
(f)	leuc/o	_____	6.	sperm cells
(g)	-log(ist)	_____	7.	chemical
(h)	-logy	_____	8.	tissue
(i)	lymph/o	_____	9.	person who studies (specialist)
(j)	-lysis	_____	10.	small
(k)	melan/o	_____	11.	specialist who views/examines
(l)	micro-	_____	12.	breakdown/ disintegration
(m)	oo-	_____	13.	poisonous/pertaining to poison
(n)	oste/o	_____	14.	cell
(o)	-pathy	_____	15.	visual examination
(p)	-scope	_____	16.	disease
(q)	-scop(ist)	_____	17.	lymph
(r)	-scopy	_____	18.	red
(s)	spermat/o	_____	19.	granule
(t)	-tox(ic)	_____	20.	viewing instrument

Score

20

Test 1B

Write the meaning of:

(a) chondrolysis   _____

(b) leucocytolysis _____

(c) histotoxic   _____

(d) osteopathy   _____

(e) lymphoblast   _____

Score

5

Test 1C

This type of test may seem difficult at first but as the terms become familiar you will improve.

Build words which mean:

(a) small cell   _____

(b) person who specializes in the   _____
     study of disease

(c) person who specializes in the   _____
     study of disease of cells

(d) scientific study of cartilage   _____

(e) pertaining to disease of cells   _____

Score

5

Check answers to Self-Assessment Tests on page 251.

2 The digestive system

Objectives

Once you have completed Unit 2 you should be able to:

- understand the meaning of medical words relating to the digestive system
- build medical words relating to the digestive system
- associate medical terms with their anatomical position
- understand medical abbreviations relating to the digestive system.

Exercise Guide

Use this list of word components and their meanings to complete the word exercises in this unit.

Prefixes

a-	without
endo-	inside/within
mega-	large
para-	beside
peri-	around

Suffixes

-aemia	condition of blood
-al	pertaining to
-algia	condition of pain
-clysis	infusion/injection into
-ectomy	removal of
-emia (Am.)	condition of blood
-gram	X-ray/tracing/recording
-graphy	technique of recording/making X-ray
-ia	condition of
-iasis	abnormal condition
-ist	specialist
-itis	inflammation of
-lith	stone
-lithiasis	abnormal condition of stones
-logist	specialist who studies ...
-logy	study of
-lysis	breakdown/disintegration
-megaly	enlargement
-oma	tumour/swelling
-pathy	disease of
-scope	instrument to view/examine
-scopy	technique of viewing/examining
-stomy	formation of an opening into ...
-tomy	incision into
-toxic	pertaining to poisoning
-uria	condition of the urine

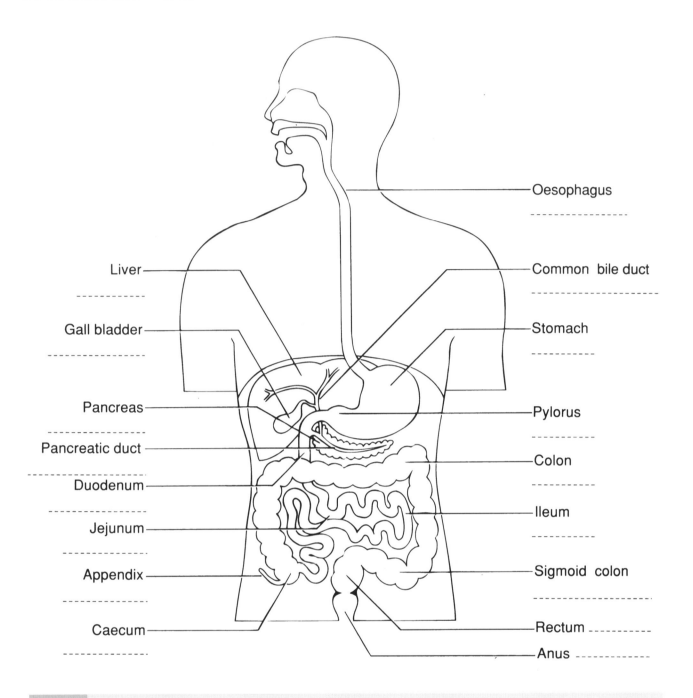

Figure 6   The digestive system

ANATOMY EXERCISE

When you have finished Word Exercises 1–12, look at the word components listed below. Complete Figure 6 by writing the appropriate combining form on each dotted line. (You can check their meanings in the Quick Reference box on page 22.)

Appendic/o	Gastr/o	Pancreatic/o
Caec/o, Cec/o (Am.)	Hepat/o	Proct/o
Cholecyst/o	Ile/o	Pylor/o
Choledoch/o	Jejun/o	Rect/o
Col/o	Oesophag/o, Esophag/o (Am.)	Sigmoid/o
Duoden/o	Pancreat/o	

The digestive system

The organs which compose the digestive system digest, absorb and process nutrients taken in as food. Material which is not absorbed into the lining of the intestine is known as faeces and it leaves the body by the anus.

Our study of the digestive system begins at the point where food leaves the mouth and enters the gullet or oesophagus.

Use the Exercise Guide at the beginning of this unit to complete Word Exercises 1–12 unless you are asked to work without it.

Root	**Oesophag** *(From a Greek word* **oisophagos,** *meaning oesophagus or gullet.)*
Combining forms	**Oesophag/o** **Esophag/o** *(Am.)*

 ## WORD EXERCISE 1

Using your Exercise Guide, find the meaning of:

(a) **oesophago**scope _____
     (Am. esophagoscope)

Remember that, to understand the meaning of these medical terms, we read the components from the suffix towards the beginning of the word.

(b) **oesophag**ectomy _____
     (Am. esophagectomy)

(c) **oesophago**tomy _____
     (Am. esophagotomy)

(d) **oesophag**itis _____
     (Am. esophagitis)

Once you have learnt the suffixes in Word Exercise 1, it is easy to work out the meaning of other words with similar endings. Now we will use the same suffixes again with a different word root.

Root	**Gastr** *(From a Greek word* **gaster,** *meaning belly or stomach.)*
Combining forms	**Gastr/o**

 # WORD EXERCISE 2

Without using your Exercise Guide, write the meaning of:

(a) **gastro**scope _____

(b) **gastr**ectomy _____

(c) **gastro**tomy _____

(d) **gastr**itis _____

Using your Exercise Guide, build words which mean:

(e) disease of the stomach _____

(f) study of the stomach _____

Remember, when building words the combining vowel is usually dropped if the suffix begins with a vowel.

Root	**Enter** *(From a Greek word* **enteron,** *meaning intestine or gut.)*
Combining forms	**Enter/o**

 # WORD EXERCISE 3

Without using your Exercise Guide, write the meaning of:

(a) **enter**itis _____

(b) **entero**pathy _____

(c) **entero**tomy _____

Using your Exercise Guide, find the meaning of:

(d) **entero**stomy _____

Note. Here you need to note the difference between:

-stomy
This means a mouth or opening. Usually a stoma is formed by surgery, e.g. a colostomy is an opening or the formation of an opening into the colon. This word component also refers to an operation to form an opening/communication (or anastomosis) between two parts (Fig. 7). A stoma can be temporary or permanent.

-tomy
This refers to an incision as at the beginning of an operation.

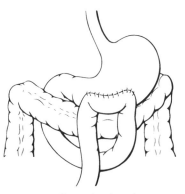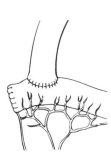

Stomach to intestine
(side to side)

Intestine to intestine
(side to end)

Figure 7   Surgical anastomoses

(e) **entero**lith _____

Without using your Exercise Guide, build words which mean:

(f)   study of the intestine _____

(g)   a person who studies the intestines _____

Now we can put two roots together to make a larger word. Although these words look complicated it is now quite easy to understand their meaning.

Without using your Exercise Guide, write the meaning of:

(h)   gastro**entero**logy _____

(i)   gastro**entero**pathy _____

(j)   gastro**enter**itis _____

(k)   gastro**entero**scopy _____

Note.   When the two roots **gastr/o** and **enter/o** are joined the combining vowel is retained.

Between the stomach and the small intestine there is a sphincter muscle known as the **pylorus**. This acts as a valve which opens periodically to allow digested food to leave the stomach.

Root   **Pylor**
*(From a Greek word **pylouros**, meaning gate-keeper. It is used to mean the pylorus.)*

Combining forms   **Pylor/o**

WORD EXERCISE 4

Without using your Exercise Guide, write the meaning of:

(a)   **pyloro**gastrectomy _____

(b)   **pyloro**scopy _____

The small intestine

Now let us examine the small intestine which consists of three parts, the **duodenum**, **jejunum** and **ileum**. The duodenum is concerned mainly with digestion of food while the jejunum and ileum are specially adapted for the absorption of nutrients.

Note.   Although the root enter refers generally to intestines, it is often used to mean the small intestine. However, there are special roots which describe the different regions of the intestine. We shall use these in the next three exercises.

Root   **Duoden**
*(From a Latin word **duodeni**, meaning twelve. It refers to the duodenum, which is the first 12 inches of the small intestine.)*

Combining forms   **Duoden/o**

Root   **Jejun**
*(From a Latin word **jejunus**, meaning empty. It refers to the jejunum, part of the intestine between the duodenum and ileum approx 2.4 m in length.)*

Combining forms   **Jejun/o**

Ile
*(From a Latin word **ilia,** meaning flanks. We use it here to mean the lower three-fifths of the small intestine.)*

Combining forms   **Ile/o**

WORD EXERCISE 5

Without using your Exercise Guide, write the meaning of:

(a) **duodeno**enterostomy   _____

(b) **jejunojejuno**stomy   _____

Using your Exercise Guide, find the meaning of:

(c) **duodenojejun**al   _____

Without using your Exercise Guide, build words which mean:

(d) formation of an opening into the ileum   _____

(e) inflammation of the ileum   _____

Note.   Exception – two vowels together.

A permanent opening or **ileostomy** is made when the whole of the large intestine has been removed. This acts as an artificial anus. The ileum opens directly on to the abdominal wall and the liquid discharge from it is collected in a plastic **ileostomy bag** (Fig. 8).

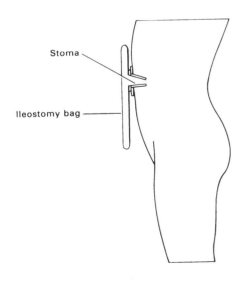

Stoma

Ileostomy bag

Figure 8   Ileostomy

After passing through the small intestine, any remaining material passes into the large intestine or large bowel.

The large intestine

The large intestine has a wider diameter than the small intestine and it is shorter. Its main function is to absorb water from the materials which remain after digestion and form faeces (Am. feces) which are ejected from the body during defaecation. The large intestine is made up of the **caecum** (Am. cecum), **appendix**, **colon**, **rectum** and **anus** (Fig. 9).

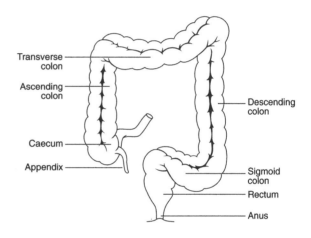

Transverse colon
Ascending colon
Descending colon
Caecum
Appendix
Sigmoid colon
Rectum
Anus

Figure 9   The large intestine

The next six roots refer to the large intestine:

Caec
*(From a Latin word **caecus** meaning blind. It refers to a blindly ending pouch, the caecum attached to the vermiform appendix and separated from the ileum by a valve, the ileocaecal valve.)*

Combining forms   **Caec/o**
Cec/o *(Am.)*

Appendic
*(From a Latin word **appendix,** meaning appendage.)*

Combining forms   **Appendic/o**
Append/o *(Am.)*

Root   **Col**
(From a Greek word **kolon,** *meaning colon, the large bowel extending from caecum to rectum.)*

Combining forms   **Col/o, colon/o**

 WORD EXERCISE 6

Using your Exercise Guide, find the meaning of:

(a) mega**colon**   _____

Without using your Exercise Guide, write the meaning of:

(b) **appendic**itis   _____

(c) **col**ectomy   _____

(d) **colo**stomy   _____
(see Fig. 10)

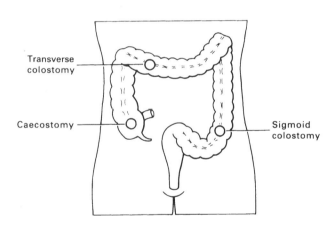

Transverse colostomy

Caecostomy

Sigmoid colostomy

Figure 10   Common sites of stomas of large bowel

Without using your Exercise Guide, build words which mean:

(e) formation of an opening into the   _____
caecum (Am. cecum)

(f) removal of the appendix   _____

(g) formation of an opening   _____
(anastomosis) between the colon
and stomach

Root   **Sigm**
(From a Greek word **sigma –** *meaning the letter* **S.** *It refers to the last part of the descending colon which resembles an S-shape and is called the sigmoid colon.)*

Combining forms   **Sigmoid/o**

Root   **Rect**
(From a Latin word **rectus,** *meaning straight. Here it refers to the last part of the large intestine, the rectum, which is straight.)*

Combining forms   **Rect/o**

Root   **Proct**
(From a Greek word **proktos,** *meaning anus. It is used to mean the rectum or anus.)*

Combining forms   **Proct/o**

WORD EXERCISE 7

Using your Exercise Guide, find the meaning of:

(a) **sigmoido**scopy   _____

(b) para**rect**al   _____

(c) peri**proct**itis   _____

(d) **procto**clysis   _____

(e) **proct**algia   _____

Without using your Exercise Guide, build words which mean:

(f) instrument to view anus/rectum   _____

(g) formation of an opening between   _____
the caecum and anus

(h) formation of an opening between   _____
the sigmoid colon and caecum

Sometimes the lining of the intestine develops enlarged pouches or sacs. Each is known as a **diverticulum** (pl. **diverticulae**). These can become inflamed as in **diverticulitis** and may have to be removed by **diverticulectomy**.

The outer layer of the intestines and the lining of the cavity in which they lie consist of serous membrane. This secretes a serum-like fluid, serous fluid which acts as a lubricant. A film of serous fluid allows organs to slide over each other as they move by peristalsis.

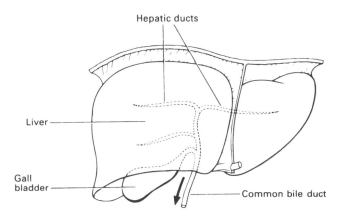

Root	**Peritone** *(From a Greek word **peri**, meaning around, and **teinein**, meaning to stretch. It refers to the peritoneum, the serous membrane lining the abdominal and pelvic cavities, which covers all abdominal organs.)*
Combining forms	**Periton/e/o**

Figure 11 The liver and bile ducts

WORD EXERCISE 8

Without using your Exercise Guide, write the meaning of:

(a) **periton**itis _____

(b) **peritoneo**clysis _____

Accessory organs of the digestive system

The pancreas

This gland is found beneath the stomach (see Fig. 6). Its function is to produce **pancreatic juice** which is passed to the duodenum where it neutralizes acid and digests food. It can also produce the hormones **insulin** and **glucagon** which are secreted directly into the blood.

Root	**Pancreat** *(From a Greek word **pankreas**, meaning the pancreas.)*
Combining forms	**Pancreat/o** *A combining form **pancreatic/o** is also derived from this root. It is used to mean pancreatic duct. This duct transfers pancreatic juice containing digestive enzymes from the pancreas to the duodenum.*

The liver

The liver is the largest abdominal organ (Fig. 11). It is located just beneath the diaphragm. It processes nutrients which it receives from the intestine, stores materi-

als and excretes wastes in the form of **bile** back into the intestine.

Root	**Hepat** *(From a Greek word **hepatos**, meaning the liver.)*
Combining forms	**Hepat/o** *A combining form **hepatic/o** is also derived from this root and is used to mean the hepatic bile duct.*

WORD EXERCISE 9

Using your Exercise Guide, find the meaning of:

(a) **Pancreato**lysis _____

(b) **Hepato**megaly _____

(c) **Hepat**oma _____

(d) **Hepato**toxic _____

Without using your Exercise Guide, write the meaning of:

(e) **Hepatico**gastrostomy _____

(f) **Pancreatico**duodenal _____

Root	**Chol** *(From a Greek word **chole**, meaning bile.)*
Combining forms	**Chol/e**

Liver cells produce a yellowish-brown waste known as bile. This drains through small canals and hepatic ducts into a sac known as the gall bladder. Bile leaves the gall bladder through the common bile duct and enters the intestine. Although bile is a waste product, the bile salts it contains help to emulsify lipids (fats) in the intestine. The structures in which bile is transported are sometimes referred to as the **biliary** system.

WORD EXERCISE 10

Using your Exercise Guide, find the meaning of:

(a) a**chol**ia   _____

(b) **chole**lith   _____

(c) **chole**lithiasis   _____

(d) **chol**aemia (Am. cholemia)   _____

(e) **chol**uria   _____

A word root which is commonly combined with **chol/e** is **cyst/o,** meaning bladder. **Cholecyst/o** refers specifically to the gall bladder, i.e. bile bladder.

Without using your Exercise Guide, write the meaning of:

(f) **cholecysto**tomy   _____

(g) **cholecyst**ectomy   _____

(h) **cholecysto**lithiasis   _____

A second word root often combined with **chol/e** is **angi/o** meaning vessel. **Cholangi/o** therefore refers to the bile vessels/ducts.

Using your Exercise Guide, find the meaning of:

(i) **cholangio**gram   _____

(j) **cholangio**graphy   _____

A third word root which is often combined with **chol/e** is **doch/o,** meaning to receive. **Choledoch/o** refers to the common bile duct, i.e. that which receives the bile.

Without using your Exercise Guide, write the meaning of:

(k) **choledocho**lithiasis   _____

(l) **choledocho**lithotomy   _____

Note. Here we need to distinguish between three suffixes which often cause some confusion:

> **-gram**
> This refers to a tracing. In practice in medicine it usually refers to an X-ray picture, paper recording or to a trace on a screen.
>
> **-graphy**
> This refers to the technique or process of making a recording, e.g. an X-ray or tracing. It can also refer to a written description.
>
> **-graph**
> This means a description or writing but more often it is used in medicine for the name of an instrument which carries out a recording. Occasionally it is used to mean the recording itself.

     Root   **Lapar**
(From a Greek word **lapara,** _meaning soft part between the ribs and hips, i.e. the flank/abdominal wall.)_

Combining forms   **Lapar/o**

WORD EXERCISE 11

Without using your Exercise Guide, write the meaning of:

(a) **laparo**scopy   _____

(b) **laparo**tomy   _____

Laparotomy is performed when a diagnosis of an abdominal problem is uncertain. It is a type of exploratory operation. The laparoscope is passed through a small opening into the abdominal cavity to view the internal organs (viscera).

Medical equipment and clinical procedures

In this unit we have named several instruments. Let us review their names:

    gastroscope
    gastroenteroscope
    sigmoidoscope
    colonoscope

proctoscope
laparoscope

All of these instruments are used to view various parts of the digestive system. Now fibreoptic endoscopes have replaced some of the original viewing instruments. Endoscope means an instrument to view inside (**endo-** within/inside)

Endoscopes utilize flexible, fibreoptic tubes (Fig. 12) which can be inserted into body cavities or into small incisions made in the body wall. Each is provided with illumination and a system of lenses which enables the operator to view the inside of the body. The inclusion of electronic chips at the end of the fibreoptic tube allows the view to be transmitted to a video screen. Sometimes the endoscope is used for photography and it is then known as a photoendoscope.

The endoscope can be adapted to view particular areas of the body. In the case of the digestive system, the fibreoptic tube can be passed into the mouth to examine the oesophagus, stomach and intestine. Alternatively it can be passed into the anus to view the rectum and colon. Note that when an endoscope is adapted to examine the stomach it may be referred to as a gastroscope.

Often endoscopes are used to examine the oesophagus, stomach and duodenum at the same examination. This procedure is **pan**endoscopy (**pan-** means all, i.e. all the upper digestive system). Similarly, panendoscopy could be performed on all of the large intestine via the anus.

In addition to viewing cavities, endoscopes can be fitted with a variety of attachments, such as forceps and catheters, and they can then be used for special applications. One such procedure is:

ERCP or endoscopic, retrograde, cholangiopancreatography

Let us examine the words separately:

endoscopic	referring to an endoscope
retrograde	going backwards
chol	bile
angio	vessel
pancreato	pancreas
graphy	technique of making a tracing/X-ray recording

Although we cannot deduce the exact meaning from the words we can see why they have been used. Here is the meaning of ERCP:

A technique of making an X-ray (graphy) of the pancreatic vessels and bile duct (pancreat/chol/angio), by passing a catheter (tube) backwards (retrograde) into them using an endoscope. Dye is injected through the catheter to outline the vessels and ducts on the X-ray.

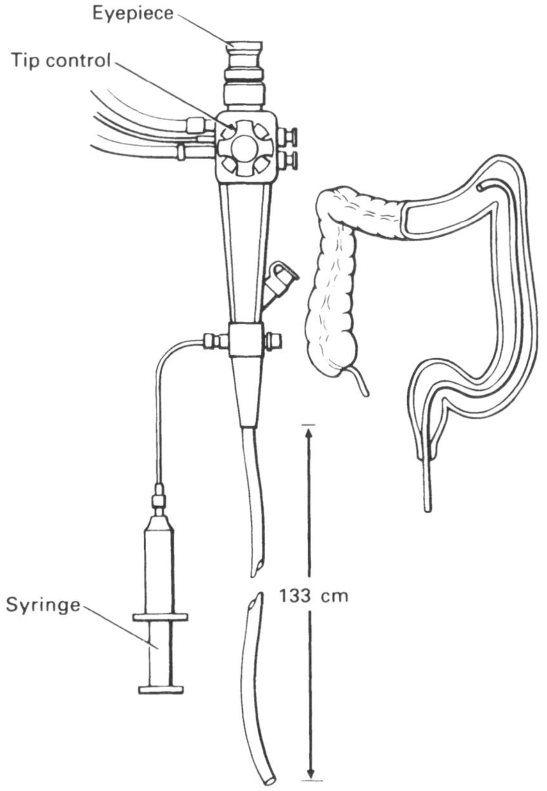

WORD EXERCISE 12

Match each term in Column A with a description from Column C by placing an appropriate number in Column B.

Column A	Column B	Column C
(a) enteroscope	_____	1. instrument to view rectum
(b) endoscope	_____	2. technique of taking photographs using an endoscope
(c) enteroscopy	_____	3. visual examination of the colon
(d) endoscopy	_____	4. instrument to view the intestine
(e) endoscopist	_____	5. visual examination of all cavities, e.g. oesophagus, stomach and duodenum
(f) colonoscopy	_____	6. instrument to view body cavities
(g) proctoscope	_____	7. visual examination of the intestine
(h) sigmoidoscopy	_____	8. person who operates an endoscope

Eyepiece

Tip control

Syringe

133 cm

Figure 12   Fibreoptic endoscope used to view the colon

Column A	Column B	Column C
(i) panendoscopy	_____	9. visual examination of body cavities
(j) photoendoscopy	_____	10. visual examination of S-colon

ANATOMY EXERCISE

Now complete the Anatomy Exercise on page 14.

Quick Reference

Medical roots relating to the digestive system:

Appendic/o	appendix
Bil/i	bile
Caec/o	caecum
Cec/o (Am.)	cecum
Chol/e	bile
Cholangi/o	bile vessel/duct
Cholecyst/o	gall bladder
Choledoch/o	common bile duct
Col/o	colon
Colon/o	colon
Diverticul/o	diverticulum
Duoden/o	duodenum
Enter/o	intestine
Esophag/o (Am.)	esophagus
Gastr/o	stomach
Hepat/o	liver
Hepatic/o	hepatic duct
Ile/o	ileum
Jejun/o	jejunum
Lapar/o	flank/abdominal wall
Oesophag/o	oesophagus
Pancreat/o	pancreas
Pancreatic/o	pancreatic duct
Peritone/o	peritoneum
Proct/o	anus/rectum
Pylor/o	pyloric sphincter
Rect/o	rectum
Ser/o	serous/serum
Sigmoid/o	sigmoid colon

Abbreviations

You should learn common abbreviations related to the digestive system. Note, however, some are not standard and their meaning may vary from one hospital to another. There is a more extensive list for reference on page 259.

Abdo	abdomen
CD	Crohn's disease
DU	duodenal ulcer
GI	gastrointestinal
GU	gastric ulcer
IUC	idiopathic ulcerative colitis
LLQ	left lower quadrant
pr/PR	per rectum
PU	peptic ulcer
RE	rectal examination
UC	ulcerative colitis
UGI	upper gastrointestinal

> ## NOW TRY THE WORD CHECK

WORD CHECK

This self-check exercise lists all the word components used in this unit. First write down the meaning of as many word components as you can. Then check your answers using the Exercise Guide and Quick Reference box or the Glossary of Word Components (pp. 269–279).

Prefixes

a-   _____

endo-   _____

mega-   _____

pan-   _____

para-   _____

peri-   _____

retro-   _____

Combining forms of word roots

angi/o _____

appendic/o _____

caec/o
(Am. cec/o) _____

chol/e _____

choledoch/o _____

col/o _____

colon/o _____

cyst/o _____

diverticul/o _____

duoden/o _____

enter/o _____

gastr/o _____

hepat/o _____

hepatic/o _____

ile/o _____

jejun/o _____

lapar/o _____

oesophag/o
(Am. esophag/o) _____

pancreat/o _____

pancreatic/o _____

peritone/o _____

proct/o _____

pylor/o _____

rect/o _____

ser/o _____

sigmoid/o _____

tox/o _____

Suffixes

-aemia
(Am. -emia) _____

-al _____

-algia _____

-clysis _____

-ectomy _____

-grade _____

-gram _____

-graph _____

-graphy _____

-ia _____

-iasis _____

-ic _____

-ist _____

-itis _____

-lith _____

-lithiasis _____

-logist _____

-logy _____

-lysis _____

-megaly _____

-oma _____

-pathy _____

-scope _____

-scopy _____

-stomy _____

-tomy _____

-toxic _____

-um _____

-uria _____

NOW TRY THE SELF-ASSESSMENT

SELF-ASSESSMENT

Test 2A

Below are some combining forms which refer to the anatomy of the digestive system. Indicate which part of the system they refer to by putting a number from the diagram (Fig. 13) next to each word. You can use a number more than once.

(a) pylor/o _____

(b) gastr/o _____

(c) proct/o _____

(d) hepat/o _____

(e) appendic/o _____

(f) choledoch/o _____

(g) col/o _____

(h) pancreat/o _____

(i) sigmoid/o _____

(j) oesophag/o _____
    (Am. esophag/o)

(k) cholecyst/o _____

(l) ile/o _____

(m) caec/o _____
    (Am. cec/o)

(n) duoden/o _____

(o) rect/o _____

Score

15

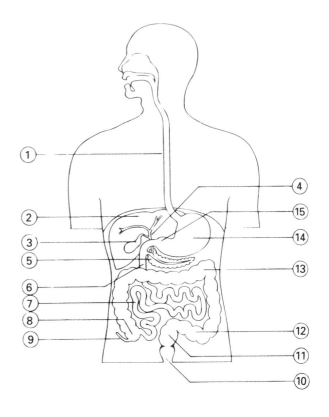

The digestive system

Column A	Column B	Column C
(a) a-	_____	1. enlargement
(b) -aemia (Am. -emia)	_____	2. condition of pain
(c) -algia	_____	3. study of
(d) -clysis	_____	4. around
(e) -ectomy	_____	5. injection/infusion
(f) endo-	_____	6. X-ray/tracing
(g) -gram	_____	7. inflammation
(h) -graph	_____	8. condition of urine
(i) -graphy	_____	9. within/inside
(j) -itis	_____	10. beside/near
(k) -lithiasis	_____	11. tumour
(l) -logy	_____	12. abnormal condition of stones
(m) mega-	_____	13. all
(n) -megaly	_____	14. without
(o) -oma	_____	15. technique of making an X-ray/tracing/record

Test 2B

Prefixes and suffixes

Match each prefix or suffix in Column A with a meaning in Column C by inserting the appropriate number in Column B.

Column A	Column B	Column C
(p) pan-	_____	16. large
(q) para-	_____	17. instrument which records
(r) peri-	_____	18. incision into
(s) -tomy	_____	19. removal of
(t) -uria	_____	20. condition of blood

Score

20

Column A	Column B	Column C
(p) peritone/o	_____	16. common bile duct
(q) proct/o	_____	17. caecum
(r) pylor/o	_____	18. pancreas
(s) rect/o	_____	19. liver
(t) sigmoid/o	_____	20. appendix

Score

20

Test 2C

Combining forms of word roots

Match each combining form of a word root from Column A with a meaning from Column C by inserting the appropriate number in Column B.

Column A	Column B	Column C
(a) angi/o	_____	1. pylorus
(b) appendic/o	_____	2. sigmoid colon
(c) caec/o (Am. cec/o)	_____	3. peritoneum
(d) chol/e	_____	4. jejunum
(e) choledoch/o	_____	5. intestine
(f) colon/o	_____	6. vessel
(g) cyst/o	_____	7. duodenum
(h) duoden/o	_____	8. colon
(i) enter/o	_____	9. rectum
(j) gastr/o	_____	10. rectum/anus
(k) hepat/o	_____	11. bladder
(l) jejun/o	_____	12. stomach
(m) lapar/o	_____	13. oesophagus
(n) oesophag/o (Am. esophag/o)	_____	14. bile
(o) pancreat/o	_____	15. abdomen/flank

Test 2D

Write the meaning of:

(a) gastroenterocolitis _____

(b) hepatography _____

(c) ileorectal _____

(d) proctosigmoidoscope _____

(e) pancreatomegaly _____

Score

5

Test 2E

Build words which mean:

(a) inflammation of the duodenum _____

(b) condition of pain in the stomach _____

(c) incision into the liver _____

(d) study of the anus/rectum _____

(e) formation of an opening/ anastomosis between the anus and the ileum _____

Score

5

Check answers to Self-Assessment Tests on page 251.

3 The breathing system

Objectives

Once you have completed Unit 3 you should be able to:

- understand the meaning of medical words relating to the breathing system

- build medical words relating to the breathing system

- associate medical terms with their anatomical position

- understand medical abbreviations relating to the breathing system.

Exercise Guide

Use this list of word components and their meanings to complete the word exercises in this unit.

Prefixes

a-	without
dys-	difficult/painful
hyper-	above/excessive
hypo-	below/low
inter-	between
tachy-	fast

Roots/Combining forms

chondr/o	cartilage
esophag/o (Am.)	esophagus
gastr/o	stomach
haem/o	blood
hem/o (Am.)	blood
hepat/o	liver
myc/o	fungus
oesophag/o	oesophagus
radi/o	radiation/X-ray

Suffixes

-al	pertaining to
-algia	condition of pain
-ary	pertaining to
-centesis	surgical puncture to remove fluid
-desis	fixation/bind together by surgery/sticking together
-dynia	condition of pain
-eal	pertaining to
-ectasis	dilatation/stretching
-ectomy	removal of
-genic	pertaining to formation/originating in
-gram	X-ray/tracing/recording
-graphy	technique of recording/making X-ray
-ia	condition of
-ic	pertaining to
-itis	inflammation of
-logy	study of
-meter	measuring instrument
-metry	process of measuring
-osis	abnormal condition/disease of
-pathy	disease of
-plasty	surgical repair/reconstruction
-pexy	surgical fixation/fix in place
-plegia	condition of paralysis
-rrhaphy	suture/stitch/suturing
-rrhea (Am.)	excessive discharge/flow
-rrhoea	excessive discharge/flow
-scope	an instrument to view/examine
-scopy	technique of viewing/examining
-stenosis	abnormal condition of narrowing
-stomy	formation of an opening into …
-tomy	incision into
-us	thing/a structure (indicates an anatomical part)

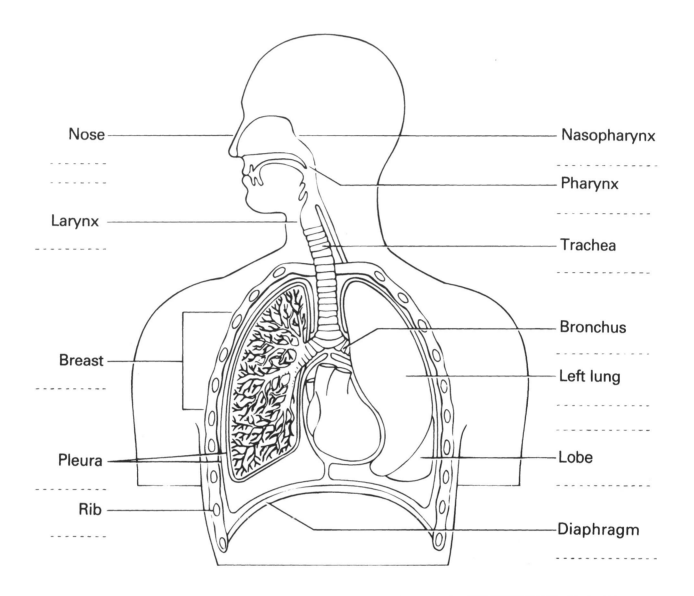

Nose

Nasopharynx

Pharynx

Larynx

Trachea

Breast

Bronchus

Left lung

Pleura

Lobe

Rib

Diaphragm

Figure 14 The breathing system

ANATOMY EXERCISE

When you have finished Word Exercises 1–16, look at the word components listed below. Complete Figure 14 by writing the appropriate combining form on each dotted line – more than one component may relate to the same position. (You can check their meanings in the Quick Reference box on p. 34.)

Bronch/o	Nasopharyng/o	Pulmon/o
Cost/o	Pharyng/o	Rhin/o
Laryng/o	Phren/o	Steth/o
Lob/o	Pleur/o	Trache/o
Nas/o	Pneumon/o	

The breathing system

Humans breathe air into paired lungs through the nose and mouth during inspiration. Whilst air is in the lungs gaseous exchange takes place. In this process oxygen enters the blood in exchange for carbon dioxide. During expiration, air containing less oxygen and more carbon dioxide leaves the body. The oxygen obtained through gaseous exchange is required by body cells for cellular respiration, a process which releases energy from food.

We will begin this unit at the point where air enters the body, the nose.

Use the Exercise Guide at the beginning of this unit to complete Word Exercises 1–16 unless you are asked to work without it.

Root	**Rhin** *(From a Greek word **rhinos**, meaning nose.)*
Combining forms	**Rhin/o**

 WORD EXERCISE 1

Using your Exercise Guide, find the meaning of:

(a) **rhino**scopy _____

(b) **rhino**pathy _____

(c) **rhin**algia _____

(d) **rhin**itis _____

(e) **rhino**rrhoea _____
     (Am. rhinorrhea)

(f) **rhino**plasty _____

Root	**Nas** *(From a Latin word **nasus**, meaning nose.)*
Combining forms	**Nas/o**

 WORD EXERCISE 2

Using your Exercise Guide, find the meaning of:

(a) **naso**gastric tube _____

(b) **naso**-oesophageal tube _____
     (Am. naso-esophageal)

Root	**Pharyng** *(From a Greek word **pharynx**, meaning throat.)*
Combining forms	**Pharyng/o**

 WORD EXERCISE 3

Without using your Exercise Guide, write the meaning of:

(a) **pharyng**algia _____

(b) **pharyngo**rrhoea _____
     (Am. pharyngorrhea)

Without using your Exercise Guide, build words which mean:

(c) surgical repair of the pharynx _____

(d) inflammation of the nose and _____
     pharynx (use rhin/o)

Root	**Laryng** *(From a Greek word **larynx** which refers to the voice box.)*
Combining forms	**Laryng/o**

 WORD EXERCISE 4

Using your Exercise Guide, find the meaning of:

(a) **laryngo**logy _____

(b) **laryngo**pharyngectomy _____

Without using your Exercise Guide, build words which mean:

(c) technique of viewing the larynx _____

(d) the study of the nose and larynx _____
     (use rhin/o).

When swallowing, food is prevented from falling into the larynx by the **epiglottis**, a thin flap of cartilage lying above the glottis and behind the tongue. When the epiglottis moves, it covers the opening into the larynx and sound-producing glottis. **Epiglott/o** is the combining form derived from epiglottis. Inflammation of the epiglottis may produce **epiglott**itis and tumours may be removed by **epiglott**ectomy.

Root   **Trache**
*(From Greek **tracheia**, meaning rough. Note that it refers to the rough appearance of the rings of cartilage in the windpipe. It is used to mean trachea or windpipe.)*

Combining forms   **Trache/o**

WORD EXERCISE 5

Using your Exercise Guide, find the meaning of:

(a) **tracheo**tomy

(b) **tracheo**stomy (operation used to maintain the airway; see Fig. 15)

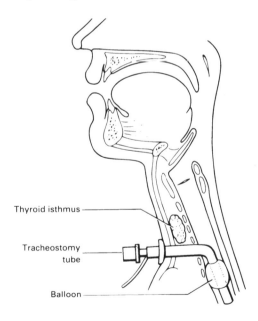

Thyroid isthmus

Tracheostomy tube

Balloon

Figure 15   Tracheostomy

Root   **Bronch**
*(From a Greek word **bronchos**, meaning bronchus or windpipe.)*

Combining forms   **Bronch/i, bronch/o**

WORD EXERCISE 6

Using your Exercise Guide, build words which mean:

(a) discharge/excessive flow of mucus   _____
    from bronchi

(b) an X-ray of the bronchus   _____

(c) technique of making an X-ray of   _____
    the bronchi

(d) an instrument for the visual   _____
    examination of the bronchi

Using your Exercise Guide, find the meaning of:

(e) **bronch**us   _____

(f) **broncho**plegia   _____

(g) **bronch**orrhaphy   _____

(h) **bronchi**ectasis   _____

(i) **broncho**mycosis   _____

(j) **broncho**genic   _____

(k) tracheo**bronchi**al   _____

Without using your Exercise Guide, write the meaning of:

(l) laryngotracheo**bronch**itis   _____

(m) **bronch**oesophagostomy   _____
    (Am. bronchesophagostomy)

Note.   The combining form **bronchiol/o** is used when referring to the very small subdivisions of the bronchi known as **bronchioles**, e.g. **bronchiol**itis for inflammation of the bronchioles.

The smallest bronchioles end in microscopic air sacs known as **alveoli** (from Latin *alveus*, meaning hollow cavity). Alveoli form a large surface area of the lungs across which the gases oxygen and carbon dioxide are exchanged. They play an essential role in maintaining life. The combining form is **alveol/o** but few terms are in use, e.g. **alveol**itis.

Root   **Pneumon**
(A Greek word, meaning lung.)

Combining forms   **Pneumon/o**

WORD EXERCISE 7

Without using your Exercise Guide, write the meaning of:

(a) **pneumono**tomy   _____

(b) **pneumono**rrhaphy   _____

(c) **pneumon**osis   _____

Without using your Exercise Guide, build words which mean:

(d) removal of a lung   _____

(e) disease of a lung   _____

Using your Exercise Guide, find the meaning of:

(f) **pneumono**centesis   _____

(g) **pneumono**pexy   _____

Root	Pneum
	(From a Greek word **pneumatos,** *meaning breath, air, gas and lung. Here we are using it to mean gas/air.)*
Combining forms	**Pneum/a, Pneum/o, Pneumat/o**

We should include here the word **pneumothorax**. The components of this word refer to air and thorax (chest) but the meaning of the word is not obvious. It is used to mean air or gas in the pleural cavity, i.e. the space between the wall of the thorax and the lungs. A pneumothorax is formed by puncture of the chest wall; this can be caused by a stab wound or made as part of a surgical procedure.

WORD EXERCISE 8

Using your Exercise Guide, find the meaning of:

(a) **pneumo**haemothorax   _____
(Am. pneumohemothorax; see Fig. 16)

(b) **pneumo**radiography   _____
(This term does not refer specifically to the breath-

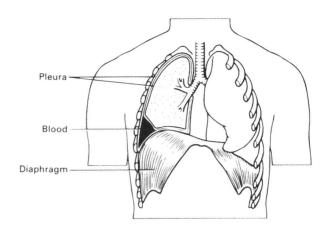

Pleura

Blood

Diaphragm

Figure 16	Haemothorax

ing system. It is a technique which is used to enhance the contrast of X-rays of body cavities by injecting air into them.)

Note.   A combining form -**pnoea**, meaning breathing, is also derived from this root (Am. -pnea).

Using your Exercise Guide, find the meaning of:

(c) a**pnoea**   _____
(Am. apnea)

(d) dys**pnoea**   _____
(Am. dyspnea)

(e) hyper**pnoea**   _____
(Am. hyperpnea)

(f) hypo**pnoea**   _____
(Am. hypopnea)

(g) tachy**pnoea**   _____
(Am. tachypnea)

Root	Lob
	(From a Greek word **lobos,** *meaning a rounded section of an organ. In the lungs, lobes are formed by fissures or septa which divide the right lung into three lobes and the left lung into two. Note that other organs in the body are lobar.)*
Combining forms	**Lob/o**

WORD EXERCISE 9

Without using your Exercise Guide, build words which mean:

(a) incision into a lobe _____

(b) removal of a lobe _____

Pulmon
*(From a Latin word **pulmonis**, meaning lung.)*

Combining forms   **Pulmon/o**

 WORD EXERCISE 10

Using your Exercise Guide, find the meaning of:

(a) **pulmon**ic _____

(b) **pulmon**ary _____

Pleur
*(From a Greek word **pleura**, meaning rib or side. It is used to mean the shiny membranes covering the lungs and internal surfaces of the thorax. The space in between the membranes is the pleural cavity.)*

Combining forms   **Pleur/o**

 WORD EXERCISE 11

Without using your Exercise Guide, write the meaning of:

(a) **pleur**itis (also called pleurisy) _____

(b) **pleuro**centesis _____

Without using your Exercise Guide, build a word which means:

(c) technique of making an X-ray
      of pleural cavity _____

Using your Exercise Guide, find the meaning of:

(d) **pleuro**dynia _____

(e) **pleuro**desis _____

Phren
(A Greek word, meaning midriff or diaphragm.)

Combining forms   **Phren/o**

 WORD EXERCISE 12

Using your Exercise Guide, find the meaning of:

(a) **phreno**gastric _____

(b) **phreno**hepatic _____

(c) **phreno**plegia _____

Thorac
*(From a Greek word **thorax**, meaning chest.)*

Combining forms   **Thorac/o, -thorax**

 WORD EXERCISE 13

Without using your Exercise Guide, build words which mean:

(a) any disease of thorax _____

(b) incision into chest _____

Without using your Exercise Guide, write the meaning of:

(c) **thoraco**centesis _____

(d) **thoraco**scope _____

Using your Exercise Guide, find the meaning of:

(e) **thoraco**stenosis _____

Root

Cost
(From a Latin word **costa**, meaning rib.)

Combining forms   **Cost/o**

WORD EXERCISE 14

Using your Exercise Guide, find the meaning of:

(a) inter**cost**al   _____

(b) **costo**genic   _____

(c) **costo**chondritis   _____

Medical equipment and clinical procedures

In this unit we have named several instruments used to examine the breathing system. Some of those mentioned may be modified fibreoptic endoscopes. Let us review their names:

rhinoscope
pharyngoscope
laryngoscope   } All of these are used for visual examination of parts of the breathing system.
bronchoscope
thoracoscope

The nose and pharynx can be superficially examined using a source of illumination with a tongue depressor and a nasal speculum (Figs 17 and 18).

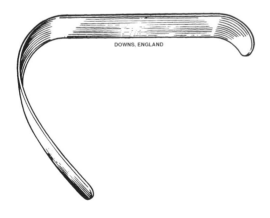

Figure 17   Tongue depressor

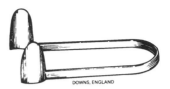
DOWNS, ENGLAND

Figure 18   Nasal speculum

Note.   The word **speculum** refers to an instrument used to hold the walls of a cavity apart so that the interior can be examined visually.

Other instruments which are used in investigating the breathing system include:

Stethoscope
(From a Greek word *stethos*, meaning breast, and *skopein*, meaning to examine.) Although this word ends in scope, which usually refers to an instrument for visual examination, it is used to listen to the sounds from the chest.

Spirograph
(From a Latin word *spirare*, meaning to breathe.) Instrument which records breathing movements of lungs.

Spirometer
Instrument which measures the capacity of the lung. The technique for using this instrument is spirometry (synonymous with pneumatometry).

Note.   Here we need to distinguish between the suffixes:

-meter
an instrument which measures.

-metry
the technique of measuring, i.e. using a measuring instrument.

Now revise the names and uses of all instruments and examinations mentioned in this unit and then try Exercises 15 and 16.

WORD EXERCISE 15

Match each term in Column A with a description from Column C by placing an appropriate number in Column B.

Column A	Column B	Column C
(a) bronchoscope	_____	1. person who may use a nasal speculum
(b) laryngoscopy	_____	2. instrument to examine the vocal cords
(c) rhinoscope	_____	3. instrument to examine the bronchi
(d) pharyngoscope	_____	4. visual examination of the vocal cords
(e) bronchoscopy	_____	5. device used to allow air through tracheal wall
(f) rhinologist	_____	6. instrument to view the back of the mouth
(g) tracheostomy tube	_____	7. visual examination of the bronchi
(h) laryngoscope	_____	8. instrument to view nasal cavities

WORD EXERCISE 16

Match each term in Column A with a description from Column C by placing an appropriate number in Column B.

Column A	Column B	Column C
(a) thoracoscope	_____	1. instrument to open nostril
(b) stethoscope	_____	2. technique of making X-ray of pleura
(c) spirometer	_____	3. technique of recording breathing movements

Column A	Column B	Column C
(d) spirography	_____	4. technique of measuring capacity of lungs
(e) nasal speculum	_____	5. instrument to view thorax
(f) nasogastric tube	_____	6. instrument which measures capacity of lungs
(g) pleurography	_____	7. instrument to examine/listen to breast
(h) spirometry	_____	8. tube inserted into stomach via nose

ANATOMY EXERCISE

Now complete the Anatomy Exercise on page 28.

Quick Reference

Medical roots relating to the breathing system:

Alveol/o	alveolus
Bronch/o	bronchus
Bronchiol/o	bronchiole
Chondr/o	cartilage
Cost/o	rib
Epiglott/o	epiglottis
Laryng/o	larynx
Lob/o	lobe
Nas/o	nose
Pharyng/o	pharynx
Phren/o	diaphragm
Pleur/o	pleura
Pneum/o	gas/air/lung
Pneumon/o	lung/air
-pnoea	breathing
-pnea (Am.)	breathing
Pulmon/o	lung
Rhin/o	nose
Spir/o	to breathe
Thorac/o	thorax
Trache/o	trachea

Abbreviations

You should learn common abbreviations related to the breathing system. Note, however, some are not standard and their meaning may vary from one hospital to another. There is a more extensive list for reference on page 259.

BRO   bronchoscopy
COAD   chronic obstructive airways disease
CXR   chest X-ray
ET   endotracheal
FVC   forced vital capacity
LLL   left lower lobe
PE   pulmonary embolism
PEFR   peak expiratory flow rate
PFts   pulmonary function tests
RSV   respiratory syncytial virus
SOBE   shortage of breath on exertion
URTI   upper respiratory tract infection

> ## NOW TRY THE WORD CHECK <

 ## WORD CHECK

This self-check exercise lists all the word components used in this unit. First write down the meaning of as many word components as you can. Then check your answers using the Exercise Guide and Quick Reference box or the Glossary of Word Components (pp. 269–279).

Prefixes

a-

dys-

hyper-

hypo-

inter-

tachy-

Combining forms of word roots

alveol/o

bronch/o

bronchiol/o

chondr/o

cost/o

epiglott/o

gastr/o

haem/o
(Am. hem/o)

hepat/o

laryng/o

lob/o

myc/o

nas/o

oesophag/o
(Am. esophag/o)

pharyng/o

phren/o

pleur/o

pneum/o

pneumon/o

-pnoea
(Am. -pnea)

pulmon/o

radi/o

rhin/o

spir/o

sten/o

thorac/o

trache/o

Suffixes

-al

-algia

-ary

-centesis

-desis

-dynia

-ectasis   _____

-ectomy   _____

-genic   _____

-gram   _____

-graphy   _____

-ia   _____

-ic   _____

-itis   _____

-logy   _____

-meter   _____

-metry   _____

-osis   _____

-pathy   _____

-pexy   _____

-plasty   _____

-plegia   _____

-rrhaphy   _____

-rrhoea
(Am. -rrhea)   _____

-scope   _____

-scopy   _____

-stomy   _____

-tomy   _____

-us   _____

(a)   bronch/o   _____

(b)   nasopharyng/o   _____

(c)   phren/o   _____

(d)   lob/o   _____

(e)   pleur/o   _____

(f)   pneum/o   _____

(g)   trache/o   _____

(h)   laryng/o   _____

(i)   pharyng/o   _____

(j)   rhin/o   _____

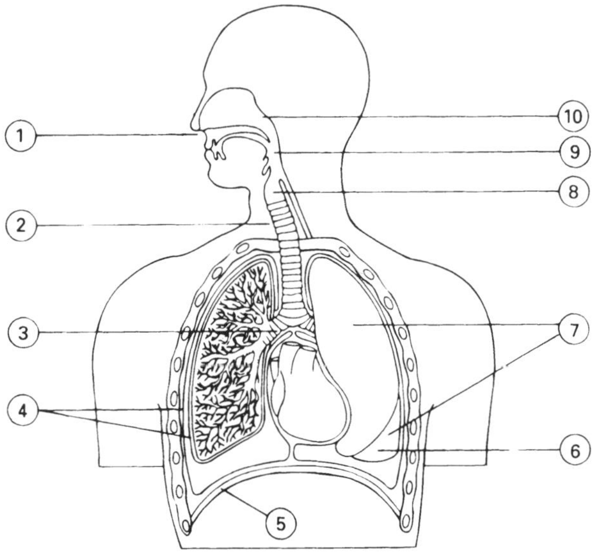

Figure 19   The breathing system

Score

10

> **NOW TRY THE SELF-ASSESSMENT**

 SELF-ASSESSMENT

Test 3A

Below are some combining forms which refer to the anatomy of the breathing system. Indicate which part of the system they refer to by putting a number from the diagram (Fig. 19) next to each word. You can use a number more than once.

Test 3B

Prefixes and suffixes

Match each prefix and suffix in Column A with a meaning in Column C by inserting the appropriate number in Column B.

Column A	Column B	Column C
(a) -centesis	_____	1. measuring instrument

Column A	Column B	Column C
(b) -desis	_____	2. pertaining to originating in/formation
(c) -dynia	_____	3. opening into/connection between two parts
(d) dys-	_____	4. between
(e) -ectomy	_____	5. abnormal condition/disease of
(f) -genic	_____	6. fixation (by surgery)
(g) hyper-	_____	7. condition of pain
(h) hypo-	_____	8. removal of
(i) inter-	_____	9. excessive flow/discharge
(j) -meter	_____	10. fast
(k) -metry	_____	11. above
(l) -osis	_____	12. difficult/painful
(m) -pexy	_____	13. surgical repair
(n) -plasty	_____	14. puncture
(o) -plegia	_____	15. condition of paralysis
(p) -rrhaphy	_____	16. to bind together
(q) -rrhoea (Am. -rrhea)	_____	17. incision into
(r) -stomy	_____	18. below
(s) -tachy	_____	19. technique of measuring
(t) -tomy	_____	20. suturing/stitching

Score

20

Column A	Column B	Column C
(a) bronch/o	_____	1. larynx
(b) cost/o	_____	2. diaphragm
(c) enter/o	_____	3. bronchus
(d) epiglott/o	_____	4. thorax
(e) gastr/o	_____	5. intestine
(f) hepat/o	_____	6. pleural membranes
(g) laryng/o	_____	7. stomach
(h) lob/o	_____	8. trachea
(i) myc/o	_____	9. breathing (wind)
(j) nas/o	_____	10. nose (i)
(k) pharyng/o	_____	11. nose (ii)
(l) phren/o	_____	12. fungus
(m) pleur/o	_____	13. lobule
(n) pneum/o	_____	14. pharynx
(o) pneumon/o	_____	15. liver
(p) -pnoea (Am. -pnea)	_____	16. gas/air/wind
(q) rhin/o	_____	17. lung
(r) sten/o	_____	18. epiglottis
(s) thorac/o	_____	19. rib
(t) trache/o	_____	20. narrowing

Score

20

Test 3C
Combining forms of word roots

Match each combining form in Column A with a meaning in Column C by inserting the appropriate number in Column B.

Test 3D

Write the meaning of:

(a) bronchogenic _____

(b) tracheostenosis _____

(c) pulmonologist _____

(d) phrenograph _____

(e) laryngoplegia _____

Score

5

Test 3E

Build words which mean:

(a) surgical repair of the bronchus   _____

(b) technique of visually   _____
     examining bronchi

(c) suturing of the trachea   _____

(d) study of the nose (use rhin/o)   _____

(e) pertaining to the diaphragm   _____
     and ribs

Score

5

Check answers to Self-Assessment Tests on page 251.

The cardiovascular system

Objectives

Once you have completed Unit 4 you should be able to:

- understand the meaning of medical words relating to the cardiovascular system

- build medical words relating to the cardiovascular system

- associate medical terms with their anatomical position

- understand medical abbreviations relating to the cardiovascular system.

Exercise Guide

Use this list of word components and their meanings to complete the word exercises in this unit.

Prefixes

a-	without
brady-	slow
dextro-	right
electro-	electrical
endo-	within/inside
pan-	all
peri-	around
tachy-	fast

Roots/Combining forms

dynam/o	force
ech/o	echo/reflected sound
lith/o	stone
man/o	pressure
my/o	muscle
necr/o	death, dead
phon/o	sound/voice

Suffixes

-algia	condition of pain
-ar	pertaining to
-centesis	surgical puncture to remove fluid
-clysis	infusion/injection/irrigation
-ectasis	dilatation/stretching
-ectomy	removal of
-genesis	capable of causing/pertaining to formation
-gram	X-ray/tracing/recording
-graph	usually an instrument that records
-graphy	technique of recording/making X-ray
-ia	condition of
-itis	inflammation of
-logy	study of
-lysis	breakdown/disintegration
-megaly	enlargement
-meter	measuring instrument
-metry	process of measuring
-oma	tumour/swelling
-osis	abnormal condition/disease of
-pathy	disease of
-plasty	surgical repair/reconstruction
-pexy	surgical fixation/fix in place
-plegia	condition of paralysis
-poiesis	formation
-rrhaphy	suture/stitch/suturing
-sclerosis	abnormal condition of hardening
-scope	an instrument to view/examine
-spasm	involuntary contraction of muscle
-stasis	stopping/controlling/cessation of movement
-stenosis	abnormal condition of narrowing
-tome	cutting instrument
-tomy	incision into
-um	thing/a structure/anatomical part
-us	thing/a structure/anatomical part

Heart

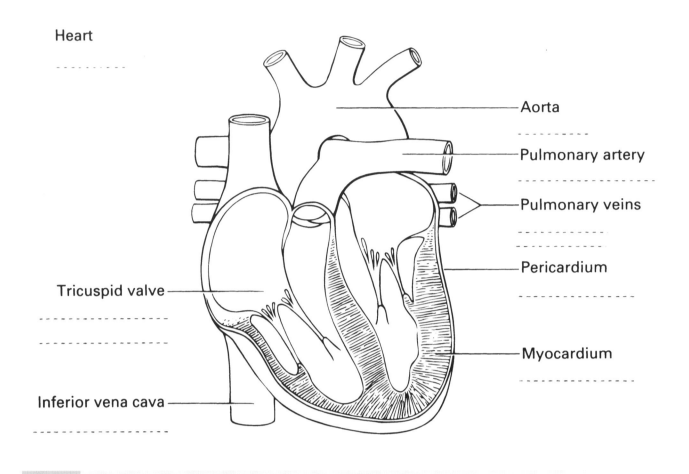

Aorta

Pulmonary artery

Pulmonary veins

Pericardium

Tricuspid valve

Myocardium

Inferior vena cava

Figure 20   The heart

![icon] **ANATOMY EXERCISE**

When you have finished Word Exercises 1–16, look at the word components listed below. Complete Figure 20 by writing the appropriate combining form on each dotted line – more than one component may relate to the same position. (You can check their meanings in the Quick Reference box on p. 47.)

Aort/o	Pericardi/o	Venacav/o
Arteri/o	Phleb/o	Ven/o
Cardi/o	Valv/o	
Myocardi/o	Valvul/o	

The cardiovascular system

In order to remain alive, cells within the body need a continuous supply of oxygen and nutrients for their metabolism. Any metabolic wastes excreted by these cells must be transported to the excretory organs where they can be removed from the body. The cardiovascular system provides a transport system for supply and removal of materials to and from the tissue cells, it consists of the heart and blood vessels.

The heart

The heart is a four-chambered, muscular pump whose function is to pump blood continuously through the body systems. The heart muscle (myocardium), is stimulated to contract rhythmically by a special patch of tissue called the sino-atrial node (SAN) or 'pacemaker'. Although the SAN gives the heart the ability to contract by itself, its rate of contraction is determined by nerve impulses from centres in the brain.

The heart muscle receives a supply of fully oxygenated blood from branches of the aorta known as the coronary arteries.

Use the Exercise Guide at the beginning of this unit to complete Word Exercises 1–16 unless you are asked to work without it.

Root   **Card**
*(From a Greek word **kardia**, meaning heart.)*

Combining forms   **Card, cardi/o**

WORD EXERCISE 1

Using your Exercise Guide, find the meaning of:

(a) **cardi**algia   _____

(b) **cardio**scope   _____

(c) **cardio**graph   _____

(d) **cardio**gram   _____

(e) tachy**card**ia   _____

Using your Exercise Guide, build words using cardi/o which mean:

(f) enlargement of the heart   _____

(g) surgical repair of the heart   _____

(h) disease of the heart   _____

(i) study of the heart   _____

Using your Exercise Guide, find the meaning of:

(j) myo**cardi**um   _____

(k) **cardio**myopathy   _____

(l) **cardio**rrhaphy   _____

(m) electro**cardio**graph   _____

(n) endo**card**itis   _____

(o) pan**card**itis   _____

(p) brady**card**ia   _____

(q) dextro**card**ia   _____

(r) phono**cardio**graphy   _____

(s) echo**cardio**graphy   _____

(t) electro**cardio**gram   _____

To make an electrocardiogram (ECG; Fig. 21) electrodes are attached to the skin at various sites on the body. The heart muscle generates electrical impulses which can be detected at the surface of the body, amplified and converted into a trace on a screen or paper. The P wave appears when the atria are stimulated, the QRS complex when the impulse passes to the ventricles and the T wave is generated when the ventricles contract. Abnormal electrical activity and changes in heart rate seen in coronary heart disease can be detected from the ECG.

The heart is continuously supplied with blood through coronary arteries. Narrowing of these vessels results in **ischaemia**, a deficient blood supply (*ischia* means to check), which produces pain in the chest known as **angina pectoris**. If the flow of blood to the heart muscle is interrupted, the muscle dies; this is a **myocardial infarction** or heart attack. Heart muscle deprived of oxygen produces a rapid, uncoordinated, quivering contraction known as **fibrillation**. Normal rhythm can sometimes be restored by applying an electric shock with an instrument known as a **defibrillator**.

Around the heart there is a double membranous sac known as the **pericardium** (peri-, prefix meaning

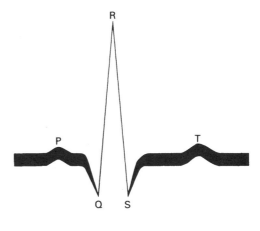

Figure 21   Electrocardiogram

around). Between the membranes is a pericardial cavity containing a small amount of fluid. The combining forms of pericardium are **pericard/o** and **pericardi/o**.

WORD EXERCISE 2

Without using your Exercise Guide, build a word which means:

(a) inflammation of the pericardium _____

Using your Exercise Guide, find the meaning of:

(b) cardio**pericardio**pexy _____

(c) **pericardio**centesis _____

(d) **pericardi**ectomy _____

Blood flow through the heart is controlled by **valves**. Between the right atrium and the right ventricle there is a **tricuspid valve** (with three flaps or cusps) which allows blood to flow from the right atrium to the right ventricle but not in the opposite direction. Similarly there is a valve on the left side of the heart which allows blood to flow from the left atrium to the left ventricle. This is known as the **bicuspid valve** or the **mitral valve** (with two flaps or cusps).

Root
Valv
*(From Latin **valva**, meaning fold. In medicine it refers to a valve, i.e. a fold or membrane in a tube or passage permitting flow in one direction only.)*

Combining forms   **Valv/o**

WORD EXERCISE 3

Without using your Exercise Guide, build words which mean:

(a) surgical repair of a heart valve _____

(b) removal of a heart valve _____

Valvul/o is a New Latin combining form also derived from *valva*; using your Exercise Guide, find the meaning of:

(c) cardio**valvulo**tome _____

Note.   -tome comes from *tomon*, meaning cutter.

(d) **valvul**ar _____

(e) **valvo**tomy _____

The blood vessels

Blood circulates through a closed system of blood vessels throughout the body. It flows away from the heart in arteries which divide into smaller arterioles and then into capillaries. Blood flows back to the heart through venules and then into larger vessels known as veins.

The system which supplies blood to the tissues is known as the **arterial system** and that which takes it away the **venous system.** Now we will look at some of the terms concerned with these blood vessels.

Root
Vas
(A Latin word, meaning vessel. Here it refers to blood vessels of any type.)

Combining forms   **Vas/o**
Vascul/o, *also derived from vas, has the same meaning.*

WORD EXERCISE 4

Using your Exercise Guide, find the meaning of:

(a) **vaso**spasm _____

Blood vessels can widen (**vaso**dilatation) and they can narrow (**vaso**constriction) because of the activity of muscles in their walls. If a vessel widens then the blood pressure within it falls. Some drugs are designed to stimulate this action, i.e. reducing blood pressure. They are known as **vasodilators**.

(b) a**vascul**ar _____

Without using your Exercise Guide, build words using vascul/o which mean:

(c) inflammation of blood vessels _____

(d) disease of blood vessels _____

Root

Angi
*(From a Greek word **angeion**, meaning vessel, in this case a blood vessel.)*

combining forms   **Angi/o**

WORD EXERCISE 5

Without using your Exercise Guide, write the meaning of:

(a) **angio**gram _____

(b) **angio**cardiogram _____

(c) **angio**cardiography _____

Digital subtraction angiography

Angiography is the technique of making X-rays or images of blood vessels. Both arteries and veins can be made visible on radiographic film following the injection of a contrast medium. This results in an X-ray film on which the injected vessels cast a shadow showing their size, shape and location.

Digital subtraction angiography (DSA) is very similar, except, instead of having an X-ray film, the X-rays are detected electronically and a computer builds an image of the blood vessels on a television monitor.

One problem in visualizing blood vessels is that overlying tissues cast an image on the picture. To eliminate these unwanted images, an X-ray is taken before and after dye is injected. A computer then subtracts the first image from the second, removing the interfering image. The picture produced by DSA is superior to a film-based angiogram.

Without using your Exercise Guide, build words which mean:

(d) study of blood vessels _____

(e) surgical repair of blood vessels _____

A common surgical repair is a balloon angioplasty. In this procedure a catheter containing an inflatable balloon is inserted into a narrowed vessel (see Fig. 22). When the balloon is inflated and moved along the lining any fatty plaques are displaced and the flow of blood through the vessel is restored.

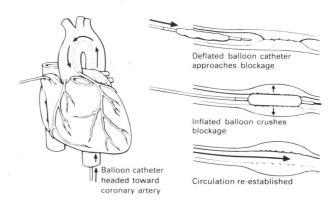

Deflated balloon catheter approaches blockage

Inflated balloon crushes blockage

Circulation re-established

Balloon catheter headed toward coronary artery

Figure 22   Balloon angioplasty

Using your Exercise Guide, find the meaning of:

(f) **angi**oma _____

(g) **angi**ectasis _____

(h) **angio**poiesis _____

(i) **angio**sclerosis _____

The above roots refer generally to blood vessels. Now we will look at those which refer to a specific type of vessel.

Root

Aort
*(From Greek **aorte**, meaning great vessel. It refers to the largest artery in the body. This vessel leaves the left ventricle of the heart and divides into smaller arteries which supply all body systems with oxygenated blood.)*

Combining forms   **Aort/o**

WORD EXERCISE 6

Without using your Exercise Guide, build words which mean:

(a) any disease of the aorta _____

(b) technique of X-raying the aorta _____

Root   **Arter**
(From a Greek word **arteria***,
meaning artery. The function of
arteries is to move blood away from
the heart. They divide into smaller
arterioles and then into capillaries
which exchange materials with the
tissue cells.)*

Combining forms   **Arter/i, arteri/o**

WORD EXERCISE 7

Without using your Exercise Guide, build words using
arteri/o which mean:

(a) suturing of an artery   _____

(b) condition of hardening of arteries   _____

Using your Exercise Guide, find the meaning of:

(c) end**arter**ectomy   _____
      (In this procedure fatty deposits are removed from
      the lining of the artery.)

(d) **arterio**necrosis   _____

(e) **arterio**stenosis   _____

Root   **Vena cav**
(From Latin words **vena cavum***,
meaning hollow vein.)*

Combining forms   **Venacav/o**

Venae cavae are the great veins of the body, i.e. the
superior vena cava which drains blood from the head
and the **inferior vena cava** which drains blood from the
lower parts of the body. The **venae cavae** pass their
blood into the right atrium of the heart.

 ## WORD EXERCISE 8

Without using your Exercise Guide, write the meaning
of:

(a) **venacavo**gram   _____

(b) **venacavo**graphy   _____

Root   **Ven**
(From a Latin words **vena***, meaning
vein. The function of veins is to
transfer blood back to the heart.
Capillaries are drained by small
vessels called venules, these join and
form larger veins. Unlike arteries,
veins contain valves which prevent
the backflow of blood.)*

Combining forms   **Ven/o**

WORD EXERCISE 9

Using your Exercise Guide, find the meaning of:

(a) **Ven**ectasis   _____

(b) **veno**clysis   _____

Without using your Exercise Guide, build words which
mean:

(c) X-ray picture of a vein (after   _____
      injection of opaque dye)

(d) technique of making an   _____
      X-ray of a vein
      (venous system)

 Root   **Phleb**
(From a Greek word **phlebos***,
meaning vein.)*

Combining forms   **Phleb/o**

WORD EXERCISE 10

Without using your Exercise Guide, write the meaning of:

(a) **phleb**arteriectasis   _____

(b) **phlebo**clysis   _____

(c) **phlebo**tomy   _____

Using your Exercise Guide, find the meaning of:

(d) **phlebo**stasis   _____

(e) **phlebo**manometer   _____   _____

(f) **phlebo**lith   _____

Root **Thromb**
*(From a Greek word **thrombos**, meaning a clot. Clots are formed mainly of platelets, fibrin and blood cells. They can block blood vessels, restricting or stopping the flow of blood.)*

Combining forms **Thromb/o**

WORD EXERCISE 11

Without using your Exercise Guide, write the meaning of:

(a) **thrombo**poiesis _____

(b) **thrombo**phlebitis _____

(c) **thrombo**endarterectomy _____

Without using your Exercise Guide, build words which mean:

(d) abnormal condition of having a clot _____

(e) removal of a clot _____

Using your Exercise Guide, find the meaning of:

(f) **thrombo**genesis _____

(g) **thrombo**lysis _____

The sudden blocking of an artery by a clot is referred to as an **embolism**. Emboli can be caused by thrombi as well as other foreign materials, such as fat, air and infective material. The combining form **embol/o** is used when referring to an **embolus**, e.g. as in **embol**ectomy.

Thrombolytic therapy

Recently developed enzymes are being used to dissolve blood clots in situ. The drug streptokinase, extracted from bacteria, can be injected into the coronary vessels to lyse a clot and thereby restore blood in the coronary system.

Atheroma is used to refer to another very common disorder of the blood vessels. The meaning of this word is

 Root **Ather**
*(From a Greek word **athere**, meaning porridge. Used to mean fatty plaques on walls of vessels.)*

Combining forms **Ather/o**

a porridge-like tumour but it is used to describe the yellow plaques of fatty material which are deposited in the lining of the arteries. The presence of such deposits is believed to be partly related to diets rich in certain types of fat. Atheroma in coronary arteries increases the chance of their becoming blocked, thus predisposing the heart to myocardial infarction (death of heart muscle due to lack of oxygen, i.e. a heart attack).

WORD EXERCISE 12

Without using your Exercise Guide, write the meaning of:

(a) **athero**genesis _____

(b) **athero**embolus _____

Atherosclerosis refers to the hardening of arteries and to the presence of atheroma.

 Root **Aneurysm**
*(From Greek **aneurysma**, meaning a dilatation. Here it is used to refer to a dilated vessel, usually an artery. It is due to a local fault in the wall through defect, disease or injury. An aneurysm appears as a pulsating swelling which can rupture.)*

Combining forms **Aneurysm/o**

WORD EXERCISE 13

Without using your Exercise Guide, write the meaning of:

(a) **aneurysmo**plasty _____

(b) **aneurysmo**rrhaphy _____

Root

Sphygm

*(From a Greek word **sphygmos**, meaning pulsation. We use it to refer to the pulse which can be felt wherever an artery is near to the surface of the body. The pulsation is due to the heart forcing blood into the arterial system at ventricular systole (contraction). Pulse rate is therefore a measure of heart rate.)*

Combining forms **Sphygm/o**

WORD EXERCISE 14

Using your Exercise Guide, find the meaning of:

(a) **sphygmo**dynamometer _____

(b) **sphygmo**manometer _____

(c) **sphygmo**metry _____

Without using your Exercise Guide, write the meaning of:

(d) **sphygmo**graph _____

(e) **sphygmo**gram (refers to movements created by arterial pulse) _____

(f) **sphygmo**cardiograph _____

Note. Mano comes from Greek *manos*, meaning rare. Manometers were first used for measuring rarefied air, i.e. gases. The combining form **man/o** is now used to mean pressure.

Figure 23 is a drawing of an instrument which uses a manometer to measure blood pressure. Two pressures are measured: the **systolic** pressure when the ventricles of the heart are forcing blood into the circulation, and the **diastolic** pressure which is the pressure within the vessels when the heart is dilating and refilling.

The sphygmomanometer can be used to detect **hyper**tension, i.e. a persistently high arterial blood pressure, or **hypo**tension, an abnormally low blood pressure. Both of these conditions have a variety of causes.

The **stethoscope** (Fig. 24) is used in conjunction with the sphygmomanometer. It is used to listen to the sounds made by blood flowing through the brachial artery when recording the blood pressure.

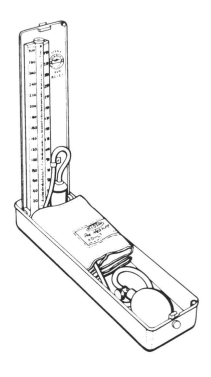

Figure 23 Sphygmomanometer

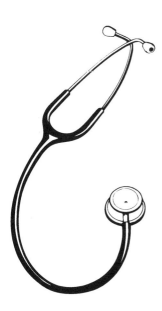

Figure 24 Stethoscope

Note. In medicine the suffix -scope is usually used to refer to an instrument for visual examination. Here we are using the stethoscope to listen to sounds. Scope comes from the Greek word *skopein* which also means to examine. **Steth/o** means breast. Stethoscope therefore means an instrument to examine the breast.

Medical equipment and clinical procedures

In this unit we have named many instruments used for examining the cardiovascular system. Two new combining forms have been used with them and we will revise them before completing the next exercise.

> **mano**
> means pressure. In sphygmo**mano**meter it refers to the pressure of the pulse, i.e. arterial blood pressure.
>
> **dynam**
> means power. In sphygmo**dynam**ometer it refers to the force of the pulse (volume and pressure).

Note. Words ending in **-graph** usually refer to a recording instrument and those ending in **-scope** usually to a viewing instrument (except for the stethoscope which is used for listening).

Revise the names of all instruments mentioned in this unit and then complete Exercises 15 and 16.

 ## WORD EXERCISE 15

Match each term in Column A with a description from Column C by placing an appropriate number in Column B.

Column A	Column B	Column C
(a) cardioscope	_____	1. instrument which measures arterial blood pressure (pressure of the pulse)
(b) cardiograph	_____	2. instrument used to cut a heart valve
(c) electro-cardiograph	_____	3. technique of X-raying heart and blood vessels after injection of radio-opaque dye
(d) cardioval-votome	_____	4. instrument which records heart (beat)
(e) angiocardio-graphy	_____	5. instrument which records the electrical activity of the heart
(f) sphygmo-manometer	_____	6. instrument to view the heart

 ## WORD EXERCISE 16

Match each term in Column A with a description from Column C by placing an appropriate number in Column B.

Column A	Column B	Column C
(a) echocardio-graphy	_____	1. recording of heart sounds
(b) sphygmocar-diograph	_____	2. instrument used to listen to sounds within the chest
(c) stethoscope	_____	3. tracing or recording of the electrical activity of the heart
(d) phonocardio-gram	_____	4. instrument which measures the pressure within a vein
(e) electrocardio-gram	_____	5. instrument which records pulse and heart beat
(f) phlebomano-meter	_____	6. technique of recording heart using reflected ultrasound

 ## ANATOMY EXERCISE

Now complete the Anatomy Exercise on page 40.

Quick Reference

Medical roots relating to the cardiovascular system:

Aneurysm/o	aneurysm
Angi/o	vessel
Aort/o	aorta
Arteri/o	artery
Ather/o	atheroma
Cardi/o	heart
Embol/o	embolism
My/o	muscle
Pericardi/o	pericardium
Phleb/o	vein
Sphygm/o	pulse
Steth/o	breast
Thromb/o	thrombus/clot
Valv/o	valve

Quick Reference (contd.)

Medical roots relating to the cardiovascular system:

Valvul/o	valve
Vas/o	vessel
Vascul/o	vessel
Ven/o	vein
Venacav/o	vena cava

Abbreviations

You should learn common abbreviations related to the cardiovascular system. Note, however, some abbreviations are not standard and their meaning may vary from one hospital to another. There is a more extensive list for reference on page 259.

AAA	abdominal aortic aneurysm
AF	atrial fibrillation
AMI	acute myocardial infarction
CABG	coronary artery bypass grafting
CAD	coronary artery disease
CCU	coronary care unit
CPR	cardiopulmonary resuscitation
CT	coronary thrombosis
ECG	electrocardiogram
iv	intravenous
MI	myocardial infarction
MS	mitral stenosis

NOW TRY THE WORD CHECK

WORD CHECK

This self-check exercise lists all word components used in this unit. First write down the meaning of as many word components as you can. Then check your answers using the Exercise Guide and Quick Reference box or the Glossary of Word Components (pp. 269–279).

Prefixes

a- _____

bi- _____

brady- _____

dextro- _____

electro- _____

endo- _____

hyper- _____

hypo- _____

pan- _____

peri- _____

tachy- _____

tri- _____

Combining forms of word roots

aneurysm/o _____

angi/o _____

aort/o _____

arteri/o _____

ather/o _____

cardi/o _____

ech/o _____

embol/o _____

dynam/o _____

man/o _____

my/o _____

necr/o _____

pericardi/o _____

phleb/o _____

phon/o _____

sphygm/o _____

sten/o _____

steth/o _____

thromb/o _____

valv/o _____

valvul/o _____

vas/o _____

vascul/o _____

ven/o _____

venacav/o _____

Suffixes

-algia _____

-ar _____

-centesis _____

-clysis _____

-ectasis _____

-ectomy _____

-genesis _____

-gram _____

-graph _____

-graphy _____

-ia _____

-itis _____

-ium _____

-lith _____

-logy _____

-lysis _____

-megaly _____

-meter _____

-metry _____

-oma _____

-osis _____

-pathy _____

-pexy _____

-plasty _____

-poiesis _____

-rrhage _____

-rrhaphy _____

-sclerosis _____

-scope _____

-stasis _____

-tome _____

-tomy _____

-um _____

❯ NOW TRY THE SELF-ASSESSMENT

SELF-ASSESSMENT

Test 4A

Below are some combining forms which refer to the anatomy of the cardiovascular system. Indicate which part of the system they refer to by putting a number from the diagram (Fig. 25) next to each word.

(a) aort/o _____

(b) venacav/o _____

(c) endocardi/o _____

(d) valv/o _____

(e) pericardi/o _____

(f) myocardi/o _____

Score

| 6 |

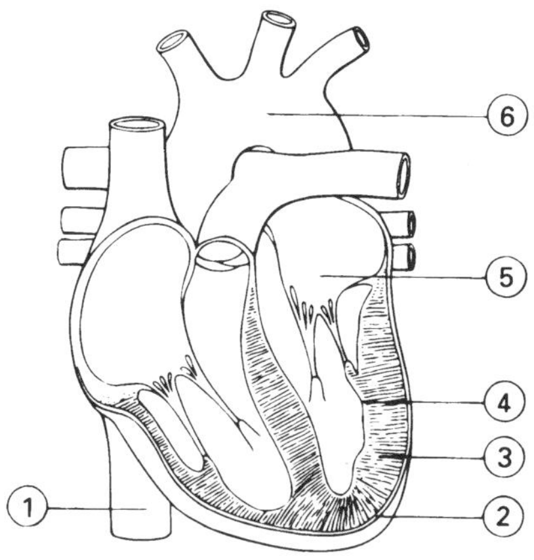

Figure 25 The heart

Test 4B

Prefixes and suffixes

Match each prefix or suffix in Column A with a meaning in Column C by inserting the appropriate number in Column B.

	Column A	Column B	Column C
(a)	a-	_____	1. to hold back/check
(b)	bi-	_____	2. formation (i)
(c)	brady-	_____	3. formation (ii)
(d)	-clysis	_____	4. infusion/injection
(e)	dextro-	_____	5. two
(f)	-ectasis	_____	6. fast
(g)	electro-	_____	7. dilatation
(h)	endo-	_____	8. without
(i)	-genesis	_____	9. fixation
(j)	isch-	_____	10. right
(k)	-megaly	_____	11. around
(l)	pan-	_____	12. electrical
(m)	peri-	_____	13. stopping/cessation
(n)	-pexy	_____	14. hardening
(o)	-poiesis	_____	15. slow
(p)	-sclerosis	_____	16. tissue/thing
(q)	-stasis	_____	17. three
(r)	tachy-	_____	18. all
(s)	tri-	_____	19. enlargement
(t)	-um	_____	20. inside

Score

20

Test 4C

Combining forms of word roots

Match each combining form in Column A with a meaning in Column C by inserting the appropriate number in Column B.

	Column A	Column B	Column C
(a)	aneurysm/o	_____	1. echo/reflected sound
(b)	angi/o	_____	2. artery
(c)	aort/o	_____	3. death/corpse
(d)	arteri/o	_____	4. sound
(e)	ather/o	_____	5. valve
(f)	cardi/o	_____	6. aorta
(g)	dynam/o	_____	7. porridge (yellow plaque on wall of blood vessel)
(h)	ech/o	_____	8. heart
(i)	man/o	_____	9. vessel (i)
(j)	my/o	_____	10. vessel (ii)
(k)	necr/o	_____	11. force
(l)	phleb/o	_____	12. aneurysm (swelling)
(m)	phon/o	_____	13. pressure/rare
(n)	sphygm/o	_____	14. muscle
(o)	sten/o	_____	15. vein (i)
(p)	steth/o	_____	16. vein (ii)
(q)	thromb/o	_____	17. clot
(r)	valv/o	_____	18. narrowing
(s)	vas/o	_____	19. pulse
(t)	ven/o	_____	20. breast

Score

20

Test 4D

Write the meaning of:

(a) cardiovalvulitis   _____

(b) aortorrhaphy   _____

(c) angioscope   _____

(d) phlebostenosis   _____

(e) thromboendarteritis   _____

Score

5

Test 4E

Build words which mean:

(a) Inflammation of an artery   _____
    associated with a thrombosis

(b) Puncture of the heart   _____

(c) Disease of an artery   _____

(d) Removal of a vein   _____

(e) Study of heart and blood   _____
    vessels (use angi/o)

Score

5

Check answers to Self-Assessment Tests on page 252.

5 The Blood

Objectives

Once you have completed Unit 5 you should be able to:

- understand the meaning of medical words relating to the blood

- build medical words relating to blood

- associate medical terms with the components of blood

- understand medical abbreviations relating to the blood.

Exercise Guide

Use this list of word components and their meanings to complete the word exercises in this unit.

Prefixes

a-	without
an-	without/not
aniso-	unequal
ellipto-	shaped like an ellipse
hyper-	above/abnormal increase
hypo-	below/abnormal decrease
macro-	large
micro-	small
peri-	around
poikil/o	varied/irregular
poly-	many

Roots/Combining forms

cyt/e/o	cell
dynam/o	force
fibr/o	fibre
path/o	disease
pericardi/o	pericardium
septic/o	sepsis/infection/putrefaction

Suffixes

-aemia	condition of blood
-apheresis	removal
-blast	germ cell/embryonic/immature
-chromia	condition of colour/haemoglobin
-crit	separate/device for measuring cells
-cytosis	increased number of cells
-emia (Am.)	condition of blood
-genesis	capable of causing/pertaining to formation
-globin	protein
-ia	condition of
-ic	pertaining to
-ium	structure/anatomical part
-logy	study of
-lysis	breakdown/disintegration
-meter	measuring instrument
-oma	tumour/swelling
-osis	abnormal condition/disease of
-penia	condition of lack of/deficiency
-poiesis	formation
-rrhage	bursting forth (of blood/bleeding)
-stasis	stopping/controlling/cessation of movement
-toxic	pertaining to poisoning
-um	thing/structure/anatomical part
-uria	condition of urine

Blood (a stained smear)

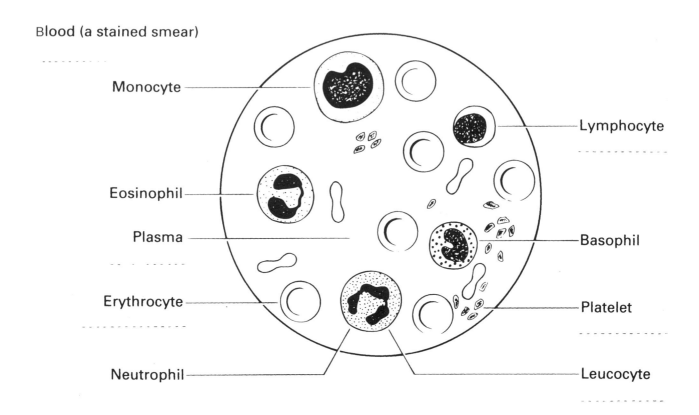

Monocyte

Eosinophil

Plasma

Erythrocyte

Neutrophil

Lymphocyte

Basophil

Platelet

Leucocyte

Figure 26   Blood

ANATOMY EXERCISE

When you have finished Word Exercises 1–7, look at the word components listed below. Complete Figure 26 by writing the appropriate combining form on each dotted line – more than one component may relate to the same position. (You can check their meanings in the Quick Reference box on p. 58.)

Erythr/o	Leuc/o	Plasma-
Haem/o	Lymph/o	Thrombocyt/o

The blood

Blood is a complex fluid which is classified as a connective tissue because it contains cells, plus an intercellular matrix known as plasma. Here we can see the main components of whole blood:

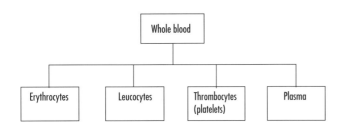

The blood cells carry out a variety of functions: erythrocytes (red blood cells) transport gases whilst leucocytes (white blood cells) defend the body against invasion by microorganisms and foreign antigens. Thrombocytes, or platelets, are actually fragments of larger cells. They are concerned with the formation of blood clots following injury.

The plasma carries nutrients, wastes, hormones, antibodies and blood-clotting proteins. The study of blood is very important in medicine for the diagnosis of disease.

Use the Exercise Guide at the beginning of the unit to complete Word Exercises 1–7 unless you are asked to work without it.

Root   **Haem**
(From a Greek word **haima**, *meaning blood.)*

Combining forms   **Haem/o, haemat/o, -aemia, -haemia**
Hem/o, hemat/o, -emia, -hemia *(Am.)*

WORD EXERCISE 1

Using your Exercise Guide, find the meaning of:

(a) **haemato**logy
(Am. hematology)   _____

(b) **haemo**pathology
(Am. hemopathology)   _____

(c) **haemo**dynamics
(Am. hemodynamics)   _____

(d) **haemo**poiesis
(Am. hemopoiesis)   _____

(e) **haemo**stasis
(Am. hemostasis)   _____

(f) **haemo**pericardium (Fig. 27)   _____
(Am. hemopericardium)

Using your Exercise Guide, build words which mean:

(g) Tumour/swelling containing blood   _____

(h) Breakdown/disintegration of blood   _____

(i) Condition of blood in the urine   _____

(j) Bursting forth of blood   _____

Using your Exercise Guide, find the meaning of:

(k) polycyt**haemia**
(Am. polycythemia)   _____

(l) an**aemia**
(Am. anemia)   _____

(m) septic**aemia**
(Am. septicemia)   _____

Haemoglobin is a red pigment found inside red blood cells, it functions to transport oxygen and carbon dioxide. The amount of haemoglobin present in the blood is of great importance to the efficiency of gaseous trans-

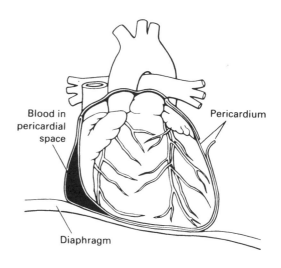

Blood in pericardial space   Pericardium

Diaphragm

Figure 27   Haemopericardium

port within the body. Several types of investigation are performed to estimate the amount of haemoglobin in the blood. Here are some terms which relate specifically to haemoglobin (globin means protein). The combining form **haemoglobin/o** refers to haemoglobin.

Using your Exercise Guide, find the meaning of:

(n) **haemoglobino**meter   _____
(Am. hemoglobin)

Without using your Exercise Guide, write the meaning of:

(o) **haemoglobin**   _____
(Am. hemoglobin)

(p) **haemoglobin**uria   _____
(Am. hemoglobinuria)

The amount of haemoglobin within red blood cells can be estimated and abnormal levels are found in some patients. Terms describing these conditions have been formed from the suffix **-chromia** (from Greek *chromos*, meaning colour). Here the colour refers to the red pigment haemoglobin.

Using your Exercise Guide, find the meaning of:

(q) hypo**chromia**   _____

(r) hyper**chromia**   _____

Another common term related to the colour of haemoglobin is **cyanosis**. **Cyan/o** means blue. In the absence of oxygen, haemoglobin develops a bluish tinge. Nailbeds, lips and skin show signs of cyanosis when oxygenation of the blood is deficient. Tissues deprived of oxygen can also be described as **anoxic**.

Now we will examine word roots which refer to the different types of blood cells. All of these cells are suspended in the liquid matrix of the blood known as plasma.

Root	**Erythr**
	*(From a Greek word **erythros**, meaning red. Here it is used to refer to red blood cells, i.e. erythrocytes.)*
Combining forms	**Erythr/o**

WORD EXERCISE 2

Using your Exercise Guide, find the meaning of:

(a) **erythro**penia   _____

(b) **erythro**genesis   _____

(c) **erythro**blast   _____
(This refers to the cell which eventually forms the mature erythrocyte.)

Without using your Exercise Guide, write the meaning of:

(d) **erythro**poiesis   _____

(e) **erythrocyto**lysis   _____

(f) **erythrocyt**haemia   _____
(Am. erythrocythemia)

This last condition is synonymous with erythrocytosis which means an abnormal condition of red cells, i.e. too many red cells. This condition is usually a physiological response to low levels of oxygen circulating in the blood. Besides changes in number, individual erythrocytes can suffer from various abnormalities, some of which are listed below.

Using your Exercise Guide, find the meaning of:

(g) micro**cytosis**   _____
(NB: Cytosis is used in (g) to (k) to mean too many red blood cells.)

(h) macro**cytosis**   _____

(i) ellipto**cytosis**   _____

(j) aniso**cytosis**   _____

(k) poikilo**cytosis**   _____

Root	**Reticul**
	*(From a Latin word **reticulum**, meaning small net. Here it refers to a very young erythrocyte lacking a nucleus, its cytoplasm giving a net-like appearance with basic dyes.)*
Combining forms	**Reticul/o**

WORD EXERCISE 3

Without using your Exercise Guide, build words which mean:

(a) an immature erythrocyte   _____

(b) condition of too many immature erythrocytes   _____

(c) condition of deficiency of reticulocytes   _____

Root	**Leuc**
	*(From a Greek word **leukos**, meaning white. Here it is referring to white blood cells, i.e. leucocytes.)*
Combining forms	**Leuc/o, leuk/o**
	(Leuc/o is more commonly used in the UK, leuk/o in America.)

WORD EXERCISE 4

Without using your Exercise Guide, build words which mean:

(a) condition of deficiency of white cells   _____

(b) the formation of white blood cells   _____

Without using your Exercise Guide, write the meaning of:

(c) **leuco**cytogenesis   _____
(Am. leukocytogenesis)

(d) **leuk**aemia   _____
(Am. leukemia. This is a malignant condition, i.e. a type of cancer.)

(e) **leuco**cytosis   _____
(Am. leukocytosis. This refers to an excess of white cells as seen during infection.)

(f) **leuco**cytoma   _____
(Am. leukocytoma)

(g) **leuco**blast   _____
(Am. leukoblast)

(h) **leuco**blastosis   _____
(Am. leukoblastosis)

Using your Exercise Guide, find the meaning of:

(i) **leuco**toxic   _____
(Am. leukotoxic)

Leucocyte is a general term meaning white cell but there are many types of white cell. Some leucocytes contain granules and are known as **granulocytes**, those without granules are called **agranulocytes** (*a*- without).

Among the commonest granulocytes are polymorphonuclear granulocytes or polymorphs. These all have nuclei which show many shapes (*poly* – many, *morpho* – shape). There are three types of polymorph:

Neutrophils
From *neutro*, meaning neither, and *philein*, meaning to love. These cells stain well with (love) **neutral** dyes. Neutrophils engulf microorganisms which have entered the blood and destroy them. These cells are sometimes referred to as phagocytes (*phago* means eat, i.e. cells which eat). The process of engulfing particles is known as phagocytosis.

Basophils
These cells stain well with **basic** (alkaline) dyes.

Eosinophils
These cells stain well with acid dyes like **eosin**, a red dye.

Among the agranular leucocytes are lymphocytes and large monocytes (*mono* means single). The latter can leave the blood and wander to the site of infections. Lymphocytes will be studied in Unit 6.

Root

Myel
*(From a Greek word **myelos**, meaning marrow. Here it is used to refer to the bone marrow which gives rise to the granulocyte, a type of white blood cell.)*

Combining forms   **Myel/o**

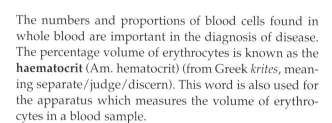

WORD EXERCISE 5

Without using your Exercise Guide, write the meaning of:

(a) **myelo**cyte   _____

(b) **myelo**fibrosis   _____

Without using your Exercise Guide, build words which mean: _____

(c) germ cell of the marrow   _____

(d) tumour of myeloid tissue   _____

WORD EXERCISE 6

We have already used the combining form **thromb/o** which means clot but here it is combined with cyte. It refers to fragments of cells which are concerned with the clotting of blood, i.e. platelets or **thrombocytes**.

Without using your Exercise Guide, write the meaning of:

(a) **thrombocyto**penia   _____

(b) **thrombocyto**poiesis   _____

(c) **thrombocyto**lysis   _____

(d) **thrombocyto**pathy   _____

The numbers and proportions of blood cells found in whole blood are important in the diagnosis of disease. The percentage volume of erythrocytes is known as the **haematocrit** (Am. hematocrit) (from Greek *krites*, meaning separate/judge/discern). This word is also used for the apparatus which measures the volume of erythrocytes in a blood sample.

Now write down what is meant by:

(e) **thrombocyto**crit   _____

The number of blood cells can be counted using a device known as a **haemocytometer**. The simplest type of counter consists of a specially designed microscope slide which holds a precise volume of blood and a grid for the manual counting of cells. Today, the process of counting cells is performed automatically in a Coulter counter. A doctor may request particular types of cell count to aid diagnosis, e.g.:

Blood count
This is a count of the number of red cells, white cells or platelets in 1 mm³ blood.

Differential count
This is a count of the proportions of different types of cells in stained smears.

Platelet count
This is a count of the number of platelets in 1 mm³ blood.

Techniques have been developed to take blood from a donor, remove wanted or unwanted components from it and return the cells in fresh or frozen plasma back into the body. When plasma is removed the technique is known as **plasmapheresis**. Plasma refers to the liquid matrix of the blood in which cells are suspended and nutrients and wastes dissolved. Apheresis is from the Greek *hairein*, meaning take/remove.

Without using your Exercise Guide, write the meaning of:

(f) erythrocyt**apheresis**   _____

(g) thrombocyt**apheresis**   _____

(h) leuc**apheresis**   _____

Medical equipment and clinical procedures

Revise the names of all instruments and procedures mentioned in this unit and then complete Exercise 7.

WORD EXERCISE 7

Match each term in Column A with a description from Column C by placing an appropriate number in Column B.

Column A	Column B	Column C
(a) plasmapheresis	_____	1. count of numbers of blood cells in 1 mm³ blood

Column A	Column B	Column C
(b) differential count	_____	2. instrument which estimates the percentage volume of red cells in blood, or the actual value (as a percentage of the volume) of red cells in blood
(c) haematocrit	_____	3. estimate of proportions of white cells in a stained smear
(d) haemoglobinometer	_____	4. continuous removal of plasma from blood and retransfusion of cells
(e) blood count	_____	5. instrument which measures amount of haemoglobin in a sample

ANATOMY EXERCISE

Now complete the Anatomy Exercise on page 54.

Quick Reference

Medical roots relating to the blood:

Cyt/o	cell
Erythr/o	red
Fibr/o	fibre
Globin/o	protein
Granul/o	granule
Haem/o	blood
Hem/o (Am.)	blood
Leuc/o	white
Leuk/o (Am.)	white
Morph/o	shape/form
Myel/o	marrow
Phag/o	eating/consuming
Reticul/o	immature erythrocyte
Thromb/o	clot
Thrombocyt/o	platelet

Abbreviations

You should learn common abbreviations related to the blood. Note, however, some abbreviations are not standard and their meaning may vary from one hospital to another. There is a more extensive list for reference on page 259.

ALL	acute lymphocytic leukaemia
AML	acute myeloid leukaemia
Diff	differential blood count (of cell types)
ESR	erythrocyte sedimentation rate
FBC	full blood count
Hb	haemoglobin (Am. hemoglobin)
Hct	haematocrit (Am. hematocrit)
MCH	mean corpuscular haemoglobin
MCHC	mean corpuscular haemoglobin concentration
PCV	peaked cell volume
RBC	red blood cell/count
WBC	white blood cell/count

> ## NOW TRY THE WORD CHECK

WORD CHECK

This self-check exercise lists all the word components used in this unit. First write down the meaning of as many word components as you can. Then check your answers using the Exercise Guide and Quick Reference box or the Glossary of Word Components (pp. 269–279).

Prefixes

a- _____

an- _____

aniso- _____

basi- _____

ellipto- _____

eosino- _____

hyper- _____

hypo- _____

macro- _____

micro- _____

neutro- _____

peri- _____

poikil/o _____

poly- _____

Combining forms of word roots

cardi/o _____

cyan/o _____

cyt/o _____

dynam/o _____

erythr/o _____

fibr/o _____

globin/o _____

granul/o _____

haem/o (Am. hem/o) _____

leuc/o (Am. leuk/o) _____

morph/o _____

myel/o _____

ox/y _____

path/o _____

phag/o _____

reticul/o _____

sept/i _____

thromb/o _____

thrombocyt/o _____

Suffixes

-aemia (Am. -emia) _____

-apheresis _____

-blast _____

-chromia   _____

-crit   _____

-genesis   _____

-ic   _____

-ium   _____

-logy   _____

-lysis   _____

-meter   _____

-oma   _____

-osis   _____

-penia   _____

-phil   _____

-poiesis   _____

-rrhage   _____

-stasis   _____

-toxic   _____

-um   _____

-uria   _____

> ## NOW TRY THE SELF-ASSESSMENT ◁

SELF-ASSESSMENT

Test 5A

Below are some combining forms which relate to the components of blood. Indicate which part of the blood they refer to by putting a number from the diagram (Fig. 28) next to each word. You may use a number more than once.

(a) plasma-   _____

(b) erythr/o   _____

(c) haemoglobin/o   _____
    (Am. hemoglobin/o)

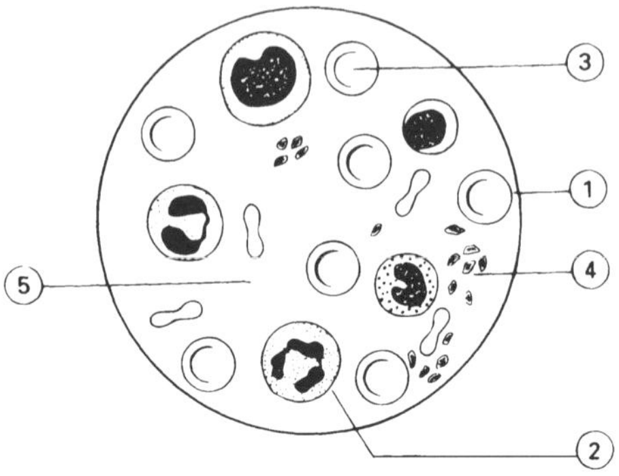

Figure 28   Blood

(d) leucocyt/o   _____
    (Am. leukocyt/o)

(e) thrombocyt/o   _____

Score

5

Test 5B

Prefixes, suffixes and combining forms of word roots

Match each word component in Column A with a meaning in Column C by inserting the appropriate number in Column B.

Column A	Column B	Column C
(a) -aemia (Am. -emia)	_____	1. condition of urine
(b) an-	_____	2. disintegration/breakdown
(c) aniso-	_____	3. red
(d) baso-	_____	4. measuring instrument
(e) -blast	_____	5. abnormal condition/disease of
(f) -chromia	_____	6. basic/alkaline
(g) ellipt/o	_____	7. white
(h) eosin/o	_____	8. clot
(i) erythr/o	_____	9. unequal
(j) granul/o	_____	10. condition of blood
(k) leuc/o (Am. leuk/o)	_____	11. disease

	Column A	Column B	Column C
(l)	-lysis	_____	12. granule
(m)	macro-	_____	13. germ cell
(n)	-meter	_____	14. cessation of flow
(o)	micro-	_____	15. affinity for/loving
(p)	neutr/o	_____	16. condition of deficiency/lack of
(q)	-osis	_____	17. not/without
(r)	-pathy	_____	18. small
(s)	-penia	_____	19. condition of colour/ haemoglobin
(t)	-phil	_____	20. oval/elliptoid
(u)	sept/i	_____	21. large
(v)	-stasis	_____	22. eosin (acid dye)
(w)	thromb/o	_____	23. neutral
(x)	-uria	_____	24. decay/sepsis/ infection

Score

24

Test 5C

Write the meaning of:

(a) leucocyturia
(Am. leukocyturia)   _____

(b) myelocytosis   _____

(c) erythrocyturia   _____

(d) thrombocythaemia   _____
(Am. thrombocythemia)

(e) phagocytolysis   _____

Score

5

Test 5D

Build words which mean:

(a) any disease of blood
(use haem/o, Am. hem/o)   _____

(b) condition of deficiency in
the number of red cells   _____

(c) a physician who specializes
in the study of blood
(use haemat/o, Am. hemat/o)   _____

(d) pertaining to the poisoning
of blood   _____

(e) condition of deficiency in the
number of neutrophils   _____

Score

5

Check answers to Self-Assessment Tests on page 252.

6 The lymphatic system

Objectives

Once you have completed Unit 6 you should be able to:

- understand the meaning of medical words relating to the lymphatic system

- build medical words relating to the lymphatic system

- associate medical terms with their anatomical position

- understand medical abbreviations relating to the lymphatic system.

Exercise Guide

Use this list of word components and their meanings to complete the word exercises in this unit.

Prefixes

auto-   self

Roots/Combining forms

aden/o	gland
angi/o	vessel
cyt/e/o	cell
helc/o	ulcer

hepat/o	liver
path/o	disease
pharyng/o	pharynx
port/o	portal vein

Suffixes

-aemia	condition of blood
-cele	swelling/protrusion/hernia
-cytosis	abnormal increase in cells
-eal	pertaining to
-ectasis	dilatation/stretching
-ectomy	removal of
-emia (Am.)	condition of blood
-genesis	pertaining to formation
-genic	pertaining to formation/ originating in
-globulin	protein
-gram	X-ray/tracing/recording
-graphy	technique of recording/making X-ray
-ic	pertaining to
-itis	inflammation of
-logy	study of
-lysis	breakdown/disintegration
-malacia	condition of softening
-megaly	enlargement
-oma	tumour/swelling
-osis	abnormal condition/disease of
-pathy	disease of
-pexy	surgical fixation/fix in place
-poiesis	formation
-rrhagia	condition of bursting forth
-rrhea (Am.)	excessive discharge/flow
-rrhoea	excessive discharge/flow
-tome	cutting instrument

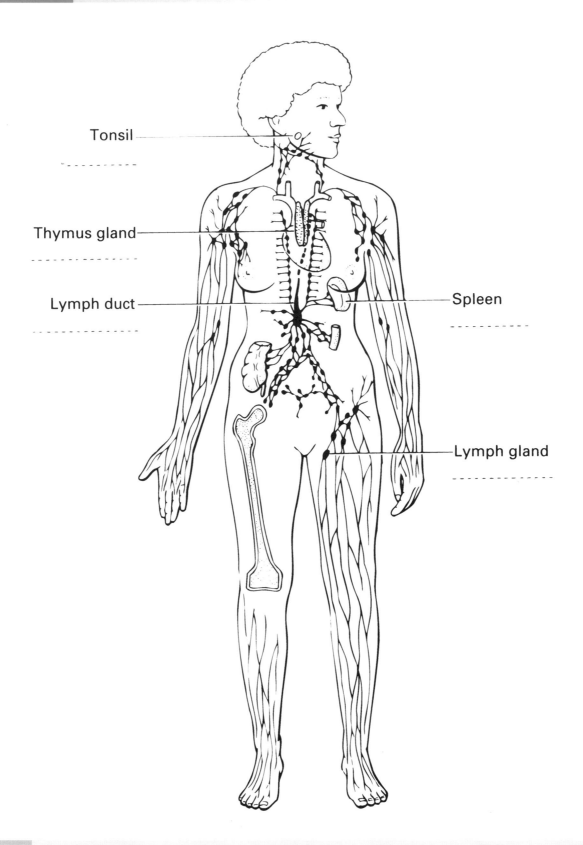

Tonsil

Thymus gland

Lymph duct

Spleen

Lymph gland

Figure 29   The lymphatic system

ANATOMY EXERCISE

When you have finished Word Exercises 1–8, look at the word components listed below. Complete Figure 29 by placing the appropriate combining form on each dotted line. (You can check their meanings in the Quick Reference box on p. 68.)

Lymphaden/o   Splen/o   Tonsill/o

Lymphangi/o   Thym/o

The lymphatic system

The lymphatic system consists of capillaries, vessels, ducts and nodes which transport a fluid known as lymph. Lymph is formed from tissue fluid which surrounds all tissue cells and performs three important functions: (i) transportation of lymphocytes which defend the body against infection and foreign antigens, (ii) transportation of lipids and (iii) by its formation, the drainage of excess fluid from the tissues.

Let us begin by examining the terms associated with the cells and components of the system. Distinct patches of lymphatic tissue have been given specific names; the familiar ones mentioned here include tonsils, adenoids, spleen and thymus.

Use the Exercise Guide at the beginning of this unit to complete Word Exercises 1–8 unless you are asked to work without it.

	Lymph
Root	*(From Greek **lympha**, meaning water. It is used to mean the fluid lymph or lymphatic tissue.)*
Combining forms	**Lymph/o**

WORD EXERCISE 1

Using your Exercise Guide, find the meaning of:

(a) **lymph**ocytosis   _____

(b) **lymph**orrhagia   _____

(c) **lymph**angiography   _____

(d) **lymph**angiogram   _____

(e) **lymph**angiectasis   _____

(f) **lymph**adenoma   _____

(g) **lymph**adenectomy   _____

(h) **lymph**adenopathy   _____

(i) **lymph**adenitis   _____

Lymph nodes (glands) consist of lymphatic channels held in place by fibrous connective tissue which forms a capsule. The nodes contain lymphocytes and special cells called **macrophages** (large-eaters) which, like neutrophils, can engulf foreign substances and microorganisms (by phagocytosis). Lymph nodes often trap malignant cells as well as microorganisms, some of which are also destroyed. During infection lymphocytes and macrophages multiply rapidly, causing the lymph nodes to swell. They may become inflamed and sore. Lymphocytes and macrophages can enter the lymph and blood from nodes.

The macrophages which line the lymph organs are part of a large system of cells known as the **reticuloendothelial system** or macrophage system. Cells which form this network have a common ancestry and carry out phagocytosis (Fig. 30) in the liver, bone marrow, lymph nodes, spleen, nervous system, blood and connective tissues. Macrophages found in connective tissues are known as **histiocytes** (i.e. tissue cells). If there is an increase in the number of histiocytes without infection this is known as a **histiocytosis**.

	Splen
Root	*(A Greek word, meaning spleen. This organ has four main functions: destruction of old blood cells, blood storage, blood filtration and participation in the immune response.)*
Combining forms	**Splen/o**

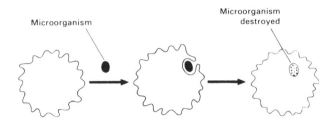

Figure 30   Phagocytosis

 WORD EXERCISE 2

Using your Exercise Guide, find the meaning of:

(a) **spleno**megaly   _____

(b) **spleno**hepatomegaly   _____

(c) **spleno**pexy   _____

(d) **spleno**cele   _____

(e) **spleno**malacia   _____

(f) **spleno**lysis   _____

Without using your Exercise Guide, write the meaning of:

(g) **spleno**gram   _____

(h) **spleno**portogram   _____

(**Port/o** refers to the portal vein which drains blood from the intestines, stomach, pancreas and spleen into the liver.)

Root	**Tonsill**
	*(From Latin **tonsillae**, meaning tonsils. These form a ring of lymphoid tissue at the back of the mouth and nasopharynx. They are thought to be important in the formation of antibodies and lymphocytes.)*
Combining forms	**Tonsill/o**

 WORD EXERCISE 3

Without using your Exercise Guide, build words which mean:

(a) inflammation of the tonsils   _____

(b) removal of the tonsils   _____

Using your Exercise Guide, find the meaning of:

(c) **tonsillo**pharyngeal   _____
     (Look up suffix -eal.)

(d) **tonsillo**tome   _____

Note.   An enlarged nasopharyngeal tonsil is known as an **adenoid**. Sometimes these obstruct the passage of air or interfere with hearing. Removal of the adenoids is known as an **adenoid**ectomy.

Root	**Thym**
	*(From a Greek word **thymos**, meaning soul/emotion. It is used to mean the thymus gland which lies high in the chest above the aorta. It controls the development of the immune system in early life.)*
Combining forms	**Thym/o, thymic/o**

 WORD EXERCISE 4

Without using your Exercise Guide, build words using thym/o which mean:

(a) a cell of the thymus   _____

(b) disease of the thymus   _____

(c) protrusion/swelling of   _____
     the thymus

Using your Exercise Guide, find the meaning of:

(d) **thym**elcosis (Look up helc.) _____

(e) **thymico**lymphatic   _____

Immun
*(From Latin **immunis**, meaning exempt from public burden. In medicine it means exemption from disease, i.e. immunity.)*

Combining forms   **Immun/o**

Immunity

This is the condition of being immune to infectious disease and antigenic substances which might harm the body. Immunity is brought about by the production of antibodies and cells which destroy invading pathogens. During our lifetime we acquire an immunity to common disease-producing organisms, such as viruses, which cause colds and influenza. We can also acquire an immunity to more serious diseases by vaccination.

Antibody
An antibody is a substance which circulates in the blood and can destroy or precipitate foreign substances which have entered the body. (Anti means against, body is an Anglo-Saxon word, in this case referring to a foreign body.)

Antigen
An antigen is any foreign substance that enters the body and stimulates antibody production.

WORD EXERCISE 5

Using your Exercise Guide, build words which mean:

(a) the study of immunity   _____

(b) branch of medicine   _____
concerned with the study
of immune reactions
associated with disease

Using your Exercise Guide, find the meaning of:

(c) **immuno**genesis   _____

(d) auto**immun**ity   _____

(e) **immuno**globulin   _____

Immunity is brought about by two basic types of lymphocyte:

T-cells (thymic cells)

These are formed in the thymus and then move to other parts of the lymphatic system. They are responsible for the **cell-mediated response**. These cells can multiply rapidly, producing a clone of cells which are active in the destruction of viruses, bacteria and skin grafts. They can also produce chemicals that stimulate macrophages to attack foreign cells.

B-cells

These are named after the site in birds where they are produced, the Bursa of Fabricius. In humans B-cells may differentiate in the fetal liver. These cells transform into large **plasma cells** when confronted with an antigen. They then multiply to form a large clone of plasma cells (**plasmacytosis**) which secrete antibody to the antigen. This is known as the **humoral response**. Some antibodies activate protein in the blood. Known as **complement**, this aids the antibody in destroying antigen. (Plasma means to mould or form.)

Ser
*(From a Latin word **serum**, meaning whey. It is used in medicine to mean the clear portion of any liquid separated from its more solid elements. Blood serum is the supernatant liquid formed when blood clots. This serum can be used as a source of antibodies.)*

Combining forms   **Ser/o**

WORD EXERCISE 6

Without using your Exercise Guide, build a word which means:

(a) the scientific study of sera   _____

Serum investigations can lead to a patient being seronegative or seropositive for the presence of a particular antibody.

Seronegative
means a lack of antibody.

Seropositive
means a high level of antibody.

Root **Py**
(From a Greek word **pyon,** *meaning pus.)*

Combining forms **Py/o**

Pus is a yellow, protein-rich liquid, composed of tissue fluids containing bacteria and leucocytes. When a wound is forming or discharging pus it is said to be suppurating. Pus is formed in response to certain types of infection.

WORD EXERCISE 7

Using your Exercise Guide, find the meaning of:

(a) **py**aemia
    (Am. pyemia) _____

(b) **pyo**genic _____

(c) **pyo**rrhoea
    (Am. pyorrhea) _____

(d) **pyo**poiesis _____

The immune response of the lymphatic system not only resists invasion by infective organisms but also functions to identify and destroy everything described as 'non-self', i.e. foreign antigens which have entered the body, such as in transplanted organs or body cells which have changed their form, such as malignant cells.

Patients infected with microorganisms, such as those present in tonsillitis, experience swollen lymph glands, and blood counts will indicate an increase in the number of circulating white blood cells. Once the foreign cells have been destroyed, the lymph glands will return to their normal size.

An important feature of some lymphocytes which make the initial response to an infection is that they become memory cells. This means that they retain the ability to respond very rapidly to the same organism should it enter the body again. This process is the basis of immunity.

Medical equipment and clinical procedure

The lymphatic system is investigated by radiological examination and few specific instruments are used to examine it. Revise the meaning of **-gram** and **-graphy** and then try Exercise 8.

WORD EXERCISE 8

Match each term in Column A with a description from Column C by placing an appropriate number in Column B.

Column A	Column B	Column C
(a) lymphography	_____	1. X-ray picture of portal veins and spleen
(b) lymphangio-graphy	_____	2. X-ray picture of lymphatic system
(c) lymphadeno-graphy	_____	3. instrument for cutting tonsils
(d) lymphogram	_____	4. technique of making an X-ray of lymph vessels
(e) splenoportogram	_____	5. the technique of making an X-ray of the lymphatic system
(f) tonsillotome	_____	6. technique of making an X-ray of lymph glands/nodes

ANATOMY EXERCISE

Now complete the Anatomy Exercise on page 65.

Quick Reference

Medical roots relating to the lymphatic system:

Aden/o	gland
Adenoid/o	adenoid
Cyt/e/o	cell
-globulin	protein
Hist/i/o	tissue
Immun/o	immune
Lymph/o	lymph
Lymphaden/o	lymph gland (node)
Lymphangi/o	lymph vessel
Phag/o	eating/consuming
Plasma-	plasma cell
Py/o	pus
Ser/o	serum
Splen/o	spleen
Thym/o	thymus gland
Thymic/o	thymus gland
Tonsill/o	tonsil

Abbreviations

You should learn common abbreviations related to the lymphatic system. Note, however, some are not standard and their meaning may vary from one hospital to another. There is a more extensive list for reference on page 259.

AIDS	acquired immune deficiency syndrome
ALL	acute lymphocytic leukaemia (Am. leukemia)
BM (T)	bone marrow (trephine)
CLL	chronic lymphocytic leukaemia (Am. leukemia)
HLA	human leucocyte antigen
Ig	immunoglobulin
LAS	lymphadenopathy syndrome
Lymphos	lymphocytes
T & A	tonsils and adenoids
TD	thymus-dependent cells
TI	thymus-independent cells
TLD	thoracic lymph duct

> ## NOW TRY THE WORD CHECK

WORD CHECK

This self-check exercise lists all the word components used in this unit. First write down the meaning of as many word components as you can. Then check your answers using the Exercise Guide and Quick Reference box or the Glossary of Word Components (pp. 269–279).

Prefixes

anti- _____

auto- _____

macro- _____

Combining forms of word roots

aden/o _____

angi/o _____

cyt/o _____

-globulin _____

helc/o _____

hepat/o _____

hist/i/o _____

immun/o _____

lymph/o _____

lymphaden/o _____

lymphangi/o _____

phag/o _____

pharyng/o _____

plasm/a _____

port/o _____

py/o _____

reticul/o _____

ser/o _____

splen/o _____

thym/o _____

tonsill/o _____

Suffixes

-aemia
(Am. -emia) _____

-cele _____

-eal _____

-ectasis _____

-ectomy _____

-genesis _____

-genic _____

-gram _____

-graphy _____

-ia _____

-ic _____

-itis _____

-logy _____

-lysis   _____

-malacia   _____

-megaly   _____

-oma   _____

-osis   _____

-pathy   _____

-pexy   _____

-poiesis   _____

-rrhagia   _____

-rrhoea
(Am. -rrhea)   _____

-tome   _____

> ## NOW TRY THE SELF-ASSESSMENT

SELF-ASSESSMENT

Test 6A

Below are some medical terms which refer to the anatomy of the lymphatic system. Indicate which part of the system they refer to by putting a number from the diagram (Fig. 31) next to each word.

(a) lymphaden/o   _____

(b) splen/o   _____

(c) thym/o   _____

(d) tonsill/o   _____

(e) lymphangi/o   _____

Score

5

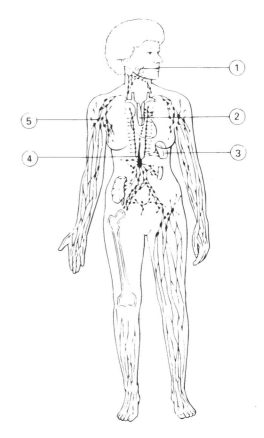

Figure 31   The lymphatic system

Test 6B

Prefixes, suffixes and combining forms of word roots

Match each word component in Column A with a meaning in Column C by inserting the appropriate number in Column B.

Column A	Column B	Column C
(a) aden/o	_____	1. protein/ball
(b) angi/o	_____	2. swelling/hernia/ protrusion
(c) anti-	_____	3. immune
(d) auto-	_____	4. self
(e) -cele	_____	5. vessel
(f) -globin	_____	6. pus
(g) -gram	_____	7. cutting instrument
(h) helc/o	_____	8. against
(i) immun/o	_____	9. spleen
(j) lymph/o	_____	10. ulcer

Column A	Column B	Column C
(k) -lysis	_____	11. serum
(l) -malacia	_____	12. tonsil
(m) port/o	_____	13. lymph
(n) py/o	_____	14. gland
(o) -rrhoea (Am. -rrhea)	_____	15. excessive flow
(p) ser/o	_____	16. picture/tracing/ recording
(q) splen/o	_____	17. condition of softening
(r) thym/o	_____	18. disintegration/ breakdown
(s) -tome	_____	19. portal vein
(t) tonsill/o	_____	20. thymus gland

Score

20

Test 6C

Write the meaning of:

(a) lymphorrhoea (Am. lymphorrhea) _____

(b) splenic _____

(c) lymphadenectasis _____

(d) thymolysis _____

(e) serologist _____

Score

5

Test 6D

Build words which mean:

(a) tumour of lymph (tissue) _____

(b) X-ray examination of the lymph system _____

(c) removal of the spleen _____

(d) condition of bleeding/ bursting forth of the spleen _____

(e) tumour of a lymph vessel _____

Score

5

Check answers to Self-Assessment Tests on page 252.

The urinary system

Objectives

Once you have completed Unit 7 you should be able to:

* understand the meaning of medical words relating to the urinary system

* build medical words relating to the urinary system

* associate medical terms with their anatomical position

* understand medical abbreviations relating to the urinary system.

Exercise Guide

Use this list of word components and their meanings to complete the word exercises in this unit.

Prefixes

dys-	difficult/painful
intra-	within/inside
oligo-	deficiency/few/little
poly-	many/much

Roots/Combining forms

albumin/o	albumin/albumen
azot/o	urea
col/o	colon
enter/o	intestine
gastr/o	stomach
haemat/o	blood
hemat/o (Am.)	blood
hydr/o	water
lith/o	stone
metr/o	a measure
proct/o	anus/rectum
py/o	pus
sigmoid/o	sigmoid colon
trigon/o	trigone of the bladder

Suffixes

-al	pertaining to
-algia	condition of pain
-cele	swelling/protrusion/hernia
-clysis	infusion/injection/irrigation
-dynia	condition of pain
-ectasis	dilatation/stretching
-ectomy	removal of
-ferous	pertaining to carrying/bearing
-genesis	capable of causing/pertaining to formation
-gram	X-ray/tracing/recording
-graphy	technique of recording/making an X-ray
-ia	condition of
-iasis	abnormal condition
-ic	pertaining to
-itis	inflammation of
-lapaxy	empty/wash out/evacuate
-lithiasis	abnormal condition of stones
-logist	specialist who studies
-lysis	breakdown/disintegration
-meter	measuring instrument
-metry	process of measuring
-osis	abnormal condition/disease of
-ous	pertaining to
-pathy	disease of
-pexy	surgical fixation/fix in place
-phyma	tumour/boil
-plasty	surgical repair/reconstruction
-ptosis	falling/diplacement/prolapse
-rrhagia	condition of bursting forth of blood/bleeding
-rrhaphy	suture/stitch
-sclerosis	hardening
-scope	instrument to view
-scopy	visual examination
-stenosis	abnormal condition of narrowing
-stomy	to form a new opening or outlet
-tome	cutting instrument
-tomy	incision into
-tripsy	act of crushing
-triptor	instrument to crush/fragment (using shock waves)
-trite	instrument to crush/fragment
-uresis	excrete in urine/urinate

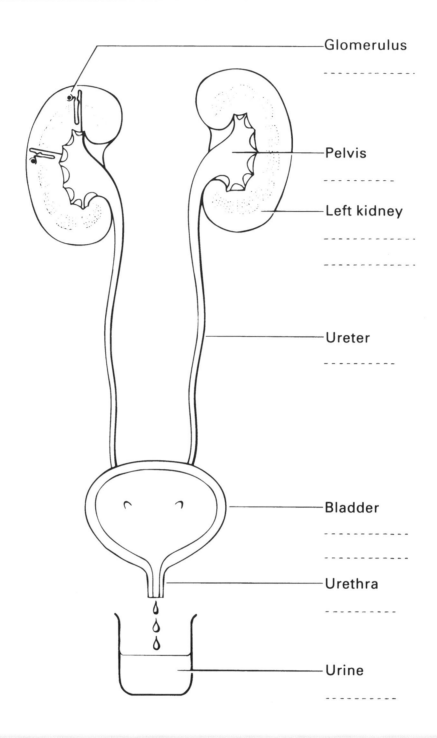

Glomerulus

- - - - - - - - - - - -

Pelvis

- - - - - - - - -

Left kidney

- - - - - - - - - - - - -

- - - - - - - - - - - - -

Ureter

- - - - - - - - -

Bladder

- - - - - - - - - - - -

- - - - - - - - - - - -

Urethra

- - - - - - - - -

Urine

- - - - - - - - -

Figure 32   The urinary system

ANATOMY EXERCISE

When you have finished Word Exercises 1–11, look at the word components listed below. Complete Figure 32 by writing the appropriate combining form on each dotted line – more than one component may relate to the same position. (You can check their meanings in the Quick Reference box on p. 81.)

Cyst/o	Ren/o	Urin/o
Glomerul/o	Ureter/o	Vesic/o
Nephr/o	Urethr/o	
Pyel/o		

The urinary system

The main components of the urinary system are the kidneys, which remove metabolic wastes from the blood by forming them into urine. This yellow liquid is then passed to the urinary bladder where it is stored before being passed out of the body in the process of urination.

Besides removing waste substances which could be toxic to tissue cells, the kidneys maintain the volume of water in the blood and regulate its salt concentration and pH. The kidneys are therefore involved in homeostasis, i.e. maintaining constant conditions within the tissue fluids of the body. The continuous activity of the kidneys is required to maintain life.

Use the Exercise Guide at the beginning of this unit to complete Word Exercises 1–11 unless you are asked to work without it.

Root   **Ren**
*(A Latin word **ren**, meaning kidney.)*

Combining forms   **Ren/o**

WORD EXERCISE 1

Using your Exercise Guide, find the meaning of:

(a) **reno**gastric   _____

(b) **reno**gram   _____

(c) **reno**graphy   _____

Renography may show up renal calculus (from Latin *calcis* – small stone), i.e. a kidney stone. The presence of stones in the ureter leads to severe pain and is referred to as **renal colic**. Renal colic can also be caused by disorder and disease within a kidney.

Radioisotope renograms which are used to compare kidney function can be made following injection of radioisotopes into the bloodstream.

Root   **Nephr**
*(From a Greek word **nephros**, meaning kidney.)*

Combining forms   **Nephr/o**

WORD EXERCISE 2

Using your Exercise Guide, find the meaning of:

(a) **nephro**ptosis   _____

(b) hydro**nephro**sis   _____

(c) **nephro**cele   _____

(d) **nephr**algia   _____

Using your Exercise Guide, build words which mean:

(e) surgical fixation of a kidney (e.g. floating kidney)   _____

(f) surgical repair of a kidney   _____

(g) incision into a kidney   _____

(h) condition of stones in the kidney   _____

(i) removal of a kidney   _____

Within each kidney are approximately one million kidney tubules or nephrons which do the work of the kidney. At the beginning of each nephron is a **glomerulus**; this is a ball of capillaries surrounded by porous membranes which filter metabolic wastes from the blood. Glomeruli can undergo pathological change and this will affect the functioning of the kidney.

Using your Exercise Guide, find the meaning of:

(j) **glomerul**itis (suppurative)   _____

(k) **glomerulo**pathy   _____

(l) **glomerulo**sclerosis   _____

Infections and disorders of kidneys sometimes lead to kidney failure. This results in the waste products of metabolism increasing in concentration within the blood and a failure to regulate water, mineral metabolism and pH; these changes will lead to death. The patient with kidney failure can be kept alive if one of the following procedures is applied:

Haemodialysis

This involves diverting the patient's blood through a dialyser, commonly called a kidney machine (Fig. 33). In the dialyser waste products are removed from the blood which is then returned to the body via another blood vessel. The patient must be connected to the dialyser for many hours per week and so cannot lead a normal life. (Dialysis means separating, i.e. separating wastes from the blood.)

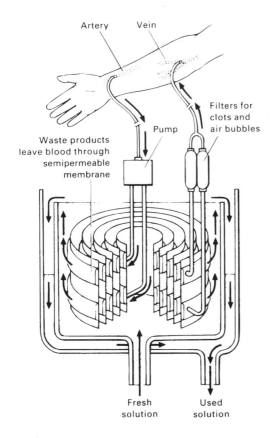

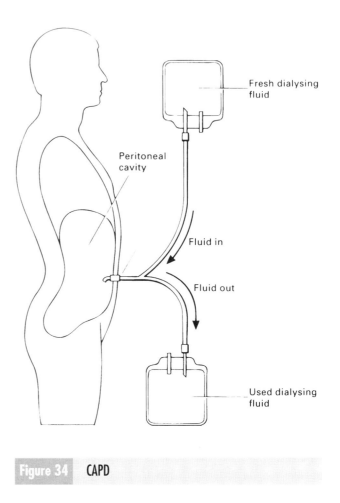

Figure 34   CAPD

Kidney transplant

A kidney can be transplanted between two individuals of the same species, i.e. between two humans who are not closely related. This type of transplant or graft is known as a homotransplant or homograft (*homo* meaning the same, synonymous with allograft). The donor could be living, and survive with his/her one remaining kidney, or a victim of a fatal accident. A transplant may keep a patient alive for many years and avoids the inconvenience and dangers associated with CAPD and dialysis. Transplants between genetically identical twins are more successful. These are known as isografts (*iso* means same/equal).

Figure 33   Haemodialysis

CAPD (continuous ambulatory peritoneal dialysis)

The patient is fitted with a peritoneal catheter (tube) (Fig. 34). Every 6 hours approximately 2 litres of dialysing fluid is passed into the peritoneum. Toxic wastes diffuse into the dialysing fluid and are removed from the body when the fluid is changed. This procedure is repeated four times a day, 7 days a week. CAPD has been used on a long-term basis but there is danger from peritonitis caused by infection.

Root	**Pyel** *(From a Greek word **pyelos**, meaning trough. Here it refers to the space inside a kidney, the renal pelvis in which urine collects after its formation.)*
Combining forms	**Pyel/o** *(Do not confuse these with py/o – meaning pus.)*

WORD EXERCISE 3

Without using your Exercise Guide, write the meaning of:

(a) **pyelo**nephritis _____
(This is often due to a
bacterial infection.)

(b) **pyelo**lithotomy _____

(c) **pyelo**nephrosis _____

Without using your Exercise Guide, build words which mean:

(d) surgical repair of the renal pelvis _____

(e) X-ray picture of the renal pelvis _____

The technique of making an X-ray of the renal pelvis is known as **pyelo**graphy. It involves filling the pelvis with a radio-opaque dye. There are several ways of doing this:

Intravenous pyelography
Here the dye is injected into the bloodstream and it eventually passes through the kidney pelvis (**intra** – meaning inside, **ven/o** – meaning vein).

Antegrade pyelography
Here the dye is injected into the renal pelvis (**ante** – meaning before/in front; **grad** – meaning take steps/to go (Latin)). It refers to the fact that the dye goes into the pelvis before it leaves the kidney. The dye is injected through a percutaneous catheter, i.e. through the skin.

Retrograde (or ascending) pyelography
Here the dye is injected into the kidney via the ureter, so it is being forced backwards up the ureter into the urine within the pelvis (**retro** – Latin, means backwards).

Root	**Ureter**
	*(From a Greek word **oureter**, which means the urinary canal, i.e. the narrow tube that connects each kidney to the bladder. Urine flows through the ureters assisted by muscular action.)*
Combining forms	**Ureter/o**

WORD EXERCISE 4

Without using your Exercise Guide, write the meaning of:

(a) **uretero**cele _____

(b) **uretero**celectomy _____

Using your Exercise Guide, find the meaning of:

(c) **uretero**rrhagia _____

(d) **uretero**rrhaphy _____

(e) **ureter**ectasis _____

(f) **uretero**renoscopy _____
(Note the difference between -scope and -scopy.)

(g) **uretero**stomy _____

Using your Exercise Guide, build words which mean:

(h) formation of an opening _____
between the intestine and ureter

(i) formation of an opening _____
between the colon and ureter

Root	**Cyst**
	*(From Greek **kystis**, meaning bladder.)*
Combining forms	**Cyst/o**

Note. We have already used cyst/o which means bladder. In Unit 2 we used it in combination with chol/e, meaning bile, to make cholecyst/o, i.e. the bile (gall) bladder. Here we are using **cyst/o** alone to mean the urinary bladder, the function of which is to store urine until it is expelled from the body.

WORD EXERCISE 5

Without using your Exercise Guide, write the meaning of:

(a) **cyst**itis _____
(There are many causes of this condition which may be acute or chronic. Known causes include

injury and infection. It is easy for microorganisms to enter the bladder as it is open to the external genitalia via the urethra. Sometimes infections causing cystitis are transmitted sexually, e.g. as in gonorrhoea. It is more common in women, perhaps owing to their shorter urethras.)

(b) **cysto**lithectomy   _____

(c) **cysto**pyelitis   _____

(d) **cysto**ptosis   _____

Using your Exercise Guide, find the meaning of:

(e) **cysto**scope   _____

(f) **cysto**proctostomy   _____

Meter and **metr/o** originate from Greek *metron*, meaning a measure, and **metry** from *metrein*, meaning process of measuring. Use these to build words meaning:

(g) instrument to measure bladder   _____
     (capacity or pressure within)

(h) technique of measuring the   _____
     bladder (capacities and volumes of)

(i) a trace, picture or recording of   _____
     measured volumes and capacities
     of the bladder (use metr/o)

A technique which applies an electric current to tissues, causing them to heat up, is known as **diathermy** (*dia* – meaning through and *thermy* – meaning heat). These can be combined here to make:

> **cystodiathermy**
> Which means applying an electric current to the bladder wall, the resultant heating cauterizing it.

Root **Vesic** *(From Latin **vesica**, also meaning bladder.)*

Combining forms **Vesic/o**

WORD EXERCISE 6

Without using your Exercise Guide, build words which mean:

(a) the formation of an opening   _____
     into the bladder

(b) incision into the bladder   _____

Using your Exercise Guide, find the meaning of:

(c) **vesico**clysis   _____

(d) **vesic**al   _____

(e) **vesico**sigmoidostomy   _____

Without using your Exercise Guide, write the meaning of:

(f) **vesico**ureteral   _____

Catheterization of the bladder is required following some surgical operations and when there is difficulty in emptying the bladder owing to a neuromuscular disorder or physical damage to the spinal cord. This procedure involves inserting a catheter through the urethra into the bladder (Fig. 35). A urinary **catheter** consists of a fine tube which allows urine to drain from the bladder into an external container. Some self-retaining catheters are held in position by means of an inflated balloon.

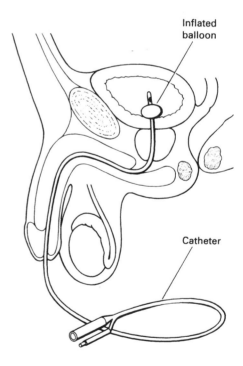

Figure 35 **Catheterization**

Root **Urethr**
*(From Greek **ourethro**, meaning urethra. It refers to the tube through which urine leaves the body from the bladder.)*

Combining forms **Urethr/o**

WORD EXERCISE 7

Without using your Exercise Guide, write the meaning of:

(a) **urethro**metry _____

(b) **urethro**trigonitis _____
(Trigone refers to a triangular area at the base of the bladder, bounded by the openings of the ureters at the back and the urethral opening at the front.)

(c) **urethro**pexy _____

Without using your Exercise Guide, build words which mean:

(d) condition of pain in the urethra _____

(e) condition of flow of blood from the urethra _____

(f) visual examination of the urethra _____

Using your Exercise Guide, find the meaning of:

(g) **urethro**phyma _____

(h) **urethro**tome _____

(i) **urethro**stenosis _____

(j) **urethro**dynia _____

| Root | **Urin**
(From a Latin word **urina**, meaning urine, the excretory product of the kidneys.) |
| --- | --- |
| Combining forms | **Urin/a, urin/o, urin/i** |

WORD EXERCISE 8

Using your Exercise Guide, find the meaning of:

(a) **urin**iferous _____

(b) **urin**alysis _____

(This word refers to all the techniques of analysing urine. Detailed urinalysis is a valuable aid to the diagnosis of disease, e.g. the presence of high concentrations of glucose in the urine may indicate diabetes. Other components which are commonly analysed are colour, pH, specific gravity, ketone bodies, phenylketones, protein, bilirubin and solid casts of varying composition.)

Without using your Exercise Guide, write the meaning of:

(c) **urino**meter _____
(This is usually used to estimate specific gravity of urine which changes in illness.)

| Root | **Ur**
(From a Greek word **ouron**, also meaning urine.) |
| --- | --- |
| Combining forms | **Ur/o**
(These forms are also used to refer to the urinary tract and urination.) |
| | **-uria**
(This means a condition of the urine.) |

WORD EXERCISE 9

Without using your Exercise Guide, write the meaning of:

(a) **uro**graphy _____
(Synonymous with intravenous pyelogram (IVP). The above procedure is also performed by injecting dye directly into the urinary tract rather than into a vein.)

Using your Exercise Guide, find the meaning of:

(b) **uro**logist _____

(c) **uro**genesis _____

(d) olig**uria** _____

(e) albumin**uria** _____

(f) azot**uria** _____

(g) poly**uria** _____

(h) dys**uria** _____

(i) haemat**uria** _____
(Am. hematuria)

(j) py**uria** _____

Note. The act of passing urine is known as micturition (from Latin *micturire*, meaning to pass water.)

Root	Lith
	*(From a Greek word **lithos**, meaning stone.)*
Combining forms	**Lith/o**

Here *lithos* refers to a kidney stone, which is a hard mass composed mainly of mineral matter present in the urinary system. Remember a stone is sometimes called a **renal calculus** (pl. **calculi**). Stones can prevent the passage of urine, causing pain and kidney damage. They need to be removed or they will seriously affect the functioning of the kidneys.

WORD EXERCISE 10

Without using your Exercise Guide, write the meaning of:

(a) **litho**nephritis _____

(b) uro**lith**iasis _____

(c) **litho**genesis _____

Using your Exercise Guide, find the meaning of:

(d) **litho**trite _____

(e) **litho**lapaxy _____

(f) **litho**triptor _____
(This instrument focuses high energy shock waves generated by a high voltage spark on to a kidney stone. No surgery is required, as the stone disintegrates within the body and is passed in the urine. The procedure for using this instrument is called extra-corporeal shock wave lithotripsy (ECSL), *extra* meaning outside, *corporeal* meaning body.)

(g) **litho**tripsy _____

(h) **lith**uresis _____

Medical equipment and clinical procedures

Before completing Exercise 11, check the names of instruments and techniques of examination of the urinary system mentioned in this unit. Revise -scope, -scopy, -tome, -metry, -meter and -thermy.

WORD EXERCISE 11

Match each term in Column A with a description from Column C by placing an appropriate number in Column B.

Column A	Column B	Column C
(a) diathermy	_____	1. instrument for crushing stones
(b) cystoscope	_____	2. device which separates wastes from the blood
(c) lithotriptor	_____	3. instrument for cutting the urethra
(d) urinometer	_____	4. visual examination of the ureter
(e) haemodialyser (Am. hemodialyzer)	_____	5. instrument which measures the pressure and capacity of the bladder
(f) ureteroscopy	_____	6. instrument to view the urethra
(g) urethrotome	_____	7. device which destroys stones using shock waves
(h) cystometer	_____	8. technique of heating a tissue by applying an electric current
(i) urethroscope	_____	9. instrument for measuring specific gravity of urine
(j) lithotrite	_____	10. instrument to view the bladder

ANATOMY EXERCISE

Now complete the Anatomy Exercise on page 74.

Quick Reference

Medical roots relating to the urinary system:

Albumin/o	albumin/albumen
Azot/o	urea/nitrogen
Cyst/o	bladder
Glomerul/o	glomerulus
Lith/o	stone
Nephr/o	kidney
Pyel/o	pelvis of kidney
Ren/o	kidney
Trigon/o	trigone
Ureter/o	ureter
Urethr/o	urethra
Urin/o	urine
Ur/o	urine/urinary tract
Vesic/o	bladder

Abbreviations

You should learn common abbreviations related to the urinary system. Note, however, some are not standard and their meaning may vary from one hospital to another. There is a more extensive list for reference on page 259.

ARF	acute renal failure
BUN	blood urea nitrogen
CRF	chronic renal failure
CSU	catheter specimen of urine
Cysto	cystoscopy
HD	haemodialysis
	(Am. hemodialysis)
IVP	intravenous pyelogram
KUB	kidney, ureter, bladder
MSU	midstream urine
PCNL	percutaneous nephrolithotomy
U & E	urea and electrolytes
UTI	urinary tract infection

> **NOW TRY THE WORD CHECK**

WORD CHECK

This self-check exercise lists all the word components used in this unit. First write down the meaning of as many word components as you can. Then check your answers using the Exercise Guide and Quick Reference box or the Glossary of Word Components (pp. 269–279).

Prefixes

ante-   _____

dia-   _____

dys-   _____

intra-   _____

oligo-   _____

poly-   _____

retro-   _____

Combining forms of word roots

albumin/o   _____

azot/o   _____

col/o   _____

cyst/o   _____

enter/o   _____

gastr/o   _____

glomerul/o   _____

haem/o
(Am. hem/o)   _____

hydr/o   _____

lith/o   _____

nephr/o   _____

proct/o   _____

pyel/o   _____

py/o   _____

ren/o   _____

sigmoid/o _____

sten/o _____

trigon/o _____

ureter/o _____

urethr/o _____

urin/o _____

ur/o _____

ven/o _____

vesic/o _____

Suffixes

-al _____

-algia _____

-cele _____

-clysis _____

-dynia _____

-ectasis _____

-ectomy _____

-ferous _____

-genesis _____

-gram _____

-graphy _____

-iasis _____

-ic _____

-itis _____

-lapaxy _____

-lithiasis _____

-logist _____

-lysis _____

-meter _____

-metry _____

-osis _____

-ous _____

-pexy _____

-phyma _____

-plasty _____

-ptosis _____

-rrhage _____

-rrhaphy _____

-sclerosis _____

-scope _____

-scopy _____

-stomy _____

-thermy _____

-tome _____

-tomy _____

-tripsy _____

-triptor _____

-trite _____

-uresis _____

> ## NOW TRY THE SELF-ASSESSMENT ◀

SELF-ASSESSMENT

Test 7A

Below are some combining forms which refer to the anatomy of the urinary system. Indicate which part of the system they refer to by putting a number from the diagram (Fig. 36) next to each word.

(a) ureter/o _____

(b) nephr/o _____

(c) glomerul/o _____

(d) pyel/o _____

(e) urethr/o _____

(f) lith/o _____

(g) cyst/o _____

(h) urin/o _____

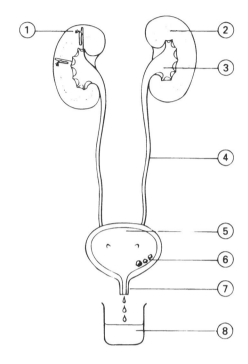

The urinary system

Score

8

Test 7B
Prefixes and suffixes

Match each prefix or suffix in Column A with a meaning in Column C by inserting the appropriate number in Column B.

Column A	Column B	Column C
(a) ante-	_____	1. technique of breaking stones with shock waves
(b) -cele	_____	2. measuring instrument
(c) -clysis	_____	3. crushing instrument
(d) dia-	_____	4. flow of urine/ excrete in urine
(e) dys-	_____	5. technique of measuring

Column A	Column B	Column C
(f) -ferous	_____	6. backward
(g) -iasis	_____	7. protrusion/ swelling/hernia
(h) intra-	_____	8. tumour/boil
(i) -lapaxy	_____	9. before
(j) -meter	_____	10. to fall/displace
(k) -metry	_____	11. pertaining to carrying
(l) oligo-	_____	12. abnormal condition of
(m) -phyma	_____	13. too little/few
(n) poly-	_____	14. difficult/painful
(o) -ptosis	_____	15. infusion/injection into
(p) retro-	_____	16. through
(q) -thermy	_____	17. within/inside
(r) -tripsy	_____	18. evacuation/ wash out
(s) -trite	_____	19. many
(t) -uresis	_____	20. heat

Score

20

Test 7C
Combining forms of word roots

Match each combining form in Column A with a meaning in Column C by inserting the appropriate number in Column B.

Column A	Column B	Column C
(a) col/o	_____	1. blood
(b) cyst/o	_____	2. kidney (i)
(c) gastr/o	_____	3. kidney (ii)
(d) glomerul/o	_____	4. sigmoid colon
(e) haemat/o (Am. hemat/o)	_____	5. pus
(f) lith/o	_____	6. trigone/base of bladder
(g) nephr/o	_____	7. urethra
(h) proct/o	_____	8. bladder (i)
(i) pyel/o	_____	9. bladder (ii)

Column A	Column B	Column C
(j) py/o	_____	10. vein
(k) ren/o	_____	11. stomach
(l) sigmoid/o	_____	12. pelvis/trough
(m) sten/o	_____	13. urine
(n) trigon/o	_____	14. urine/urinary tract
(o) ureter/o	_____	15. glomeruli (of kidney)
(p) urethr/o	_____	16. ureter
(q) urin/o	_____	17. colon
(r) ur/o	_____	18. anus/rectum
(s) ven/o	_____	19. stone
(t) vesic/o	_____	20. narrowing

Score

20

Test 7D

Write the meaning of:

(a) nephropyelolithotomy   _____

(b) ureterostenosis   _____

(c) cystourethrography   _____

(d) vesicocele   _____

(e) pyelectasis   _____

Score

5

Test 7E

Build words which mean:

(a) dilatation of a ureter   _____

(b) formation of an opening between the ureter and sigmoid colon   _____

(c) technique of making an X-ray of the bladder (use cyst/o)   _____

(d) X-ray picture of the urinary tract   _____

(e) abnormal condition of hardening of the kidney   _____

Score

5

Check answers to Self-Assessment tests on page 252.

8 The nervous system

Objectives

Once you have completed Unit 8 you should be able to:

- understand the meaning of medical words relating to the nervous system

- build medical words relating to the nervous system

- associate medical terms with their anatomical position

- understand medical abbreviations relating to the nervous system.

Exercise Guide

Use this list of word components and their meanings to complete the word exercises in this unit.

Prefixes

a-	without/not
acro-	extremities/point
agora-	open place
an-	without/not
di-	two/double
dys-	difficult/painful
electro-	electrical
epi-	above/upon/on
hemi-	half
hyper-	above
hypo-	below
macro-	large
meso-	middle
micro-	small
para-	beside/near
polio-	grey matter (of CNS)
poly-	many
post-	after/behind
pre-	before/in front of
quadri-	four
sub-	under
tetra-	four

Roots/Combining forms

aqua-	water
cancer/o	cancer
ech/o	echo/reflected sound
fibr/o	fibre
haemat/o	blood
hemat/o (Am.)	blood
hydro-	water
necr/o	death (dead tissue)
py/o	pus
somat/o	body
syring/o	pipe/tube/cavity

Suffixes

-al	pertaining to
-algia	condition of pain
-cele	swelling/protrusion/hernia
-centesis	surgical puncture to remove fluid
-cyte	cell
-ectomy	removal of
-form	having the form of
-genic	pertaining to formation/originating in
-gram	X-ray picture/tracing/recording
-graph	usually an instrument that records
-graphy	technique of recording/making an X-ray
-gyric	pertaining to circular motion
-ia	condition of
-iatr(y)	doctor/medical treatment
-ic	pertaining to
-itis	inflammation of
-logist	specialist who studies ...
-logy	study of
-malacia	condition of softening
-meter	measuring instrument
-metry	process of measuring
-oma	tumour/swelling
-osis	abnormal condition/disease of
-ous	pertaining to
-pathy	disease of
-phthisis	wasting away
-plasia	condition of growth/formation (of cells)
-rrhagia	condition of bursting forth of blood/bleeding
-schisis	cleaving/splitting/parting
-sclerosis	abnormal condition of hardening
-scopy	visual examination
-stomy	to form a new opening or outlet
-therapy	treatment
-tomy	incision into
-trauma	injury/wound
-trophy	nourishment/development
-tropic	pertaining to affinity for/stimulating/changing in response to a stimulus
-us	thing/structure

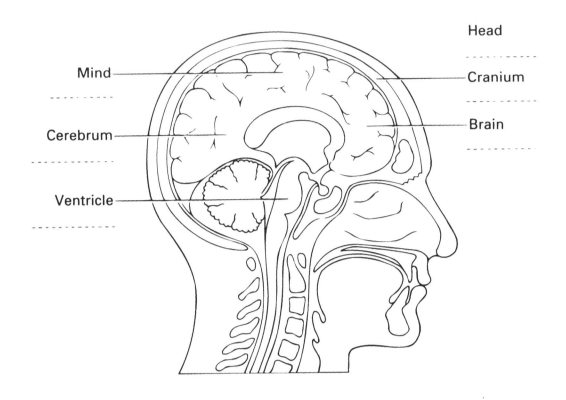

Head

Mind

Cranium

Cerebrum

Brain

Ventricle

Figure 37 Sagittal section through the head

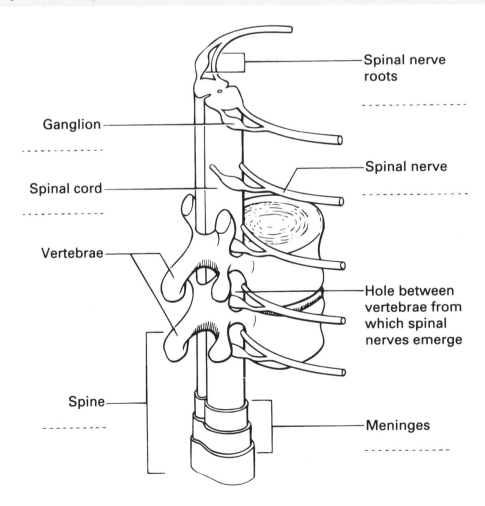

Spinal nerve roots

Ganglion

Spinal nerve

Spinal cord

Vertebrae

Hole between vertebrae from which spinal nerves emerge

Spine

Meninges

Figure 38 Section through the spine

ANATOMY EXERCISE

When you have finished Word Exercises 1–21, look at the word components listed below. Complete Figures 37 and 38 by writing the appropriate combining form on each dotted line – more than one component may relate to the same position. (You can check their meanings in the Quick Reference box on p. 96.)

Cephal/o
Cerebr/o
Crani/o
Encephal/o

Gangli/o
Mening/i/o
Myel/o
Neur/o

Psych/o
Rachi/o
Radicul/o
Ventricul/o

The nervous system

Humans have a complex nervous system with a brain which is large in proportion to their body size. The brain and spinal cord are estimated to contain at least 10^{10} cells with vast numbers of connections between them. The nervous system performs three basic functions:

- It receives, stores and analyses information from sense organs such as the eyes and ears, making us aware of our environment. This awareness enables us to think and make responses which will aid our survival in changing conditions.
- It controls the physiological activities of the body systems and maintains constant conditions (homeostasis) within the body.
- It controls our muscles, enabling us to move and speak.

Because of its complexity, the nervous system has been difficult to study and progress in understanding its common disorders has been slow. However, recently developed imaging techniques are improving the diagnosis and treatment of nervous disorders.

The structure of the nervous system

For convenience of study medical physiologists have divided the system into:

Central nervous system (CNS)
This consists of the brain and spinal cord.

Peripheral nervous system (PNS)
This is composed of 12 pairs of cranial nerves and 31 pairs of spinal nerves which connect the CNS with sense organs, muscles and glands.

Autonomic nervous system (ANS)
This describes certain peripheral nerves that send impulses to internal organs and glands.

We will begin our study of medical terms by examining the cells which form the system.

Root **Neur**
(From a Greek word **neuron**,
meaning nerve.)

Combining forms **Neur/o**

Neurons are the basic structural units of the nervous system. They are specialized cells, elongated for the transmission of nerve impulses. Each neuron consists of a cell 'body' plus long extensions known as dendrons and axons (Fig. 39).

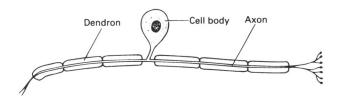

Dendron — Cell body — Axon

Figure 39 Neuron (sensory)

There are three basic types of neuron:

Sensory neuron
which transfers impulses from sense organs to the central nervous system (CNS).

Motor neuron
Which stimulates muscles and glands (motor – pertaining to action).

Connector neuron
Which connects neurons together, e.g. sensory to motor neurons.

Note. As sensory neurons are transferring information towards the CNS they are sometimes referred to as afferent neurons (from Latin *affere* – to bring). Motor neurons are sometimes referred to as efferent neurons as they carry away information from the CNS (from Latin *effere* – to carry away).

Use the Exercise Guide at the beginning of this unit to complete Word Exercises 1–21 unless you are asked to work without it.

 WORD EXERCISE 1

Using your Exercise Guide, find the meaning of:

(a) **neuro**logy   _____

(b) **neuro**pathy   _____

(c) **neur**algia   _____

(d) **neuro**fibroma   _____

(e) poly**neur**itis   _____

(f) **neuro**genic   _____

Using your Exercise Guide, build words which mean:

(g) hardening of a nerve   _____

(h) condition of softening of   _____
    a nerve

(i) person who specializes in the   _____
    study of nerves and
    their disorders

Using your Exercise Guide, find the meaning of:

(j) **neuro**phthisis _____

(k) **neuro**tropic   _____

(l) **neuro**trauma   _____

The neurons of the central nervous system are supported by another type of cell which sticks to them. These are known as neuroglia (from a Greek word *glia*, meaning glue).

Without using your Exercise Guide, write the meaning of:

(m) neuro**glio**cyte   _____

(n) neuro**gli**oma (or glioma)   _____

 Root **Plex**
(From a Latin word **plexus**, meaning a network of nerves.)

Combining forms   **Plex/o**

 WORD EXERCISE 2

Without using your Exercise Guide, write the meaning of:

(a) **plexo**pathy   _____

(b) **plexo**genic   _____

Root   **Cephal**
(From a Greek word **kephale**, meaning head.)

Combining forms   **Cephal/o**

WORD EXERCISE 3

Using your Exercise Guide, find the meaning of:

(a) **cephalo**cele   _____

(b) a**cephal**ous   _____
    (This usually refers to an abnormal, dead fetus.)

(c) **cephal**haematoma   _____
    (Am. cephalhematoma)

(d) hydro**cephal**us   _____
    (Fig. 40; this is characterized by an excess of cerebro-spinal fluid in the brain and results in enlarged head, compression of the brain and mental retardation if not corrected.)

Using your Exercise Guide, build words which mean:

(e) pertaining to a very small head   _____

(f) X-ray picture of the head   _____

(g) measurement of the head   _____

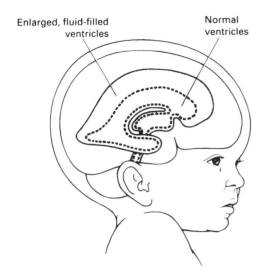

Enlarged, fluid-filled ventricles

Normal ventricles

Figure 40   Hydrocephalus

Using your Exercise Guide, find the meaning of:

(h) macro**cephal**us   _____

(i) **cephalo**gyric   _____

Root
Encephal
(From a Greek word **encephalos**,
meaning brain.)

Combining forms   **Encephal/o**

 WORD EXERCISE 4

Without using your Exercise Guide, write the meaning of:

(a) **encephal**oma   _____

Using your Exercise Guide, find the meaning of:

(b) **encephalo**pyosis   _____

(c) an**encephal**ic   _____

(d) electro**encephalo**graph   _____
     (Fig. 41)

This instrument records the electrical activity of the brain through electrodes placed on the surface of the scalp. The electroencephalogram is traced on to a recording paper and appears as a series of waves.

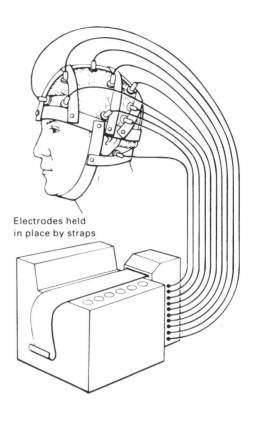

Electrodes held in place by straps

Figure 41   Electroencephalograph

Analysis of the waves can be used to diagnose epilepsy, localize intracranial lesions and confirm brain death.

Using your Exercise Guide, build a word which means:

(e) technique of X-raying/   _____
     recording the brain

Sometimes air or gas is injected into the spaces within the brain after removal of some cerebrospinal fluid. This assists in visualizing the fluid-filled spaces of the brain. A medical term which describes this process can be formed by using **pneumo-** as a prefix with the term you have just built. Remember *pneuma* means air/gas/wind.

Without using your Exercise Guide, build words which mean:

(f) technique of X-raying brain   _____
     following injection of gas into
     spaces within brain

(g) technique of making a trace/   _____
     recording of the electrical
     activity of the brain

(h) disease of the brain   _____

(i) protrusion or hernia of brain   _____

Using your Exercise Guide, find the meaning of:

(j) echo**encephalo**gram _____
   (Ultrasonic soundwaves
   are used.)

(k) mes**encephalon** _____

(l) polio**encephal**itis _____

Root	Cerebr
	*(From a Latin word **cerebrum**, meaning brain. Here it refers to the cerebral hemispheres or cerebrum of the brain.)*

Combining forms   **Cerebr/o**

WORD EXERCISE 5

Without using your Exercise Guide, build words which mean:

(a) hardening of the cerebrum _____

(b) condition of softening of _____
   the cerebrum

(c) abnormal condition/ _____
   disease of the cerebrum

Cerebrovascular accident

Disorders within blood vessels of the cerebrum can result in a **stroke** or **apoplexy**. Reduction/holding back of blood flow (ischaemia) within the cerebrum causes cells to die because of lack of oxygen and nutrients. As cells in this area control movements of many parts of the body, paralysis of limbs and loss of speech are common symptoms of strokes. The severity of symptoms depends on the area of brain tissue damaged. Sometimes there is recovery and the patient is left with slight paralysis or **paresis**.

The cerebral cortex

The outer layer of the cerebrum is known as the cerebral cortex (cortex is from Latin, meaning rind/bark). It is extensively folded into fissures, giving it a large surface area. This part of the brain contains motor and sensory areas and is the site of consciousness and intelligence.

Root	Ventricul
	*(From a Latin word **ventriculum**, meaning ventricle or chamber. Here it refers to the cavities in the brain filled with cerebrospinal fluid, the cerebral ventricles.)*

Combining forms   **Ventricul/o**

WORD EXERCISE 6

Using your Exercise Guide, build words which mean:

(a) visual examination of _____
   the ventricles

(b) incision into the ventricles _____

Without using your Exercise Guide, write the meaning of:

(c) **ventriculo**graphy _____
   (Air, gas or radio-opaque dyes
   are injected into the ventricles
   during this procedure.)

Use the Latin root **cisterna**, meaning a closed space serving as a reservoir for fluid, and your Exercise Guide, to write the meaning of the word below. The closed space referred to here is the subarachnoid space outside the brain.

(d) **ventriculo**cisternostomy _____
   (This is an operation for hydrocephalus.)

Root	Crani
	*(From Greek **kranion** and Latin **cranium**, meaning skull. The bones of the skull protect the soft brain beneath.)*

Combining forms   **Crani/o**

WORD EXERCISE 7

Without using your Exercise Guide, build words which mean:

(a) incision into the skull _____

(b) the measurement of skulls _____

Root | **Gangli**
*(From a Greek word **ganglion**, meaning swelling. Here it refers to knots of nerve cell bodies located outside the central nervous system known as ganglia.)*

Combining forms **Gangli/o, ganglion**

 # WORD EXERCISE 8

Without using your Exercise Guide, build a word using **gangli/o** which means:

(a) tumour of a ganglion   _____

Using your Exercise Guide, find the meaning of:

(b) pre**ganglion**ic   _____

(c) post**ganglion**ic   _____

(d) **ganglion**ectomy   _____

Root | **Mening**
*(From a Greek word **meningos**, meaning membrane. The meninges are three membranes which surround the brain and spinal cord.)*

Combining forms **Mening/o, mening/i**

WORD EXERCISE 9

Without using your Exercise Guide, build words using **mening/o** which mean:

(a) inflammation of the meninges   _____

(b) hernia or protrusion of the meninges   _____

(c) condition of bursting forth (of blood) from meninges   _____

Without using your Exercise Guide, write the meaning of:

(d) **meningo**encephalocele   _____

(e) **meningo**encephalitis   _____

(f) **meningo**encephalopathy   _____

(g) **meningi**oma   _____

The outer of the three membranes of the meninges is known as the dura mater. The injection of local anaesthetic into the spine above the dura, i.e. into the epidural space, is known as an epidural block. It is often used for a forceps birth or caesarean section delivery (epi- means above or upon).

Using your Exercise Guide, find the meaning of:

(h) epi**dur**al   _____

(i) sub**dur**al haematoma (Fig. 42) (Am. hematoma)   _____

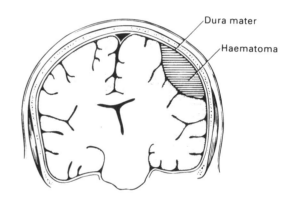

Figure 42   Subdural haematoma

This is a common condition seen by neurologists following head injuries. It requires surgery via the cranium to seal leaking blood vessels and remove the blood clot. Surgery also relieves pressure on the brain tissue and this prevents further damage.

The two inner meninges, the pia mater and the arachnoid membrane, are thin. When these are inflamed the condition is known as **leptomeningitis** (from a Greek word *leptos*, meaning thin/slender). When the thick outer dura mater is inflamed it is known as **pachymeningitis** (pachy meaning thick). When meningitis is caused by a bacterium, the coccus *Neisseria meningitidis*, it is referred to as **meningo**coccal **mening**itis.

Root | **Radicul**
*(From a Latin word **radicula**, meaning root. Here we are using it to mean the spinal nerve roots which emerge from the spinal cord.)*

Combining forms **Radicul/o**

WORD EXERCISE 10

Without using your Exercise Guide, write the meaning of:

(a) **radiculo**ganglionitis _____

(b) **radiculo**neuritis _____

Another combining form **radic/o** is also derived from this root, e.g.

(c) **radic**otomy _____

 Root

Myel
*(From a Greek word **myelos**, meaning marrow. It is used in reference to marrow within bones and also to spinal marrow, i.e. the soft spinal cord within the spine. Here we use it to mean the spinal cord.)*

Combining forms **Myel/o**

WORD EXERCISE 11

Without using your Exercise Guide, write the meaning of:

(a) **myelo**meningitis _____

(b) meningo**myelo**cele _____

(c) **myelo**radiculitis _____

(d) **myelo**encephalitis _____

(e) **myelo**phthisis _____

(f) polio**myel**itis _____

Without using your Exercise Guide, build words which mean:

(g) hardening of the spinal marrow _____

(h) condition of softening of the _____
    spinal marrow

(i) technique of making an X-ray _____
    of the spinal cord

Using your Exercise Guide, find the meaning of:

(j) **myelo**dysplasia _____

(k) **myel**atrophy _____

(l) syringo**myel**ia _____

Root

Rachi
*(From a Greek word **rhachis**, meaning spine.)*

Combining forms **Rachi/o**

WORD EXERCISE 12

Using your Exercise Guide, find the meaning of:

(a) **rachio**meter _____

(b) **rachio**centesis _____

Rachiocentesis (Fig. 43) is performed to obtain a sample of cerebrospinal fluid (CSF) from the subarachnoid space in the lumbar region of the spinal cord. This procedure is commonly known as a **lumbar puncture** or **spinal tap**.

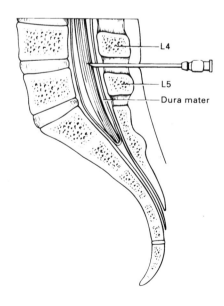

Figure 43 Lumbar puncture

Using your Exercise Guide, find the meaning of:

(c) **rachi**schisis _____
(synonymous with spina bifida)

Root **Pleg**
*(From Greek **plege**, meaning a blow, it is now used to mean a paralysis. Strokes, i.e. cerebrovascular accidents, are often the cause of this condition; these occur when a blockage or haemorrhage in the brain leads to destruction of cells which control motor activities.)*

Combining form **-plegia**

✎ WORD EXERCISE 13

Using your Exercise Guide, find the meaning of:

(a) quadri**pleg**ia _____
(paralysis of limbs)

(b) hemi**pleg**ia _____
(paralysis of right or left side of the body)

(c) para**pleg**ia _____
(paralysis of lower limbs)

(d) di**pleg**ia _____
(paralysis of like parts on either side of body)

(e) tetra**pleg**ia _____

Root **Aesthesi**
*(From Greek **aisthesis**, meaning perception or sensation.)*

Combining forms **Aesthesi/o, aesthesia, aesthetic Esthesi/o** *(Am.)*, **esthesia** *(Am.)*, **esthetic** *(Am.)*

✎ WORD EXERCISE 14

Without using your Exercise Guide, write the meaning of:

(a) an**aesthesi**a _____
(Am. anesthesia)

(b) an**aesthe**tic _____
(Am. anesthetic)

(c) an**aesthesio**logy _____
(Am. anesthesiology)

(d) an**aesthesio**logist _____
(Am. anesthesiologist)

(e) hemian**aesthes**ia _____
(Am. hemianesthesia; refers to one side of the body)

Using your Exercise Guide, find the meaning of:

(f) hypo**aesthes**ia _____
(Am. hypoesthesia)

(g) hyper**aesthes**ia _____
(Am. hyperesthesia)

The term par**aesthes**ia (Am. paresthesia) is used to mean any abnormal sensations, such as 'pins and needles' (from Greek word *para*, meaning near).

Without using your Exercise Guide, build words which mean:

(h) pertaining to following/ _____
after anaesthesia
(Am. anesthesia)

(i) pertaining to before _____
anaesthesia (Am. anesthesia)

Root **Narc**
*(From a Greek word **narke**, meaning stupor; it is used in medicine to refer to an abnormally deep sleep induced by a drug (narcotic). This is a different level of consciousness from anaesthesia; patients are not oblivious to pain and can be woken up.)*

Combining forms **Narc/o**

✎ WORD EXERCISE 15

Without using your Exercise Guide, write the meaning of:

(a) **narco**sis _____

Using your Exercise Guide, find the meaning of:

(b) **narco**therapy   _____

Root	**Alges**
	*(From a Greek word **algesis**, meaning a sense of pain.)*
Combining forms	**Algesi/o, -algesia**

WORD EXERCISE 16

Without using your Exercise Guide, write the meaning of:

(a) **algesi**a   _____

(b) an**alges**ia   _____

(c) hyper**alges**ia   _____

(d) an**alges**ic
    (a drug)   _____

Psychiatry

Disorders which interfere with the normal functioning of the brain may affect behaviour and personality, i.e. the mind. The study of the mind and treatment of its disorders is a specialist branch of medicine known as psychiatry. A psychiatrist is a person with medical qualifications who has specialized in the study and treatment of mental disease. The following terms are used by psychiatrists:

Root	**Psych**
	*(From Greek **psyche**, meaning soul or mind.)*
Combining forms	**Psych/o**

WORD EXERCISE 17

Without using your Exercise Guide, write the meaning of:

(a) **psych**ology   _____

Note. A psychologist is not usually medically qualified and cannot treat disorders by means of drugs or surgery. Psychologists study human behaviour.

(b) **psych**ic   _____

(c) **psycho**pathy   _____

Note. A psychopath is a person with a specific type of personality disorder in which he/she exhibits antisocial behaviour.

(d) **psych**osis   _____

Note. **Psychoses** originate in the mind itself, in contrast to **neuroses** which are mental conditions believed to arise because of stresses and anxieties in the patient's environment. Neurotic comes from neur + otic, otic meaning condition/disease of.

(e) **psycho**tropic drug   _____

Using your Exercise Guide, find the meaning of:

(f) **psycho**somatic   _____

(g) **psych**iatry   _____

Root	**Phob**
	*(From a Greek word **phobos**, meaning fear.)*
Combining form	**-phobia**

WORD EXERCISE 18

Using your Exercise Guide, find the meaning of:

(a) acro**phob**ia   _____

(b) agora**phob**ia   _____

(c) aqua**phob**ia   _____

(d) cancero**phob**ia   _____

(e) necro**phob**ia   _____

Root	**Epilept**
	*(From Greek **epileptikos**, meaning a seizure. It refers to epilepsy, the disordered electrical activity of the brain which produces a 'fit' and unconsciousness.)*
Combining forms	**Epilept/i, epilept/o**

WORD EXERCISE 19

Without using your Exercise Guide, write the meaning of:

(a) **epilepto**genic _____

(b) post**epileptic** _____

Using your Exercise Guide, find the meaning of:

(c) **epilepti**form _____

Modern treatments of mental disease involve drug treatments and occasionally surgery. One of the most useful physical methods of treatment which brings about improvement in depressive states, mania and stupor is **electroconvulsive therapy** (ECT). This involves the application of a high voltage to the head via electrodes placed on its surface.

Medical equipment and clinical procedures

Patients with a suspected neurological disorder are examined by a neurologist. Much information about the state of health of the nervous system can be gained from relatively simple testing of reflex actions using a tendon hammer (Fig. 44). One such test you are probably familiar with is the knee jerk reflex where the sense organs in the patella (knee cap) are tapped with a hammer. In a healthy patient the response will be that muscles in the thigh will contract, causing the leg to jerk upwards. A normal reflex action will indicate that the nerve pathway from the knee through the spinal cord is working normally.

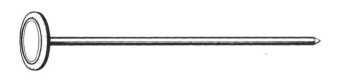

Figure 44 Tendon hammer

More detailed examinations of the nervous system require specialized equipment, e.g.:

Computerized axial tomography

This is an examination which uses a **tomograph**, i.e. an X-ray machine which can produce images of cross-sections of the body.

Electroencephalography

This technique uses an **electroencephalograph** to produce a tracing of the electrical activity of the brain. This is used to aid diagnosis of epilepsy, brain tumours and other disorders of the brain (see Fig. 41).

Magnetic resonance imaging (MRI)

This recently developed technique using nuclear magnetic resonance is particularly useful for imaging the soft tissue of the brain and spinal cord. The patient is placed in an intense magnetic field, hydrogen atoms in the nerve tissue are excited with radio waves and signals from them are detected and computed into a picture. The procedure does not have the risks associated with X-rays.

The stereotaxic instrument

This is a device that guides instruments into a precise position within the brain. It is used for neurosurgery. The stereotaxic instrument is fixed to the skull and finds its position by three-dimensional measurement. Surgeons use this to guide instruments that destroy or stimulate brain tissue which may be causing neurological or psychological problems.

Revise the names of all instruments and examinations mentioned in this unit, and then try Exercises 20 and 21.

WORD EXERCISE 20

Match each term in Column A with a description from Column C by placing an appropriate number in Column B.

Column A	Column B	Column C
(a) encephalography	_____	1. instrument for testing reflexes
(b) pneumoencephalography	_____	2. instrument which images serial sections of body using X-rays
(c) ventriculoscopy	_____	3. measurement of cranium

Column A	Column B	Column C
(d) tendon hammer	_____	4. technique for making X-ray of brain after injection of air into ventricles
(e) tomograph	_____	5. technique for making X-ray of brain
(f) craniometry	_____	6. technique for viewing ventricles

WORD EXERCISE 21

Match each term in Column A with a description from Column C by placing an appropriate number in Column B.

Column A	Column B	Column C
(a) magnetic resonance imaging	_____	1. technique of imaging serial sections of body using X-rays
(b) lumbar puncture	_____	2. technique of recording electrical activity of the brain
(c) myelography	_____	3. technique for imaging soft tissues of brain and spinal cord without using X-rays
(d) computed axial tomography	_____	4. technique of X-raying brain ventricles
(e) electroencepha-lography	_____	5. X-ray examination of spinal cord
(f) ventriculography	_____	6. technique of removing cerebrospinal fluid from spinal cord

ANATOMY EXERCISE

Now complete the Anatomy Exercise on page 87.

Quick Reference

Medical roots relating to the nervous system:

Aesthesi/o	sensation
Alges/i	sense of pain
Cephal/o	head
Cerebr/o	cerebrum/brain
Cistern/o	cistern/subarachnoid space
Crani/o	cranium
Dur/o	dura mater
Encephal/o	brain
Epilept/o	epilepsy
Esthesi/o (Am.)	sensation
Gangli/o	ganglion
Gli/o	gluelike/neuroglial cells
Mening/o	meninges
Motor	action/moving/set in motion
Myel/o	marrow/spinal cord
Narc/o	stupor/numbness
Neur/o	nerve
Plex/o	network, e.g. of nerves
Rachi/o	spine
Radicul/o	nerve root
Somat/o	body
Syring/o	tube/cavity
Ventricul/o	ventricle

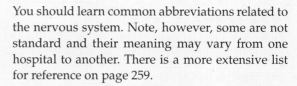

Abbreviations

You should learn common abbreviations related to the nervous system. Note, however, some are not standard and their meaning may vary from one hospital to another. There is a more extensive list for reference on page 259.

CAT	computerized axial tomography
CN	cranial nerve
CSF	cerebrospinal fluid
CVA	cerebrovascular accident
ECT	electroconvulsive therapy
EEG	electroencephalogram
ICP	intracranial pressure
KJ	knee jerk
MRI	magnetic resonance imaging
NCVs	nerve conduction velocities
PR	plantar reflex
SDH	subdural haematoma (Am. hematoma)

> NOW TRY THE WORD CHECK

WORD CHECK

This self-check exercise lists all the word components used in this unit. First write down the meaning of as many word components as you can. Then check your answers using the Exercise Guide and Quick Reference box or the Glossary of Word Components (pp. 269–279).

Prefixes

a- _____

acro- _____

agora- _____

an- _____

di- _____

dys- _____

electro- _____

epi- _____

hemi- _____

hyper- _____

hypo- _____

lepto- _____

macro- _____

meso- _____

micro- _____

pachy- _____

para- _____

polio- _____

poly- _____

post- _____

pre- _____

quadri- _____

sub- _____

tetra- _____

Combining forms of word roots

aesthesi/o
(Am. esthesi/o) _____

alges/i _____

aqua- _____

cancer/o _____

cephal/o _____

cerebr/o _____

cistern/o _____

crani/o _____

cyt/o _____

dur/o _____

ech/o _____

encephal/o _____

epilept/o _____

fibr/o _____

gangli/o _____

gli/o _____

haemat/o
(Am. hemat/o) _____

hist/o _____

hydro- _____

iatr/o _____

mening/o _____

motor _____

myel/o _____

narc/o _____

necr/o _____

neur/o _____

plex/o _____

pneum/o _____

psych/o _____

py/o _____

rachi/o _____

radicul/o _____

somat/o   _____

syring/o   _____

ventricul/o   _____

Suffixes

-al   _____

-algia   _____

-cele   _____

-centesis   _____

-cyte   _____

-ectomy   _____

-form   _____

-genic   _____

-gram   _____

-graph   _____

-graphy   _____

-gyric   _____

-ia   _____

-ic   _____

-itis   _____

-logist   _____

-logy   _____

-malacia   _____

-meter   _____

-metry   _____

-oma   _____

-osis   _____

-ous   _____

-pathy   _____

-phobia   _____

-phthisis   _____

-plasia   _____

-plegia   _____

-rrhagia   _____

-schisis   _____

-sclerosis   _____

-scopy   _____

-stomy   _____

-therapy   _____

-tomy   _____

-trauma   _____

-trophy   _____

-tropic   _____

-us   _____

▷ NOW TRY THE SELF-ASSESSMENT ◁

SELF-ASSESSMENT

Test 8A

Below are some combining forms which refer to the anatomy of the nervous system. Indicate which part of the system they refer to by putting a number from the diagrams (Figs 45 and 46) next to each word.

(a) crani/o   _____

(b) encephal/o   _____

(c) meningi/o   _____

(d) neur/o   _____

(e) rachi/o   _____

(f) gangli/o   _____

(g) ventricul/o   _____

(h) radicul/o   _____

(i) cephal/o   _____

(j) myel/o   _____

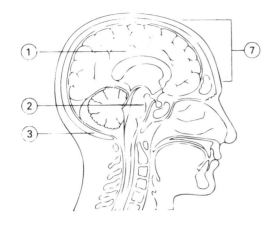

(d)	an-	_____	4. water (ii)
(e)	aqua-	_____	5. thick
(f)	di-	_____	6. large
(g)	epi-	_____	7. without/not (i)
(h)	hemi-	_____	8. without/not (ii)
(i)	hydro-	_____	9. four (i)
(j)	lepto-	_____	10. four (ii)
(k)	macro-	_____	11. before/in front of
(l)	meso-	_____	12. grey matter
(m)	micro-	_____	13. half
(n)	pachy-	_____	14. thin/slender
(o)	para-	_____	15. open space
(p)	polio-	_____	16. upon/above
(q)	post-	_____	17. small
(r)	pre-	_____	18. two/double
(s)	quadri-	_____	19. point/extremity
(t)	tetra-	_____	20. beside/near

Score

20

Figure 45   Sagittal section through the head

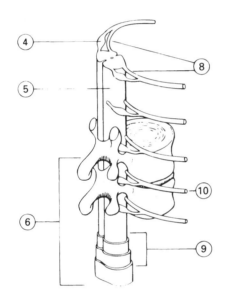

Figure 46   Section through the spine

Score

10

Test 8B
Prefixes

Match each prefix in Column A with a meaning in Column C by inserting the appropriate number in Column B

Column A	Column B	Column C
(a) a-	_____	1. after/behind
(b) acro-	_____	2. middle
(c) agora-	_____	3. water (i)

Test 8C
Combining forms of word roots

Match each combining form in Column A with a meaning in Column C by inserting the appropriate number in Column B.

Column A	Column B	Column C
(a) aesthesi/o (Am. esthesi/o)	_____	1. spine
(b) cephal/o	_____	2. mind
(c) cistern/o	_____	3. gas/wind/air
(d) crani/o	_____	4. stupor/deep sleep
(e) dur/o	_____	5. body
(f) encephal/o	_____	6. membranes of CNS
(g) epilept/o	_____	7. ganglion
(h) gangli/o	_____	8. cranium/skull
(i) gli/o	_____	9. ventricles of brain
(j) mening/o	_____	10. head

	Column A	Column B		Column C
(k)	motor	_____	11.	dura mater
(l)	myel/o	_____	12.	fit/seizure/ epilepsy
(m)	narc/o	_____	13.	cistern/reservoir/ subarachnoid space
(n)	neur/o	_____	14.	root (of spinal nerve)
(o)	pneum/o	_____	15.	nerve
(p)	psych/o	_____	16.	marrow (of spine)
(q)	rachi/o	_____	17.	pertaining to action
(r)	radicul/o	_____	18.	glue (cell)
(s)	somat/o	_____	19.	brain
(t)	ventricul/o	_____	20.	sensation

Score

20

Test 8D
Suffixes

Match each suffix in Column A with a meaning in Column C by inserting the appropriate number in Column B.

	Column A	Column B		Column C
(a)	-centesis	_____	1.	condition of paralysis
(b)	-form	_____	2.	abnormal condition/disease of
(c)	-genic	_____	3.	technique of recording/ making an X-ray
(d)	-gram	_____	4.	pertaining to the body
(e)	-graphy	_____	5.	pertaining to affinity for/ stimulating
(f)	-gyric	_____	6.	formation of an opening into …
(g)	-malacia	_____	7.	having form of

	Column A	Column B		Column C
(h)	-osis	_____	8.	condition of increase in cell formation/number of cells
(i)	-phobia	_____	9.	nourishment
(j)	-phthisis	_____	10.	hardening
(k)	-plasia	_____	11.	wasting away/decay
(l)	-plegia	_____	12.	condition of softening
(m)	-schisis	_____	13.	recording/ tracing/X-ray
(n)	-sclerosis	_____	14.	puncture
(o)	-somatic	_____	15.	treatment
(p)	-stomy	_____	16.	splitting
(q)	-therapy	_____	17.	condition of fear
(r)	-trauma	_____	18.	pertaining to movement around a centre
(s)	-trophy	_____	19.	formation/ originating in
(t)	-tropic	_____	20.	injury/shock

Score

20

Test 8E

Write the meaning of:

(a) neuromyelitis _____

(b) rachiotomy _____

(c) meningomalacia _____

(d) encephalomyelopathy _____

(e) ventriculoscope _____

Score

5

Test 8F

Build words which mean:

(a) disease of the meninges   _____

(b) instrument for measuring   _____
     the head

(c) inflammation of the spinal cord   _____
     and spinal nerve roots

(d) condition of bursting forth   _____
     (of blood) from the brain

(e) study of cells of the nervous   _____
     system

Score

5

Check answers to Self-Assessment Tests on page 253.

The eye

Objectives

Once you have completed Unit 9 you should be able to:

- understand the meaning of medical words relating to the eye

- build medical words relating to the eye

- associate medical terms with their anatomical position

- understand medical abbreviations relating to the eye.

Exercise Guide

Use this list of word components and their meanings to complete the word exercises in this unit.

Prefixes

a-	without
ambly-	dull/dim
an-	without
aniso-	unequal
bin-	two each/double
dia-	through
diplo-	double
dys-	difficult/painful
electro-	electrical
en-	in/within
ex-	out/out of/away from
hemi-	half
iso-	same/equal
mono-	one
pan-	all
presby-	old man/old age
uni-	one
xero-	dry

Roots/Combining forms

aden/o	gland
aesthesi/o	sensation
blenn/o	mucus
chromat/o	colour
cyst/o	bladder
esthesi/o (Am.)	sensation
helc/o	ulcer
lith/o	stone
motor	action
my/o	muscle
myc/o	fungus
nas/o	nose
neur/o	nerve

py/o	pus
rhin/o	nose
ton/o	tone/tension

Suffixes

-agogic	pertaining to inducing/stimulating
-al	pertaining to
-ar	pertaining to
-blast	immature germ cell/cell which forms …
-cele	swelling/protrusion/hernia
-centesis	puncture
-chalasis	slackening/loosening
-conus	cone-like protrusion
-dialysis	separating
-ectasis	dilatation/stretching
-ectomy	removal of
-edema (Am.)	swelling due to fluid
-erysis	drag/draw/suck out
-gram	X-ray/tracing/recording
-graph	usually an instrument that records
-graphy	technique of recording/making an X-ray
-gyric	pertaining to circular motion
-ia	condition of
-itis	inflammation of
-kinesis	movement
-logist	specialist who studies …
-malacia	condition of softening
-meter	measuring instrument
-metrist	specialist who measures
-metry	process of measuring
-mileusis	to carve
-nyxis	perforation/pricking/puncture
-oedema	swelling due to fluid
-oma	tumour/swelling
-osis	abnormal condition/disease/abnormal increase
-pathy	disease of
-pexy	fixation (by surgery)
-plasty	surgical repair/reconstruction
-plegia	condition of paralysis
-ptosis	falling/displacement/prolapse
-rrhaphy	suture/stitch/suturing
-rrhea (Am.)	excessive flow
-rrhoea	excessive flow
-schisis	cleavage/splitting/parting
-sclerosis	abnormal condition of hardening
-scope	viewing instrument
-scopy	visual examination
-spasm	involuntary muscle contraction
-stenosis	abnormal condition of narrowing
-stomy	formation of an opening into …
-synechia	condition of adhering together
-thermy	heat
-tome	cutting instrument
-tomy	incision into

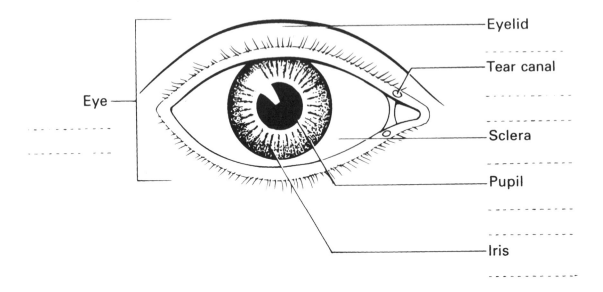

Eye

Eyelid

Tear canal

Sclera

Pupil

Iris

Figure 47 The eye

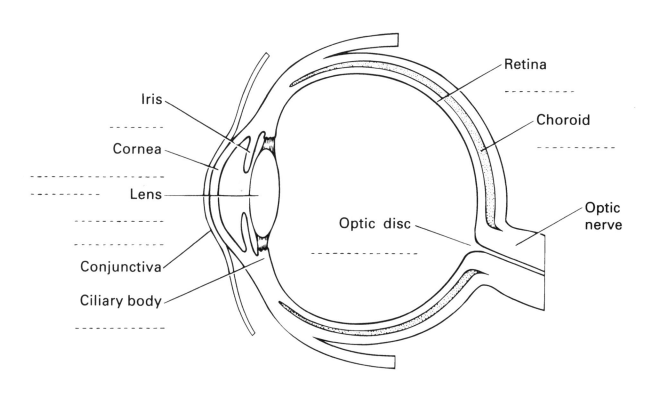

Iris

Cornea

Lens

Conjunctiva

Ciliary body

Retina

Choroid

Optic disc

Optic nerve

Figure 48 Section through the eye

ANATOMY EXERCISE

When you have finished Word Exercises 1–21, look at the word components listed below. Complete Figures 47 and 48 by writing the appropriate combining form on each dotted line – more than one component may relate to the same position. (You can check their meanings in the Quick Reference box on p. 112.)

Blephar/o	Ir/o	Papill/o
Choroid/o	Lacrim/o	Pupill/o
Corne/o	Irid/o	Phac/o
Cor/e/o	Kerat/o	Phak/o
Cycl/o	Ocul/o	Retin/o
Dacry/o	Ophthalm/o	Scler/o

The eye

The eyes are our main sense organs. Light enters the eye through the pupil and transparent cornea. It passes through the lens and is focused on to the light-sensitive retina. In the retina light stimulates receptors (rods and cones) to generate nerve impulses in sensory neurons; these impulses travel via neurons in the optic nerve to the visual areas of the brain which interpret them as an image.

Use the Exercise Guide at the beginning of this unit to complete Word Exercises 1–21 unless you are asked to work without it.

Root	**Ophthalm** *(From a Greek word* **ophthalmos**, *meaning eye.)*
Combining forms	**Ophthalm/o** *(Be careful with spelling ophth.)*

WORD EXERCISE 1

Using your Exercise Guide, build words which mean:

(a) an instrument to view the eye _____

(b) a medically qualified person who specializes in the study of the eye and its disorders _____

(c) condition of paralysis of the eye _____

(d) inflammation of the eye (synonymous with ophthalmia) _____

(e) abnormal condition of fungal infection of the eye _____

Using your Exercise Guide, find the meaning of:

(f) **ophthalmo**gyric _____

(g) **ophthalmo**neuritis _____

(h) pan**ophthalm**itis _____

(i) **ophthalmo**tonometer _____
(This instrument is used in the diagnosis of glaucoma and conditions in which there is raised pressure within the eye. Sometimes **tonometer** is used alone and **tonography** is used to mean the technique of using a tonometer.)

(j) blenn**ophthalm**ia _____

(k) xer**ophthalm**ia _____

(l) en**ophthalm**os _____

(m) ex**ophthalm**os _____

Root	**Ocul** *(From Latin* **ocularis**, *meaning of the eye.)*
Combining forms	**Ocul/o, -ocular**

WORD EXERCISE 2

Using your Exercise Guide, find the meaning of:

(a) mon**ocul**ar _____

(b) uni**ocul**ar _____

(c) bin**ocul**ar _____

(d) **oculo**motor nerve _____

(e) **oculo**nasal _____

(f) electro-**oculo**gram _____
(This is produced from an electrodiagnostic test; it also records eye position and/movement.)

Without using your Exercise Guide, write the meaning of:

(g) **oculo**gyric _____

Root	**Opt**
	*(From **optikos**, a Greek word meaning sight. The words optical and optician are derived from this root. Optical means pertaining to sight; optician refers to a person who prescribes spectacles to correct defects in sight.)*

Combining forms **Opt/o**

WORD EXERCISE 3

Without using your Exercise Guide, write the meaning of:

(a) **opto**meter _____

Using your Exercise Guide, find the meaning of:

(b) **opto**metry _____

(c) **opto**metrist _____

(d) **opto**myometer _____

(e) **opto**aesthesia _____
(Am. optoesthesia)

Orthoptics means pertaining to the study and treatment of muscle imbalances of the eye (squints). *Ortho* means straight, therefore orthoptics refers to making eyes and sight straight.

The combining form **optic/o** is also derived from the same root as **opt/o**. It also means pertaining to sight but it is sometimes used to mean optic nerve, e.g. optico-pupillary – pertaining to the pupil and optic nerve.

Root	**Op**
	*(From Greek **ops** also meaning eye. It is usually used as the suffix -opsia to mean a condition of defective vision. Many focusing defects can be corrected by prescribing appropriate spectacles.)*

Combining forms **-opia, -opsia**

WORD EXERCISE 4

Using your Exercise Guide, find the meaning of:

(a) dipl**op**ia _____

(b) presby**op**ia _____
(refers to a condition in which the lens loses its elasticity; near point approximately 1 m)

(c) ambly**op**ia _____

(d) hemiachromat**ops**ia _____

Three other common words which use -opia are difficult to understand from their word components. These are:

Hypermetropia
This is used to describe long-sightedness in which light rays are focused beyond the retina (*hyper* – beyond/above). The light rays when measured focus beyond the retina (*metr* – measure).

Myopia
This refers to short-sightedness. *My* comes from *myein*, meaning to close. Presumably the eye tends to close when trying to view a distant object.

Emmetropia
Light falls directly on to the retina in its correct position, with no errors. This word refers to normal/ideal vision (*em* meaning in, *metr* meaning measure).

(e) dys**op**ia _____

(f) hemian**op**ia _____

Root **Blephar**
(From a Greek word **blepharon***, meaning eyelid, sometimes used for eyelash.)*

Combining forms **Blephar/o**

WORD EXERCISE 5

Without using your Exercise Guide, build a word which means:

(a) condition of paralysis of _____
the eyelid

Using your Exercise Guide, build words which mean:

(b) spasm of the eyelid _____

(c) falling/displacement of _____
the eyelid

(d) suturing of an eyelid _____

Using your Exercise Guide, find the meaning of:

(e) **blephar**opyorrhoea _____
(Am. blepharopyorrhea)

(f) **blephar**oadenitis _____
(refers to meibomian glands lying in grooves on
inner surface of eyelids)

(g) **blephar**osynechia _____

(h) **blephar**ochalasis _____

Root **Scler**
(From Greek **skleros***, meaning hard. Here it is used to mean the tough, outer white part of the eye. The sclera is continuous with the transparent cornea at the front of the eye.)*

Combining forms **Scler/o**

WORD EXERCISE 6

Using your Exercise Guide, find the meaning of:

(a) **sclero**tomy _____

(b) **scler**ectasis _____

(c) **sclero**tome _____

Root **Kerat**
(From a Greek word **keras***, meaning horn. Here it is used to mean the cornea. The cornea, located at the front of the eye, provides strength, refractive power and transmits light into the eye.)*

Combining forms **Kerat/o**

WORD EXERCISE 7

Without using your Exercise Guide, write the meaning of:

(a) **sclero**keratitis _____

(b) **kerato**metry _____

(c) **kerato**tome _____

Using your Exercise Guide, find the meaning of:

(d) **kerato**plasty _____

(e) **kerato**centesis _____

(f) **kerato**helcosis _____

(g) **kerato**nyxis _____

(h) **kerato**mileusis _____
(actually an operation for correction of myopia or
short-sightedness)

(i) **kerato**conus _____

The word cornea comes from the Latin word *corneus*, also meaning horny. Corneoplasty is synonymous with keratoplasty, an operation performed to replace a diseased or damaged cornea with a corneal graft.

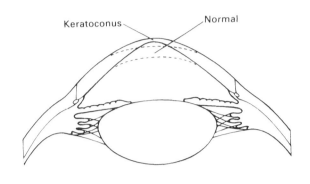

Figure 49   **Keratoconus**

Abnormal curvatures of the cornea cause light rays to focus on the retina unevenly. This is known as **astigmatism**.

The sclera and cornea are covered at the front of the eye with a delicate, transparent membrane which also lines the inner surface of the eyelids. This membrane is the **conjunctiva**, it is prone to irritation and infection, giving rise to **conjunctivitis**.

Root	**Ir**
	*(From a Greek word **iris**, meaning rainbow. It refers to the circular, coloured membrane surrounding the pupil of the eye. Contraction of its muscle fibres regulates the size of the aperture (pupil) within the iris, thereby regulating the amount of light entering the eye.)*
Combining forms	**Ir/o, irid/o**

WORD EXERCISE 8

Without using your Exercise Guide, build words using irid/o which mean:

(a) falling/displacement   _____
of the iris

(b) inflammation of the cornea   _____
and iris (use kerat/o)

Using your Exercise Guide, find the meaning of:

(c) **irido**kinesis   _____

(d) **irido**dialysis   _____

(e) **irido**cele   _____

Without using your Exercise Guide, write the meaning of:

(f) sclero**irido**dialysis   _____

(g) sclero**irido**tomy   _____

(h) kerato**iritis**   _____

Root	**Cycl**
	*(From a Greek word **kyklos** meaning circle. Here it is used to mean the circular ciliary body of the eye.)*
Combining forms	**Cycl/o**

The ciliary body, a structure composed of muscles and processes, lies behind the iris (see Fig. 48). It connects the circumference of the iris to the choroid (the middle layer of the eyeball), changes the shape of the lens and secretes a watery fluid, aqueous humor, into the anterior chamber. Study Figure 50 which shows the anterior cavity in front of the lens and the posterior cavity behind the lens. The anterior cavity is sub-divided into the anterior chamber in front of both lens and iris and the posterior chamber between the lens and iris. The ciliary body continuously secretes aqueous humor into the anterior chamber. The fluid is drained into veins in the sclera at the same rate that it is produced. A raised intraocular pressure due to the accumulation of excess aqueous humor may result in **glaucoma,** a common eye disorder which causes pain and damage. The posterior cavity is filled with vitreous humor, a soft jelly-like material which maintains the spherical shape of the eyeball.

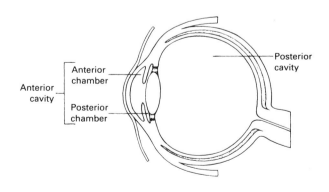

Figure 50   **Section through the eye**

WORD EXERCISE 9

Without using your Exercise Guide, write the meaning of:

(a) irido**cycl**itis _____

(b) **cyclo**plegia _____

Using your Exercise Guide, find the meaning of:

(c) **cyclo**diathermy _____

Root

Goni
*(From a Greek word **gonia**, meaning angle. Here it means the peripheral angle of the anterior chamber. This angle is observed when evaluating types of glaucoma.)*

Combining forms **Goni/o**

WORD EXERCISE 10

Without using your Exercise Guide, build words which mean:

(a) instrument to measure the angle of the anterior chamber _____

(b) instrument to view the angle of the anterior chamber _____

(c) operation to make an incision into the angle of the anterior chamber (for glaucoma) _____

Root

Pupill
*(From a Latin word **pupilla**, meaning the pupil or aperture of the eye.)*

Combining forms **Pupill/o**

WORD EXERCISE 11

Without using your Exercise Guide, write the meaning of:

(a) **pupillo**plegia _____

(b) **pupillo**metry _____

Root

Cor
*(From a Greek word **kore**, meaning pupil of eye.)*

Combining forms **Cor/o, core/o**

WORD EXERCISE 12

Using your Exercise Guide, find the meaning of:

(a) aniso**cor**ia _____

(b) **coreo**pexy _____

(c) iso**cor**ia _____

Without using your Exercise Guide, write the meaning of:

(d) **coreo**plasty _____

Root

Choroid
*(From a Greek word **choroeides**, meaning like a fetal membrane. It is used in medicine to refer to the middle pigmented vascular coat of the posterior five-sixths of the eyeball. The choroid prevents the passage of light.)*

Combining forms **Choroid/o**

WORD EXERCISE 13

Without using your Exercise Guide, write the meaning of:

(a) **choroido**cyclitis _____

(b) sclero**choroid**itis _____

The word **uvea** from Latin *uva*, meaning grape, is used when referring to the pigmented parts of the eye. These parts include the iris, ciliary body and choroid. **Uve**itis, therefore, refers to inflammation of all pigmented parts of the eye.

Root

Retin
(From a Medieval/Latin word **retina***, probably derived from rete, meaning net. It refers to the light-sensitive area of the eye. Light is focused on to the retina by the lens.)*

Combining forms **Retin/o**

WORD EXERCISE 14

Using your Exercise Guide, find the meaning of:

(a) **retino**blastoma _____

(b) **retino**malacia _____

(c) **retino**schisis _____

(d) **retino**pathy _____

(e) **retino**scopy _____

Without using your Exercise Guide, build words which mean:

(f) picture/recording of the _____
electrical activity of the retina

(g) inflammation of the _____
choroid and retina

(h) inflammation of the _____
retina and choroid

Note. The words in (g) and (h) above are synonymous. Remember, when building words, we add the components as we read the meaning, e.g. in (g) we begin with **-itis**, then add **choroid/o**, followed by **retin/o**; in (h) we begin with **-itis**, but then add **retin/o**, followed by **choroid/o**, thus making two different words which have the same meaning.

Root

Papill
(From a Latin word **papilla***, meaning nipple-shaped.)*

Combining forms **Papill/o**

Sensory neurons leaving the retina travel through the optic nerve at the back of the eye. Where the sensory neurons collect and form the optic nerve there is a disc-shaped area (visible through the pupil) in the retina. This area is known as the optic disc. **Papilla** refers to this nipple-shaped optic disc.

WORD EXERCISE 15

Using your Exercise Guide, find the meaning of:

(a) **papill**oedema _____
(Am. papilledema)

Without using your Exercise Guide, build a word which means:

(b) inflammation of the optic _____
disc and retina

Root

Phak
(From a Greek word **phakos***, meaning lentil. It refers to the lentil-shaped lens of the eye. The lens is a crystalline structure surrounded by the lens capsule. The shape of the lens and its focus are changed by ligaments connected to muscles in the ciliary body. The ability to change focus of the lens is known as accommodation.)*

Combining forms **Phac/o or phak/o**

A common disorder of the lens is the development of a cataract that is an opacity of the lens or lens capsule. There are many types of cataract. Two common ones are hard cataracts, which tend to form in the elderly, and soft cataracts, which can occur at any age. The lens can be removed by **phako-**emulsification. In this process ultrasonic vibrations liquefy the lens and it is then sucked out. The lens can be replaced with an intraocular implant, i.e. a plastic lens.

WORD EXERCISE 16

Without using your Exercise Guide, build words using phac/o which mean:

(a) condition of softening of a lens _____
(i.e. a soft cataract)

(b) instrument to view the lens _____
(actually to view changes in
its shape)

Using your Exercise Guide, build words which mean:

(c) hardening of a lens (i.e. a hard cataract) _____

(d) condition of without a lens (use a-) _____

Using your Exercise Guide, find the meaning of:

(e) **phaco**cystectomy _____

(f) **phaco**erysis _____

Root	Scot
	(From a Greek word **skotos**, *meaning darkness. It is used to refer to a scotoma, i.e. normal and abnormal blind spots in the visual field where vision is poor.)*

Combining forms **Scot/o, scotoma**

WORD EXERCISE 17

Without using your Exercise Guide, write the meaning of:

(a) **scoto**meter _____

(b) **scoto**metry _____

Using your Exercise Guide, find the meaning of:

(c) **scoto**magraph _____

Root	Lacrim
	(From a Latin word **lacrima**, *meaning tear.)*

Combining forms **Lacrim/o**

The eye is cleansed and lubricated by the lacrimal apparatus (Fig. 51) which consists of a gland, sac and ducts. This produces lacrimal fluid which is washed over the eyeball and drained into the lacrimal sac, which in turn drains into the nasolacrimal ducts. The fluid finally enters the nose from the nasolacrimal duct. Here **lacrim/o** is used to mean lacrimal apparatus (**-al** – pertaining to).

WORD EXERCISE 18

Without using your Exercise Guide, build words which mean:
(a) incision into the lacrimal _____
apparatus

Lacrimal gland
Lacrimal duct
Lacrimal sac
Nasolacrimal duct

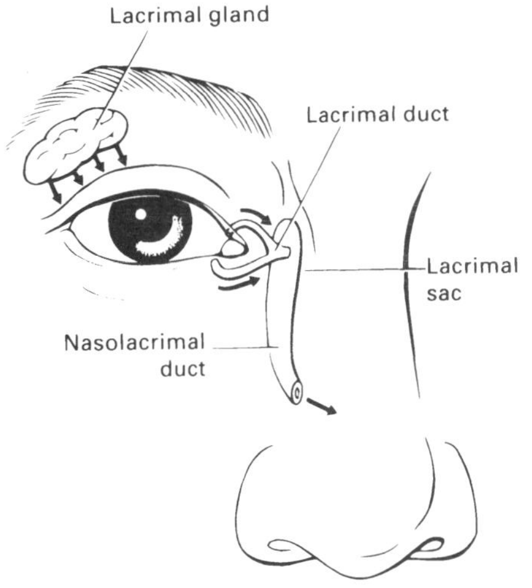

Figure 51 Lacrimal apparatus

(b) pertaining to the lacrimal _____
apparatus and nose (use nas/o)

Root	Dacry
	(From a Greek word **dakryon**, *also meaning tear or lacrimal apparatus.)*

Combining forms **Dacry/o**

WORD EXERCISE 19

Using your Exercise Guide, find the meaning of:

(a) **dacry**ocyst _____
(refers to lacrimal sac)

(b) **dacry**ocysto graphy _____

(c) **dacry**ocysto rhinostomy _____

(d) **dacry**olith _____

(e) **dacry**ostenosis _____

(f) **dacry**agogic _____

Without using your Exercise Guide, write the meaning of:

(g) **dacry**ocysto blennorrhoea _____
(Am. dacryocystoblennorrhea)

(h) **dacry**ocysto pyosis _____

Medical equipment and clinical procedures

Before completing Exercises 20 and 21, revise the names of instruments and examinations used in this unit.

 WORD EXERCISE 20

Match each term in column A with a description from column C by placing an appropriate number in Column B.

Column A	Column B	Column C
(a) ophthalmoscope	_____	1. X-ray picture of lacrimal apparatus
(b) dacryocystogram	_____	2. measurement of scotomas
(c) keratome	_____	3. instrument which measures tension within the eye
(d) pupillometry	_____	4. instrument for visual examination of the eye
(e) optometry	_____	5. instrument to cut the cornea
(f) scotometry	_____	6. instrument for measuring power of ocular muscles
(g) ophthalmotono-meter	_____	7. technique of measuring sight
(h) optomyometer	_____	8. technique of measuring pupils (width)

 WORD EXERCISE 21

Match each term in column A with a description from Column C by placing an appropriate number in Column B.

Column A	Column B	Column C
(a) sclerotome	_____	1. visual examination of retina
(b) optometer	_____	2. technique of recording raised pressure/tension in the eye

Column A	Column B	Column C
(c) keratometry	_____	3. technique of making an X-ray of tear (lacrimal) sac
(d) pupillometer	_____	4. instrument to measure sight
(e) phacoscope	_____	5. instrument to cut sclera
(f) retinoscopy	_____	6. measurement of cornea (curvature)
(g) tonography	_____	7. instrument to view the lens
(h) dacryocystography	_____	8. instrument which measures pupils (width)

 ANATOMY EXERCISE

Now complete the Anatomy Exercise on page 105.

Quick Reference

Medical roots relating to the eye:

Blephar/o	eyelid
Choroid/o	choroid
Chromat/o	colour
Conjunctiv/o	conjunctiva
Cor/e/o	pupil
Cycl/o	ciliary body
Dacry/o	tear
Goni/o	angle (of anterior chamber)
Ir/o	iris
Irid/o	iris
Kerat/o	cornea
Lacrim/o	tear
Ocul/o	eye
Ophthalm/o	eye
Optic/o	optic nerve
Opt/o	sight
Papill/o	optic disc
Phac/o	lens
Phak/o	lens
Pupill/o	pupil
Retin/o	retina
Scler/o	sclera
Scot/o	dark
Ton/o	tone/tension
Uve/o	uvea (pigmented part of eye)

Abbreviations

You should learn common abbreviations related to the eye. Note, however, some are not standard and their meaning may vary from one hospital to another. There is a more extensive list for reference on page 259.

Accom	accommodation of eye
Astigm	astigmatism of eye
Em	emmetropia/good vision
IOFB	intraocular foreign body
My	myopia/short sight
OD	oculus dexter/right eye
OS	oculus sinister/left eye
OU	oculus unitas/both eyes together
POAG	primary open angle glaucoma
PERLAC	pupils equal, react to light, accommodation consensual
VA	visual acuity
VF	visual field

> ## NOW TRY THE WORD CHECK

WORD CHECK

This self-check exercise lists all the word components used in this unit. First write down the meaning of as many word components as you can. Then check your answers using the Exercise Guide and Quick Reference box or the Glossary of Word Components (pp. 269–279).

Prefixes

a- _____

ambly- _____

an- _____

bin- _____

dia- _____

diplo- _____

dys- _____

electro- _____

em- _____

en- _____

ex- _____

hemi- _____

hyper- _____

iso- _____

mono- _____

ortho- _____

pan- _____

presby- _____

uni- _____

xero- _____

Combining forms of word roots

aesthesi/o (Am. esthesi/o) _____

aden/o _____

blast/o _____

blenn/o _____

blephar/o _____

choroid/o _____

chromat/o _____

conjunctiv/o _____

cor/e/o _____

cycl/o _____

cyst/o _____

dacry/o _____

goni/o _____

helc/o _____

ir/o _____

irid/o _____

kerat/o _____

lacrim/o _____

lith/o _____

motor _____

myc/o _____

my/o _____

my (from myein) _____

nas/o _____

neur/o _____

ocul/o _____

ophthalm/o _____

optic/o _____

opt/o _____

papill/o _____

phak/o, phac/o _____

pupill/o _____

py/o _____

retin/o _____

rhin/o _____

scler/o _____

scot/o _____

sten/o _____

ton/o _____

uve/o _____

Suffixes

-agogic _____

-al _____

-cele _____

-centesis _____

-chalasis _____

-conus _____

-desis _____

-dialysis _____

-ectasis _____

-ectomy _____

-erysis _____

-gram _____

-graph _____

-graphy _____

-gyric _____

-ia _____

-itis _____

-kinesis _____

-logist _____

-malacia _____

-meter _____

-metrist _____

-metry _____

-mileusis _____

-nyxis _____

-oedema (Am. -edema) _____

-oma _____

-opia _____

-osis _____

-pathy _____

-pexy _____

-phobia _____

-plasty _____

-plegia _____

-ptosis _____

-rrhaphy _____

-rrhoea (Am. -rrhea) _____

-schisis _____

-sclerosis _____

-scope _____

-scopy _____

-spasm _____

-synechia _____

-thermy _____

-tome   _____

-tomy   _____

> **NOW TRY THE SELF-ASSESSMENT**

SELF-ASSESSMENT

Test 9A

Below are some combining forms which refer to the anatomy of the eye. Indicate which parts of the eye they refer to by putting a number from the diagrams (Figs 52 and 53) next to each word:

(a)   irid/o   _____

(b)   scler/o   _____

(c)   pupill/o   _____

(d)   lacrim/o   _____

(e)   blephar/o   _____

(f)   phac/o   _____

(g)   papill/o   _____

(h)   retin/o   _____

(i)   kerat/o   _____

(j)   ophthalmoneur/o   _____

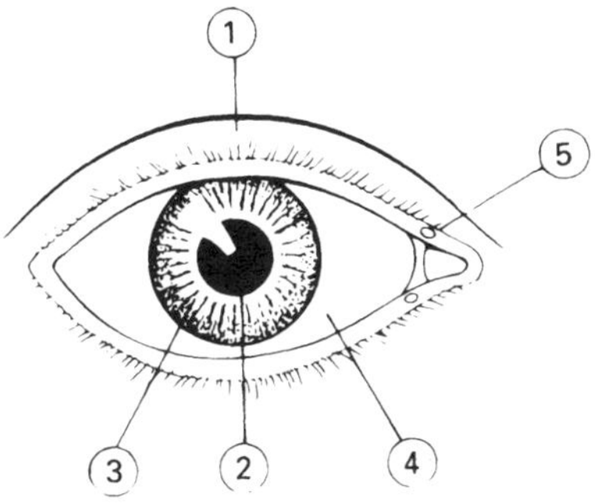

Figure 52   The eye

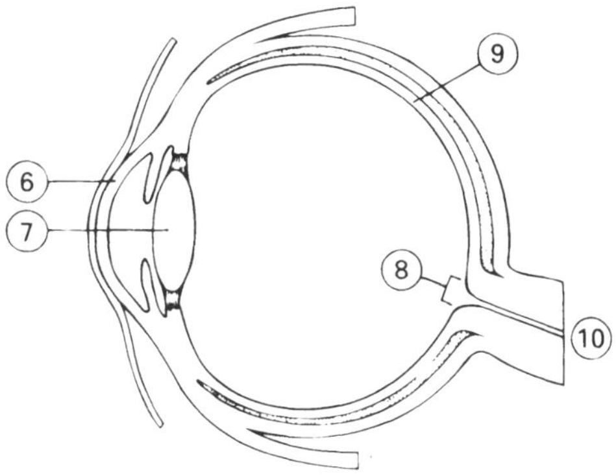

Figure 53   Section through the eye

Score

10

Test 9B
Prefixes and suffixes

Match each prefix or suffix in Column A with a meaning in Column C by inserting the appropriate number in Column B.

Column A	Column B	Column C
(a) -agogic	_____	1. dragging/ drawing/sucking out
(b) ambly-	_____	2. splitting
(c) -dialysis	_____	3. swelling (due to fluid)
(d) electro-	_____	4. one (i)
(e) -erysis	_____	5. one (ii)
(f) -graph	_____	6. person who measures
(g) -gyric	_____	7. old man, old age
(h) hemi-	_____	8. all
(i) -kinesis	_____	9. condition of sticking together
(j) -metrist	_____	10. dulled/made dim
(k) -mileusis	_____	11. condition of vision (defective)
(l) mono-	_____	12. pertaining to inducing/ stimulating

Column A	Column B	Column C
(m) -oedema (Am. -edema)	_____	13. pertaining to turning/circular movement
(n) -opia	_____	14. instrument which records
(o) pan-	_____	15. movement
(p) presby-	_____	16. to carve
(q) -rrhaphy	_____	17. suturing/stitching
(r) -schisis	_____	18. separating
(s) -synechia	_____	19. electrical
(t) uni-	_____	20. half

Score

20

Column A	Column B	Column C
(q) pupill/o	_____	17. eyelid
(r) retin/o	_____	18. conjunctiva
(s) scotom/o	_____	19. tear (i)
(t) uve/o	_____	20. tear (ii)

Score

20

Test 9C

Combining forms of word roots

Match each combining form in Column A with a meaning in Column C by inserting the appropriate number in Column B.

Column A	Column B	Column C
(a) blephar/o	_____	1. cone (shaped)
(b) choroid/o	_____	2. cornea
(c) chromat/o	_____	3. optic disc
(d) conjunctiv/o	_____	4. iris (rainbow)
(e) conus	_____	5. pupil
(f) cycl/o	_____	6. sight/vision
(g) dacry/o	_____	7. pigmented area of eye (uvea)
(h) helc/o	_____	8. retina
(i) irid/o	_____	9. colour
(j) kerat/o	_____	10. ulcer
(k) lacrim/o	_____	11. lens
(l) ocul/o	_____	12. ciliary body
(m) ophthalm/o	_____	13. darkness/blind spot
(n) optic/o	_____	14. choroid
(o) papill/o	_____	15. eye (i)
(p) phak/o	_____	16. eye (ii)

Test 9D

Write the meaning of:

(a) ophthalmoplasty _____

(b) retinopexy _____

(c) dacryopyorrhoea (Am. dacryopyorrhea) _____

(d) scleroiritis _____

(e) oculomotor nerve _____

Score

5

Test 9E

Build words which mean:

(a) visual examination of the eye _____

(b) inflammation of eyelid _____

(c) any disease of cornea _____

(d) instrument to view the retina _____

(e) condition of paralysis of iris _____

Score

5

Check answers to Self-Assessment Tests on page 253.

10 The ear

Objectives

Once you have completed Unit 10 you should be able to:

- understand the meaning of medical words relating to the ear
- build medical words relating to the ear
- associate medical terms with their anatomical position
- understand medical abbreviations relating to the ear.

Exercise Guide

Use this list of word components and their meanings to complete the word exercises in this unit.

Prefixes

bin-	two each/double
electro-	electrical
endo-	within/inside
macro-	large
micro-	small

Roots/Combining forms

laryng/o	larynx
myc/o	fungus
pharyng/o	pharynx
py/o	pus
rhin/o	nose
ten/o	tendon

Suffixes

-al	pertaining to
-algia	condition of pain
-ar	pertaining to
-centesis	puncture to remove fluid
-eal	pertaining to
-ectomy	removal of
-emphraxis	blocking/stopping up
-genic	pertaining to formation/originating in
-gram	X-ray tracing/picture/recording
-graphy	technique of recording/making an X-ray
-ia	condition of
-itis	inflammation of
-logy	study of
-meter	measuring instrument
-metry	process of measuring
-osis	abnormal condition/disease/ abnormal increase
-plasty	surgical repair/reconstruction
-rrhea (Am.)	excessive discharge/flow
-rrhoea	excessive discharge/flow
-sclerosis	abnormal condition of hardening
-scope	instrument to view
-stomy	formation of an opening/an opening
-tome	cutting instrument
-tomy	incision into

Ear

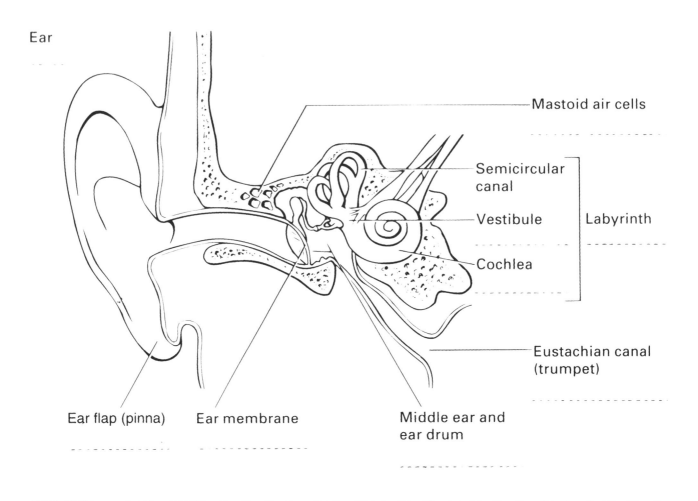

Mastoid air cells

Semicircular canal

Vestibule

Labyrinth

Cochlea

Eustachian canal (trumpet)

Ear flap (pinna)   Ear membrane   Middle ear and ear drum

Figure 54   Section through the ear

ANATOMY EXERCISE

When you have finished Word Exercises 1–14, look at the word components listed below. Complete Figure 54 by writing the appropriate combining form on each dotted line – more than one component may relate to the same position. (You can check their meanings in the Quick Reference box on p. 123.)

Auricul/o	Mastoid/o	Salping/o
Cochle/o	Myring/o	Tympan/o
Labyrinth/o	Ot/o	Vestibul/o

The ear

The ear is a major sense organ concerned with two important functions:

1. hearing
2. balance.

The ear provides an auditory input into the brain. Sound waves (vibrations) in the surrounding air are conducted to the inner ear which contains fluid and receptors. The latter generate nerve impulses in response to vibrations. These impulses are relayed via sensory nerves to auditory areas in the brain where they are interpreted as sounds. The possession of two ears provides us with the ability to sense the direction of sound.

The role of the ear in balance is achieved by receptors in the vestibular apparatus detecting changes in velocity and position of the body. Sensory neurons relay this information to centres in the cerebellum and other regions of the brain.

Use the Exercise Guide at the beginning of this unit to complete Word Exercises 1–14 unless you are asked to work without it.

 Root   **Ot**
(From a Greek word **otos**, *meaning ear.)*

Combining forms   **Ot/o**

 # WORD EXERCISE 1

Using your Exercise Guide, build words which mean:

(a) the study of the ear   _____

(b) instrument to view the ear   _____

(c) abnormal condition of
     hardening of the ear   _____
     (actually due to new bone
     formation in the middle ear)

(d) abnormal condition of pus in the ear

Using your Exercise Guide, find the meaning of:

(e) **oto**rhinolaryngology   _____

(f) **oto**mycosis   _____

(g) **oto**pyorrhoea   _____
     (Am. otopyorrhea)

(h) micr**oti**a   _____

(i) macr**oti**a   _____

The ear can be divided into three areas, the external, middle and inner ear. Infection and inflammation (**oti-tis**) can occur in any of these areas. The following terms are used to describe the position of the inflammation:

Otitis externa
    inflammation of the external ear.

Otitis media
    inflammation of the middle ear.

Otitis interna
    inflammation of the inner ear.

Infection commonly begins in the middle ear because it is connected to the **nasopharynx** by a short tube known as the **Eustachian tube** (auditory tube). This tube functions to equalize the pressure on either side of the ear drum but it also provides an entrance for microorganisms such as those present in upper respiratory tract infections.

Root   **Aur**
(From a Latin word **auris**, *meaning ear.)*

Combining forms   **Aur/i, -aural**

WORD EXERCISE 2

Without using your Exercise Guide, build a word which means:

(a) instrument to view the ear   _____
     (otoscope) (Fig. 55)

Viewing of the ear canal and tympanic membrane is improved by using an **aural speculum** (Fig. 56), a device which is inserted into the external ear before examining with an **auriscope**.

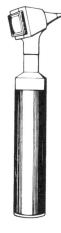

Figure 55   **Otoscope/auriscope**

The auriscope is used to examine the external ear canal and the ear membrane. Occasionally, the ear canal can become blocked by excessive wax production by the cerumenous (wax) glands in its lining. This can be

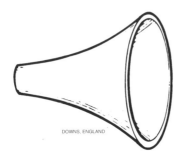

Figure 56 Aural speculum

removed by washing the ear with warm water using an aural syringe (Fig. 57). Various wax solvents can bring about cerumenolysis.

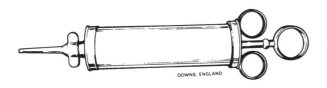

Figure 57 Aural syringe

Using your Exercise Guide, find the meaning of:

(b) bin**aur**al _____

(c) end**aur**al _____

The Latin word *auricula* refers to the ear flaps (pinnae) of the external ear.

(d) bin**auricul**ar _____

Root | **Myring**
(*A New Latin word* **myringa**, *meaning membrane. It refers to the tympanic membrane or ear membrane.*)

Combining forms **Myring/o**

 WORD EXERCISE 3

Using your Exercise Guide, build words which mean:

(a) incision into the ear membrane _____ (allows air to enter to aid drainage)

(b) instrument used to cut the _____ ear membrane

Without using your Exercise Guide, build a word which means:

(c) abnormal condition of fungal _____ infection of the ear membrane

Sometimes the tympanic membrane is surgically punctured to assist the drainage of fluid from the middle ear (as in glue ear). Once an opening is made in the membrane, fluid drains through the Eustachian tube into the nasopharynx. A small plastic grommet (Fig. 58) can be fixed into the membrane and this assists drainage for an extended period. The grommet eventually falls out and the membrane heals.

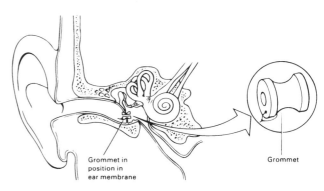

Grommet in position in ear membrane

Grommet

Figure 58 Grommet

Root | **Tympan**
(*From a Greek word* **tympanon**, *meaning drum. Here it refers to the tympanum, i.e. the cavity of the middle ear and the tympanic membrane. It is also used to mean tympanic membrane.*)

Combining forms **Tympan/o**

 WORD EXERCISE 4

Using your Exercise Guide, build words which mean:

(a) reconstructive surgery of _____ the tympanum

(b) puncture of the tympanic _____ membrane

Without using your Exercise Guide, write the meaning of:

(c) **tympan**itis _____

(d) **tympano**tomy _____

Root

Salping
*(From Greek **salpigx**, meaning trumpet tube. Here it refers to the trumpet-shaped Eustachian tube which connects the middle ear to the nasopharynx.)*

Combining forms   **Salping/o**

WORD EXERCISE 5

Using your Exercise Guide, find the meaning of:

(a) **salping**emphraxis _____

(b) **salpingo**pharyngeal _____

Within the middle ear we find the smallest bones in the body, the ear ossicles (Fig. 59). These have been named **malleus, incus** and **stapes**. Their function is to transmit vibrations from the tympanic membrane to the inner ear via the oval window. Behind the oval window is a fluid-filled structure known as the **cochlea**, the organ of hearing. Within the cochlea are sensory hair cells which respond to vibrations in the fluid by producing nerve impulses. The auditory area of the brain interprets these as sound and enables us to hear.

Root

Stapedi
*(From a Latin word **stapes**, meaning stirrup, it refers to the stirrup-shaped ear ossicle.)*

Combining forms   **Staped/o, stapedi/o**

WORD EXERCISE 6

Using your Exercise Guide, build a word which means:

(a) removal of the stapes _____

Using your Exercise Guide, find the meaning of:

(b) **stapedio**tenotomy _____

Root

Malle
*(From a Latin word **malleus**, meaning hammer. It refers to the hammer-shaped ear ossicle.)*

Combining forms   **Malle/o**

WORD EXERCISE 7

Without using your Exercise Guide, write the meaning of:

(a) **malleo**tomy _____

Root

Incud
*(From a Latin word **incus**, meaning anvil. It refers to the anvil-shaped ear ossicle.)*

Combining forms   **Incud/o, -incudal**

WORD EXERCISE 8

Without using your Exercise Guide, write the meaning of:

(a) **incudo**malleal _____

(b) **incudo**stapedial _____

(c) malleo**incud**al _____

ANATOMY EXERCISE

Write the appropriate combining form for each ossicle on the dotted lines of Figure 59.

Sometimes the ear bones are referred to in a more general way, using **ossicle**, to mean small ear bones, e.g. **ossicul**ectomy for removal of one or more ossicles, **ossiculo**tomy for incision into the ear ossicles. The ossicles can be replaced by a plastic prosthesis which will transmit vibrations to the inner ear and restore hearing.

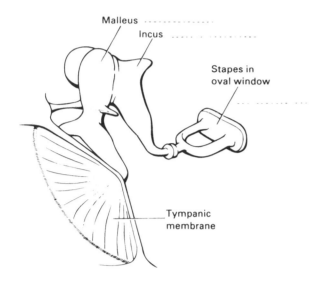

Malleus

Incus

Stapes in
oval window

Tympanic
membrane

Figure 59   Ear ossicles

Root   **Cochle**
*(From a Latin word **cochlea**, meaning snail. It refers to the spiral-shaped anterior bony labyrinth of the inner ear.)*

Combining forms   **Cochle/o**

 WORD EXERCISE 9

Using your Exercise Guide, build words which mean:

(a) an opening into the cochlea   _____

(b) technique of recording the   _____
cochlea's electrical activity

Root   **Labyrinth**
*(From a Greek word **labyrinthos**, meaning maze or anything twisted or spiral-shaped. Here it refers to the labyrinth of the inner ear.)*

Combining forms   **Labyrinth/o**

The inner ear consists of bony and membranous labyrinths. The bony labyrinth is a series of canals in the temporal bone filled with fluid. It consists of the cochlea (organ of hearing), vestibule and semicircular canals which are concerned with balance.

The membranous labyrinth lies within the bony labyrinth and is also filled with fluid. Distension of the membranous labyrinth with excess fluid gives rise to **Ménière's** disease, symptoms of which include vertigo (dizziness) and deafness.

The portions of the inner ear concerned with balance are collectively known as the vestibular apparatus.

 WORD EXERCISE 10

Without using your Exercise Guide, build words which mean:

(a) inflammation of a labyrinth   _____

(b) removal of a labyrinth   _____

Root   **Vestibul**
*(From the Latin word **vestibulum**, meaning entrance. It refers to the oval cavity in the middle of the bony labyrinth.)*

Combining forms   **Vestibul/o**

 WORD EXERCISE 11

Without using your Exercise Guide, write the meaning of:

(a) **vestibulo**tomy   _____

Using your Exercise Guide, find the meaning of:

(b) **vestibulo**genic   _____

Root   **Mast**
*(From a Greek word **mastos**, meaning breast. It refers to the nipple-shaped air cells or the air space within the mastoid process. The mastoid process is a bone located behind the external ear.)*

Combining forms   **Mastoid/o**

WORD EXERCISE 12

Using your Exercise Guide, build a word which means:

(a) condition of pain in the   _____
     mastoid region

Without using your Exercise Guide, build words which mean:

(b) incision into the mastoid bone   _____

(c) removal of tissue from   _____
     the mastoid process

(d) inflammation of the mastoid   _____
     process and tympanum

Root	**Audi** *(From a Latin word **audire**, meaning to hear.)*
Combining forms	**Audi/o**

 WORD EXERCISE 13

Without using your Exercise Guide, build a word which means:

(a) the science dealing with   _____
     the study of hearing

Using your Exercise Guide, find the meaning of:

(b) **audio**meter   _____

(c) **audio**gram   _____

(d) **audio**metry   _____

Medical equipment and clinical procedures

Revise the names of all instruments and examinations used in this unit before completing Exercise 14.

 WORD EXERCISE 14

Match each term in Column A with a description in Column C by placing an appropriate number in Column B.

Column A	Column B	Column C
(a) audiometer	_____	1. technique of measuring hearing
(b) audiometry	_____	2. instrument for viewing ear
(c) aural speculum	_____	3. technique of viewing ear
(d) auriscope	_____	4. device for removing wax from ear
(e) otoscopy	_____	5. device to aid drainage of fluid from ear
(f) aural syringe	_____	6. instrument which measures hearing
(g) grommet	_____	7. device which holds ear canal open

 ANATOMY EXERCISE

Now complete the Anatomy Exercise on page 118.

Quick Reference

Medical roots relating to the ear:

Audi/o	hearing
Aur/i	ear
Auricul/o	ear flap
Cochle/o	cochlea
Incud/o	incus (an ear ossicle)
Labyrinth/o	labyrinth (of inner ear)
Malle/o	malleus (an ear ossicle)
Mastoid/o	mastoid process
Myring/o	ear membrane (drum)
Ossicul/o	ossicle
Ot/o	ear
Salping/o	Eustachian tube
Stapedi/o	stapes (an ear ossicle)
Tympan/o	ear drum/middle ear
Vestibul/o	vestibular apparatus (of inner ear)

Abbreviations

You should learn common abbreviations related to the ear. Note, however, some are not standard and their meaning may vary from one hospital to another. There is a more extensive list for reference on page 259.

AC	air conduction
AD	auris dextra (right ear)
AS	auris sinistra (left ear)
ASOM	acute suppurative otitis media
aud	audiology
BC	bone conduction
CSOM	chronic suppurative otitis media
ENT	ear, nose and throat
ETF	Eustachian tube function
OE	otitis externa
OM	otitis media
oto	otology

NOW TRY THE WORD CHECK

WORD CHECK

This self-check exercise lists all the word components used in this unit. First write down the meaning of as many word components as you can. Then check your answers using the Exercise Guide and Quick Reference box or the Glossary of Word Components (pp. 269–279).

Prefixes

bin- _____

electro- _____

endo- _____

macro- _____

micro- _____

Combining forms of word roots

audi/o _____

aur/i _____

auricul/o _____

cochle/o _____

incud/o _____

labyrinth/o _____

laryng/o _____

malle/o _____

mastoid/o _____

myc/o _____

myring/o _____

ossicul/o _____

ot/o _____

pharyng/o _____

py/o _____

rhin/o _____

salping/o _____

stapedi/o _____

ten/o _____

tympan/o _____

vestibul/o _____

Suffixes

-al _____

-algia _____

-ar _____

-aural _____

-centesis _____

-eal _____

-ectomy _____

-emphraxis _____

-externa _____

-genic _____

-gram _____

-ia _____

-interna _____

-itis   _____

-media   _____

-logy   _____

-meter   _____

-metry   _____

-osis   _____

-plasty   _____

-rrhoea
(Am. -rrhea)   _____

-sclerosis   _____

-scope   _____

-tome   _____

-tomy   _____

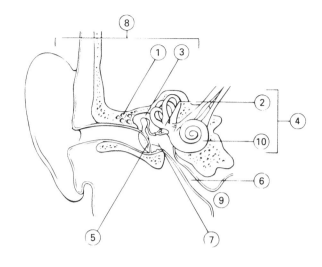

Figure 60   Section through the ear

Score

10

> **NOW TRY THE SELF-ASSESSMENT**

SELF-ASSESSMENT

Test 10A

Below are some combining forms which refer to the anatomy of the ear. Indicate which part of the system they refer to by putting a number from the diagram (Fig. 60) next to each word.

(a) ot/o   _____

(b) myring/o   _____

(c) tympan/o   _____

(d) nasopharyng/o   _____

(e) ossicul/o   _____

(f) labyrinth/o   _____

(g) cochle/o   _____

(h) mastoid/o   _____

(i) salping/o   _____

(j) vestibul/o   _____

Test 10B
Prefixes and suffixes

Match each prefix or suffix in Column A with a meaning in Column C by inserting the appropriate number in Column B.

Column A	Column B	Column C
(a) -al	_____	1. incision into
(b) -ar	_____	2. flow/discharge
(c) -aural	_____	3. external
(d) -eal	_____	4. instrument which cuts
(e) electro-	_____	5. hardening
(f) -emphraxis	_____	6. inner/internal
(g) endo-	_____	7. middle
(h) -externa	_____	8. pertaining to (i)
(i) -gram	_____	9. pertaining to (ii)
(j) -ia	_____	10. pertaining to (iii)
(k) -interna	_____	11. small
(l) macro-	_____	12. in/within
(m) -media	_____	13. abnormal condition/ disease of
(n) -metry	_____	14. pertaining to the ear

	Column A	Column B		Column C			Column A	Column B		Column C
(o)	micro-	_____	15.	picture/ X-ray/tracing		(q)	stapedi/o	_____	17.	mastoid
(p)	-osis	_____	16.	electrical		(r)	ten/o	_____	18.	ear bones/ ossicles
(q)	-rrhoea (Am. -rrhea)	_____	17.	condition of		(s)	tympan/o	_____	19.	pus
(r)	-sclerosis	_____	18.	large		(t)	vestibul/o	_____	20.	labyrinth of inner ear
(s)	-tome	_____	19.	to block/stop up						
(t)	-tomy	_____	20.	measurement						

Score

20

Score

20

Test 10C

Combining forms of word roots

Match each combining form in Column A with a meaning in Column C by inserting the appropriate number in Column B.

	Column A	Column B		Column C
(a)	audi/o	_____	1.	stapes
(b)	aur/i	_____	2.	larynx
(c)	auricul/o	_____	3.	nose
(d)	incud/o	_____	4.	Eustachian tube
(e)	labyrinth/o	_____	5.	ear (i)
(f)	laryng/o	_____	6.	ear (ii)
(g)	malle/o	_____	7.	ear flap (pinna)
(h)	mastoid/o	_____	8.	ear drum/middle ear
(i)	myc/o	_____	9.	vestibular apparatus
(j)	myring/o	_____	10.	malleus
(k)	ossicul/o	_____	11.	fungus
(l)	ot/o	_____	12.	hearing
(m)	pharyng/o	_____	13.	ear membrane
(n)	py/o	_____	14.	tendon
(o)	rhin/o	_____	15.	incus
(p)	salping/o	_____	16.	pharynx

Test 10D

Write the meaning of:

(a)   otolaryngology   _____

(b)   tympanosclerosis   _____

(c)   stapediovestibular   _____

(d)   tympanomalleal   _____

(e)   vestibulocochlear   _____

Score

5

Test 10E

Build words which mean:

(a) puncture of mastoid process   _____

(b) removal of the ear membrane   _____

(c) surgical repair of the ear   _____

(d) condition of pain in ear   _____

(e) originating in the middle ear   _____

Score

5

Check answers to Self-Assessment Tests on page 254.

11   The skin

Once you have completed Unit 11 you should be able to:

- understand the meaning of medical words relating to the skin

- build medical words relating to the skin

- associate medical terms with their anatomical position

- understand medical abbreviations relating to the skin.

Exercise Guide

Use this list of word components and their meanings to complete the word exercises in this unit.

Prefixes

a-	without
an-	without/not
auto-	self
crypto-	hidden
dys-	difficult/painful
epi-	above/upon/on
hyper-	above/excessive
hypo-	below/deficient
intra-	within/inside
pachy-	thick
para-	beside/near
sub-	under/below
xantho-	yellow
xero-	dry

Roots/Combining forms

aden/o	gland
aesthesi/i	sensation/sensitivity
esthesi/i (Am.)	sensation/sensitivity
lith/o	stone
motor	action
myc/o	fungus
schiz/o	split/cleft

Suffixes

-al	pertaining to
-auxis	increase
-cyte	cell
-ia	condition of
-ic	pertaining to
-itis	inflammation of
-lysis	breakdown/disintegration
-oma	tumour/swelling
-osis	abnormal condition/disease/ abnormal increase
-phagia	condition of eating
-phyte	plant (fungus)
-plasty	surgical repair/reconstruction
-poiesis	formation
-rrhexis	break/rupture
-rrhea (Am.)	excessive discharge/flow
-rrhoea	excessive discharge/flow
-schisis	splitting/parting/cleaving
-tome	cutting instrument
-trophy	nourishment/development
-tropic	pertaining to stimulating/ affinity for

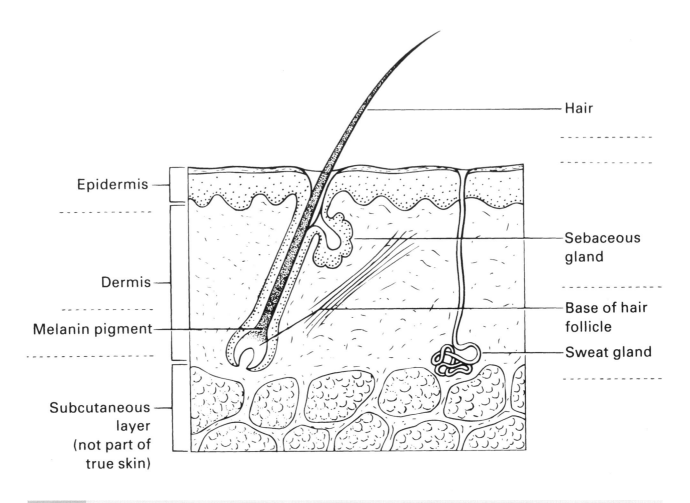

Epidermis

Dermis

Melanin pigment

Subcutaneous
layer
(not part of
true skin)

Hair

Sebaceous
gland

Base of hair
follicle

Sweat gland

Figure 61   Section through the skin

ANATOMY EXERCISE

When you have finished Word Exercises 1–9, look at the word components listed below. Complete Figure 61 by writing the appropriate combining form on each dotted line – more than one component may relate to the same position. (You can check their meanings in the Quick Reference box on p. 133.)

Derm/o   Melan/o   Seb/o
Hidraden/o   Pil/o   Trich/o
Kerat/o

The skin

The skin can be regarded as the largest organ in the body. It consists of two layers, the outer epidermis and the inner dermis. Skin is elastic; it regenerates and functions in protection, thermoregulation and secretion. In

its protective role, it prevents the body dehydrating, resists the invasion of microorganisms and protects it from the harmful effects of ultraviolet light.

Use the Exercise Guide at the beginning of this unit to complete Word Exercises 1–9 unless you are asked to work without it.

Root	Derm
	*(From a Greek word **derma**, meaning skin.)*
Combining forms	**Derm/a, dermat/o, -derma**

WORD EXERCISE 1

Using your Exercise Guide, find the meaning of:

(a) **derm**atosis _____

Actinic dermatoses are conditions in which the skin is abnormally sensitive to light (from a Greek word *aktis*, meaning ray).

(b) epi**derm**is _____

The epidermis forms the outer layer of the skin. Its function is to protect the underlying dermis. The epidermis can be subdivided into five distinct layers, the outermost forming a layer of tough dead cells (scales), known as the stratum corneum.

The cells of the epidermis fit together like the scales of a fish, so it is known as a **squamous** epithelium (from Latin *squama*, meaning scale of a fish or reptile).

(c) **dermato**phyte _____

(d) pachy**derma** _____

(e) xantho**derma** _____

(f) **dermato**autoplasty _____

(g) xero**derm**ia _____

Using your Exercise Guide, build words which mean:

(h) abnormal condition of fungi in the skin (use dermat/o and myc/o) _____

(i) an instrument to cut skin for grafts (use derm/a) _____

(j) pertaining to below the skin (use derm/a) _____

(k) pertaining to within the skin (use derm/a) _____

Note. There are a few words in use derived from *cutis*, the Latin for skin, e.g. cutaneous – pertaining to the skin; cuticle – the epidermis.

Root	Kerat
	*(From a Greek word **keras**, meaning horn. We have already used this word to mean the cornea of the eye. Here it is used to mean the outer, horny layer of the skin, i.e. the epidermis.)*
Combining forms	**Kerat/o**

There is no way of telling whether a medical term containing the root **kerat** refers to the cornea or the epidermis except by noting the context in which it is written.

The cells of the outer layer of the epidermis are said to be keratinized because they contain the waterproof protein keratin, which gives the epidermis its ability to protect the underlying dermis.

WORD EXERCISE 2

Without using your Exercise Guide, write the meaning of:

(a) actinic **kerat**osis _____
(pertaining to the sun's rays)

Using your Exercise Guide, find the meaning of:

(b) hyper**kerat**osis _____

(c) **kerat**oma _____

(d) **kerat**olysis _____

Other disorders of the epidermis include:

Ichthyosis
A disorder in which there is abnormal keratinization, giving rise to a dry scaly skin (**ichthy/o** from Greek, meaning fish, i.e. fish-like skin).

Acanthosis
A thickening of the prickle cell layer of the epidermis (**acanth/o** from Greek, meaning spike).

The skin appendages

The multiplication of cells in the basal layer of the epidermis gives rise to the appendages of the skin: hairs, sebaceous glands, sweat glands and nails. Here we use terms associated with each appendage:

Root Pil
*(From a Latin word **pilus**, meaning hair or composed of hair. Hairs grow from depressions in the epidermis known as follicles.)*

Combining forms **Pil/o**

WORD EXERCISE 3

Using your Exercise Guide, find the meaning of:

(a) **pilo**motor nerve _____
(This nerve stimulates the arrector pili muscles to contract, causing erection of the hair in cold conditions.)

A technique known as electrolysis is used to destroy hairs permanently by heating the base of a hair to destroy its dividing cells. The heating is achieved by passing an electric current through the hair follicle. This technique is also used by beauty therapists for the removal of excess hair and is known as e**pil**ation (e-meaning out from, i.e. the hair out of its follicle).

Hairs can also be removed by using a de**pil**atory paste which dissolves hair (de- meaning away). The hairs regrow following depilation as the base of the hair is not destroyed.

 Root Trich
*(From a Greek word **trichos**, meaning hair.)*

Combining forms **Trich/o**

WORD EXERCISE 4

Without using your Exercise Guide, write the meaning of:

(a) **tricho**phytosis _____

(b) **trich**osis _____

Using your Exercise Guide, find the meaning of:

(c) **tricho**aesthesia _____
(Am. trichoesthesia)

(d) schizo**trich**ia _____

(e) **trich**orrhexis _____

 Root Seb
*(From a Latin word **sebum**, meaning fat or grease. It is used to mean secretion of the sebaceous glands, i.e. sebum.)*

Combining forms **Seb/o**

The sebaceous glands can open directly on to the skin or more usually into the side of a hair follicle (a pilo**seba**ceous follicle). They produce an oily secretion, known as sebum, which lubricates and waterproofs the hair and skin. It is also mildly bacteriostatic.

Excessive production of sebum at puberty gives rise to **acne vulgaris**, a condition in which the skin becomes inflamed and develops pus-filled pimples.

WORD EXERCISE 5

Using your Exercise Guide, find the meaning of:

(a) **sebo**rrhoea _____
(Am. seborrhea)

(b) **sebo**lith _____

(c) **sebo**tropic _____

 Root Hidr
*(From a Greek word **hidros**, meaning sweat.)*

Combining forms **Hidr/o**

WORD EXERCISE 6

Without using your Exercise Guide, write the meaning of:

(a) **hidr**osis _____

(b) hyper**hidr**osis _____

Using your Exercise Guide, find the meaning of:

(c) **hidr**opoiesis _____

(d) an**hidr**osis _____

(e) hidradenitis _____

Sweat glands are also known by their Latin name of sudoriferous glands (*sudor* meaning sweat, *ferous* meaning carrying).

Root	Onych (From a Greek word **onychos**, meaning nail.)
Combining forms	**Onych/o**

WORD EXERCISE 7

Using your Exercise Guide, find the meaning of:

(a) **onycho**cryptosis _____

(b) **onych**auxis _____

(c) **onycho**dystrophy _____

(d) **onych**atrophy _____

(e) par**onychi**a _____

(f) **onycho**schisis _____

(g) **onycho**phagia _____

Without using your Exercise Guide, build words which mean:

(h) breaking down/disintegration _____
    of nails
    (Here the nail comes away from the nail bed.)

(i) fungal condition of nails _____

(j) inflammation of nails _____
    (synonymous with **onych**ia)

Without using your Exercise Guide, write the meaning of:

(k) **onycho**rrhexis _____

(l) an**onych**ia _____

(m) pachy**onych**ia _____

Root	Melan (From a Greek word **melanos**, meaning black. Here we are using it to mean melanin, a black pigment found in skin, hair and the choroid of the eye.)
Combining forms	**Melan/o**

WORD EXERCISE 8

Without using your Exercise Guide, build words which mean:

(a) a pigment cell _____

(b) abnormal condition of excessive _____
    black/pigment

Without using your Exercise Guide, write the meaning of:

(c) **melan**oma _____

Malignant melanoma is on the increase and this is believed to be the effect of solar damage caused by excessive sunbathing. Sometimes melanomas develop from pigmented naevi (moles). They are highly malignant, and once the tumour cells have spread, they become difficult to eradicate. Malignant melanoma can be fatal unless treated early in its development. 5-year survival rate can be related to the depth of the tumour in the skin at first presentation.

Note.   Naevus (pl. naevi; Am. nevus, pl. nevi)

This is a Latin word meaning a mole/mark on body. Naevi arise from pigment-producing cells or from an abnormal development of a blood vessel.

Medical equipment and clinical procedures

Suspicious lesions of skin need to be examined microscopically for signs of malignancy. Small samples of skin are removed during an excision **biopsy** (*bio* meaning life, *opsis* meaning vision, biopsy = observation of living tissue). These are then sectioned and stained in the histology laboratory. The biopsy tissue is examined by a histologist/pathologist to determine whether the cells are **benign** or **malignant** (benign means inno-cent/harmless; malignant means virulent and danger-ous to life).

Benign lesions can be removed if they are causing a problem or are unsightly. Malignant lesions threaten life and are treated by surgical excision, radiotherapy and chemotherapy.

Developments in physics have led to the development of medical **lasers** which are playing a prominent role in the treatment of skin disorders. Here we examine a selection of their applications to dermatology. First we need to understand the meaning of laser:

LASER (**L**ight **A**mplification by **S**timulated **E**mission of **R**adiation)

This is a device that produces an intense, coherent beam of monochromatic light. All the light waves in the beam are in phase and do not diverge so it can be targeted precisely.

The medical laser transfers energy in the form of light to the tissues. When the laser beam strikes living tissue it is heated and destroyed (**thermolysis**) in a fraction of a second. Some lasers can heat tissues to over 100°C, resulting in their complete vaporization.

The extent of destruction of a tissue depends on the presence of chemicals in cells that absorb the light.

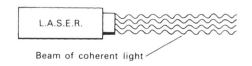

Beam of coherent light

Figure 62 Laser

These are known as **chromatophores**. There are three main chromatophores found in tissues: water, melanin and haemoglobin. A skin lesion containing a large amount of melanin, such as a mole, can be specifically targeted and destroyed by a laser with little destruction of the surrounding tissue.

There are many types of medical laser, each one emit-ting a beam of specific wavelength. The wavelength of the radiation emitted depends on the medium used by the laser, which may be a gas, liquid or solid. In the laser, the atoms of the medium are excited electrically and are stimulated to emit energy in the form of light. Here are three examples of lasers used by dermatolo-gists:

CO_2 laser

Medium	Wavelength	Chromatophore	Use in dermatology
Carbon dioxide gas	Infrared 10–600 nm	Water	Vaporizes/cuts tissue. Coagulates blood vessels. Bloodless surgery as it seals up cut vessels. Used for removing a variety of lesions

Argon laser

Medium	Wavelength	Chromatophore	Use
Ionized argon gas	Blue-green 488–514 nm	Melanin Haemoglobin	Penetrates epidermis and coagulates underlying pigments. Used to remove vascular and pigmented naevi (moles)

Dye laser

Medium	Wavelength	Chromatophore	Use
Various synthetic dyes	Can be tuned to any required wavelength	Melanin Haemoglobin	Removing tattoos. Removing pigmented tattoo inks, vascular lesions, moles, port wine stains, etc.

Besides laser light, other forms of radiation are used to treat chronic skin disorders.

Treatment of psoriasis with ultraviolet light

Psoriasis is a common chronic skin condition in which there is an increased rate of production of skin cells. The excess skin cells form plaques of silvery scales which continuously flake off, exposing erythematous skin which shows pinpoint bleeding. A large proportion of a dermatologist's time may be concerned with this disorder as it affects approximately 2% of the population. There is no cure. Therapies are aimed at reducing the scaling and inflammation. A recent innovation is the technique known as:

PUVA (**P**soralen **U**ltra **V**iolet **A** light)

This is a form of **photochemotherapy**, i.e. a procedure which uses a chemical known as a **psoralen** to sensitize the skin to light before it is irradiated with ultraviolet light (long wave A). After administration of the psoralen (orally) the patient is placed in a chamber illuminated with ultraviolet light tubes. This treatment is convenient for patients. Their skin shows dramatic improvement and the effect lasts for several months. Unfortunately there is a risk of developing skin cancer as a result of excessive exposure to UVA. This risk is being evaluated.

WORD EXERCISE 9

Match each term in Column A with a description in Column C by placing an appropriate number in Column B.

Column A	Column B	Column C
(a) excision biopsy	_____	1. removal of hair
(b) dermatome	_____	2. instrument which destroys tissue using a beam of coherent light
(c) medical laser	_____	3. destruction of tissue by heating with an electric current
(d) PUVA	_____	4. removal of living tissue from the body
(e) epilation	_____	5. instrument for cutting a thin layer of skin
(f) electrolysis	_____	6. technique of exposing photo-sensitized skin to light

ANATOMY EXERCISE

Now complete the Anatomy Exercise on page 128.

Quick Reference
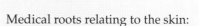

Medical roots relating to the skin:

Acanth/o	spiny
Dermat/o	skin
Hidr/o	sweat
Ichthy/o	dry/scaly/fish-like
Kerat/o	epidermis
Melan/o	melanin
Onych/o	nail
Pil/o	hair
Seb/o	sebum
Squam/o	scaly
Trich/o	hair

Abbreviations
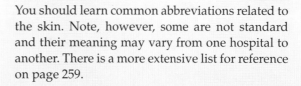

You should learn common abbreviations related to the skin. Note, however, some are not standard and their meaning may vary from one hospital to another. There is a more extensive list for reference on page 259.

bx	biopsy
Derm	dermatology
Ez	eczema
KS	Kaposi's sarcoma
SCC	squamous cell carcinoma
SED	skin erythema dose
SPF	sun protection factor
ST	skin test
STD	skin test dose
STU	skin test unit
Subcu	subcutaneous
ung	ointment (unguentum)

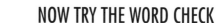

NOW TRY THE WORD CHECK

WORD CHECK

This self-check exercise lists all the word components used in this unit. First write down the meaning of as many word components as you can. Then check your answers using the Exercise Guide and Quick Reference box or the Glossary of Word Components (pp. 269–279).

Prefixes

a- _____

an- _____

auto- _____

crypto- _____

dys- _____

epi- _____

hyper- _____

hypo- _____

intra- _____

pachy- _____

para- _____

sub- _____

xantho- _____

xero- _____

Combining forms of word roots

acanth/o _____

aden/o _____

aesthesi/o
(Am. esthesi/o) _____

cyt/o _____

dermat/o _____

hidr/o _____

ichthy/o _____

kerat/o _____

lith/o

melan/o _____

motor _____

myc/o _____

onych/o _____

phyt/o _____

pil/o _____

schizo- _____

seb/o _____

squam/o _____

trich/o _____

Suffixes

-auxis _____

-ia _____

-ic _____

-itis _____

-lysis _____

-oma _____

-osis _____

-phagia _____

-plasty _____

-poiesis _____

-rrhexis _____

-rrhoea
(Am. -rrhea) _____

-schisis _____

-tome _____

-trophy _____

-tropic _____

> **NOW TRY THE SELF-ASSESSMENT**

SELF-ASSESSMENT

Test 11A

Below are some combining forms which refer to the anatomy of the skin. Indicate which part of the system they refer to by putting a number from the diagram (Fig. 63) next to each word:

(a) hidraden/o _____

(b) seb/o _____

(c) trich/o _____

(d) melan/o _____

(e) kerat/o _____

(f) dermat/o _____

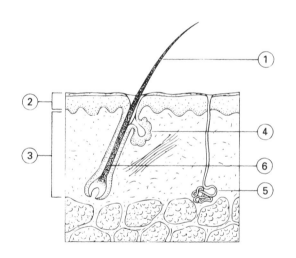

Figure 63   Section through the skin

Score

6

Test 11B
Prefixes and suffixes

Match each prefix or suffix in Column A with a meaning in Column C by inserting the appropriate number in Column B.

Column A	Column B	Column C
(a) a-	_____	1. cutting instrument
(b) auto-	_____	2. above
(c) -auxis	_____	3. breakdown/ disintegration
(d) crypto-	_____	4. within
(e) dys-	_____	5. condition of eating/swallowing
(f) hyper-	_____	6. thick
(g) hypo-	_____	7. nourishment
(h) intra-	_____	8. hidden/ concealed
(i) -lysis	_____	9. dry
(j) -oma	_____	10. formation/ making
(k) pachy-	_____	11. break/rupture
(l) -phagia	_____	12. pertaining to affinity for/ stimulating
(m) -poiesis	_____	13. difficult/painful
(n) -rrhexis	_____	14. tumour/swelling
(o) -schizo	_____	15. yellow
(p) -tome	_____	16. below
(q) -trophy	_____	17. increase
(r) -tropic	_____	18. without/not
(s) xanth/o	_____	19. self
(t) xer/o	_____	20. split

Score

20

Test 11C

Combining forms of word roots

Match each combining form in Column A with a meaning in Column C by inserting the appropriate number in Column B.

Column A	Column B	Column C
(a) aden/o	_____	1. horny/epidermis
(b) dermat/o	_____	2. pertaining to action
(c) hidr/o	_____	3. fungus
(d) kerat/o	_____	4. hair (i)
(e) lith/o	_____	5. hair (ii)
(f) motor	_____	6. nail
(g) myc/o	_____	7. skin
(h) onych/o	_____	8. plant
(i) phyt/o	_____	9. sweat
(j) pil/o	_____	10. sebum
(k) seb/o	_____	11. gland
(l) trich/o	_____	12. stone

Score

12

Test 11D

Write the meaning of:

(a) dermatophytosis   _____

(b) keratinocyte   _____

(c) trichoanaesthesia   _____
(Am. trichoanesthesia)

(d) hidradenoma   _____

(e) epidermomycosis   _____

Score

5

Test 11E

Build words which mean:

(a) inflammation of the skin   _____

(b) abnormal condition of nails   _____

(c) condition of nails blackened with melanin   _____

(d) study of skin   _____

(e) condition of thick nails   _____

Score

5

Check answers to Self-Assessment Tests on page 254.

The nose and mouth

Objectives

Once you have completed Unit 12 you should be able to:

- understand the meaning of medical words relating to the nose and mouth

- build medical words relating to the nose and mouth

- associate medical terms with their anatomical position

- understand medical abbreviations relating to the nose and mouth.

Exercise Guide

Use this list of word components and their meanings to complete the word exercises in this unit.

Prefixes

a-	without
dys-	difficult/painful
endo-	within/inside
macro-	large
ortho-	straight
peri-	around
poly-	many
prostho-	adding (replacement part)

Roots/Combining forms

aden/o	gland
aer/o	air/gas
angi/o	vessel
bronch/o	bronchi/bronchial tree
bucc/o	cheek
dynam/o	force
laryng/o	larynx
lith/o	stone
man/o	pressure
myc/o	fungus
nas/o	nose
pharyng/o	pharynx
trich/o	hair
tympan/o	middle ear/ear drum

Suffixes

-agogue	agent which induces/promotes
-al	pertaining to
-algia	condition of pain
-cele	swelling/protrusion/hernia
-dynia	condition of pain
-eal	pertaining to
-ectomy	removal of
-genic	pertaining to formation/originating in
-gram	X-ray tracing/picture/recording
-graphy	technique of recording/making an X-ray
-ia	condition of
-ic	pertaining to
-ist	specialist
-itis	inflammation of
-logy	study of
-meter	measuring instrument
-metry	process of measuring
-osis	abnormal condition/disease of
-pathy	disease of
-phagia	condition of eating
-phonia	condition of having voice
-phyma	tumour/boil
-plasty	surgical repair/reconstruction
-plegia	condition of paralysis
-rrhagia	condition of bursting forth (of blood)
-rrhaphy	suture/stitch/suturing
-rrhea (Am.)	excessive flow
-rrhoea	excessive flow
-schisis	cleaving/splitting/parting
-scope	viewing instrument
-tomy	incision into
-us	thing/structure/anatomical part

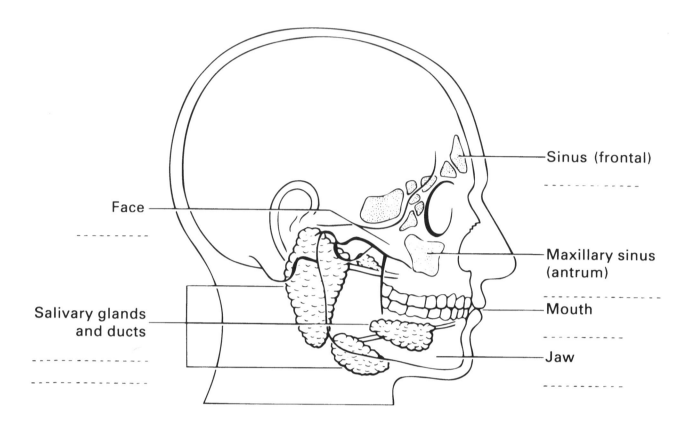

Sinus (frontal)

Face

Maxillary sinus (antrum)

Salivary glands and ducts

Mouth

Jaw

Figure 64   Sagittal section of the head showing sinuses and salivary glands

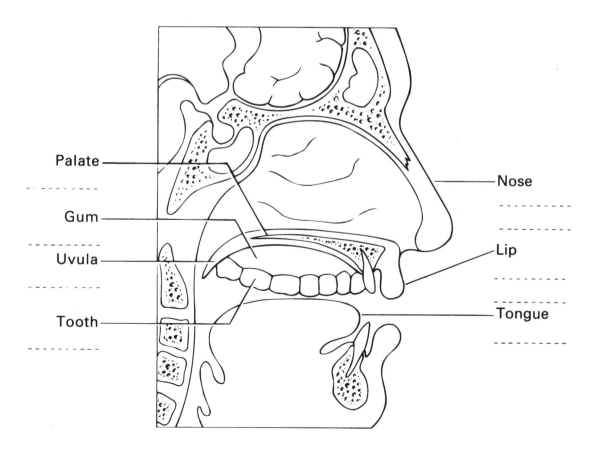

Palate

Nose

Gum

Uvula

Lip

Tooth

Tongue

Figure 65   Sagittal section of the nasal cavity

ANATOMY EXERCISE

When you have finished Word Exercises 1–18, look at the word components listed below. Complete Figures 64 and 65 by writing the appropriate combining form on each dotted line – more than one component may relate to the same position. (You can check their meanings in the Quick Reference box on p. 144.)

Antr/o	Labi/o	Sial/o
Cheil/o	Nas/o	Sin/o
Faci/o	Odont/o	Stomat/o
Gingiv/o	Palat/o	Uvul/o
Gloss/o	Ptyal/o	
Gnath/o	Rhin/o	

The nose and mouth

Receptors for the sense of smell are located in the olfactory epithelium which is in the roof of the nasal cavity. In order for us to smell a substance it must be volatile so it can be carried into the nose and then it must dissolve in the mucus covering the receptors. Humans can distinguish between 2000 and 4000 different odours.

Receptors for taste are located on the taste buds of the tongue. When a substance is eaten, four types of receptor can be stimulated, producing sensations for sweet, bitter, salty and sour. The sense of taste is known as gustation.

In this unit we will look at terms associated with the mouth and nose.

Use the Exercise Guide at the beginning of this unit to complete Word Exercises 1–18 unless you are asked to work without it.

Root	**Stomat** *(From a Greek word **stomatos**, meaning mouth.)*
Combining forms	**Stomat/o**

WORD EXERCISE 1

Using your Exercise Guide, find the meaning of:

(a) **stomato**logy _____

(b) **stomato**rrhagia _____

(c) **stomato**pathy _____

Using your Exercise Guide, build words which mean:

(d) condition of pain in the mouth _____

(e) abnormal condition of fungi in the mouth _____

Root	**Or** *(From a Latin word **oris**, meaning mouth.)*
Combining forms	**Or/o**

WORD EXERCISE 2

Using your Exercise Guide, find the meaning of:

(a) **or**al _____

(b) **oro**pharyngeal _____

(c) **oro**nasal _____

Root	**Gloss** *(From a Greek word **glossa**, meaning tongue.)*
Combining forms	**Gloss/o**

WORD EXERCISE 3

Without using your Exercise Guide, build words which mean:

(a) the study of the tongue _____

(b) condition of pain in the _____
tongue (use -dynia or -algia)

(c) pertaining to the pharynx and _____
tongue (use -eal)

Using your Exercise Guide, find the meaning of:

(d) **glosso**plegia   _____

(e) **glosso**trichia   _____

(f) **glosso**cele   _____

(g) macro**gloss**ia   _____

(h) **glosso**plasty   _____

A Latin combining form **lingu/o** is also used to mean tongue, language or relationship to the tongue, e.g. **lingu**al – pertaining to the tongue, sub**lingu**al – under the tongue.

Disorders of the mouth, tongue, pharynx and palate give rise to problems with eating, swallowing and talking, e.g.

Dysphagia
condition of difficulty in eating (from Greek *phagein* to eat).
Dyslalia
condition of difficulty in talking (from Greek *lalein* to talk).

Root   **Sial**
*(From a Greek word **sialon**, meaning saliva. It is also used to refer to salivary glands and ducts. Three pairs of salivary glands secrete saliva into the mouth. Saliva begins the digestion of starch in food.)*

Combining forms   **Sial/o**

WORD EXERCISE 4

Using your Exercise Guide, find the meaning of:

(a) **sial**adenectomy   _____

(b) **sial**angiography   _____

(c) poly**sial**ia   _____

(d) **sialo**gram   _____

Using your Exercise Guide, build a word which means:

(e) stone in the saliva (duct or gland)   _____

Using your Exercise Guide, find the meaning of:

(f) **sial**agogue   _____
(a drug)

(g) **sial**aerophagia   _____

Root   **Ptyal**
*(From a Greek word **ptyalon**, meaning saliva.)*

Combining forms   **Ptyal/o**

WORD EXERCISE 5

Using your Exercise Guide, find the meaning of:

(a) **ptyalo**genic   _____

(b) **ptyalo**rrhoea   _____
(Am. ptyalorrhea)

Without using your Exercise Guide, write the meaning of:

(c) **ptyalo**lith   _____

Root   **Gnath**
*(From a Greek word **gnathos**, meaning jaw.)*

Combining forms   **Gnath/o, -gnathic**

WORD EXERCISE 6

Without using your Exercise Guide, build words which mean:

(a) condition of pain in the jaw   _____

(b) plastic surgery of the jaw   _____

(c) science dealing with the jaw/   _____
chewing apparatus

(d) pertaining to the jaw and mouth _____

Using your Exercise Guide, find the meaning of:

(e) **gnatho**dynamometer _____

(f) **gnatho**schisis _____
(refers to upper jaw and palate – a cleft palate)

(g) **gnath**itis _____

Root **Cheil**
(From a Greek word **cheilos***,*
meaning lip.)

Combining forms **Cheil/o**

WORD EXERCISE 7

Without using your Exercise Guide, write the meaning of:

(a) **cheilo**stomatoplasty _____

(b) **cheilo**schisis _____

Using your Exercise Guide, find the meaning of:

(c) **cheilo**rrhaphy _____

Without using your Exercise Guide, build a word which means:

(d) inflammation of the lip _____

Root **Labi**
(From a Latin word **labium***, meaning*
lip.)

Combining forms **Labi/o**

WORD EXERCISE 8

Using your Exercise Guide, find the meaning of:

(a) **labio**glossolaryngeal _____

Without using your Exercise Guide, build a word which means:

(b) pertaining to pharynx, _____
tongue and lips

Root **Gingiv**
(From a Latin word **gingiva***, meaning*
gum.)

Combining forms **Gingiv/o**

WORD EXERCISE 9

Without using your Exercise Guide, build words which mean:

(a) inflammation of the gums _____

(b) removal of gum _____
(usually performed for pyorrhoea; Am. pyorrhea)

Without using your Exercise Guide, write the meaning of:

(c) labio**gingiv**al _____

Root **Palat**
(From Latin **palatum***. Here it refers*
to the palate.)

Combining forms **Palat/o**

WORD EXERCISE 10

Without using your Exercise Guide, build words which mean:

(a) condition of paralysis _____
of the soft palate

(b) pertaining to the jaw and _____
palate

(c) split palate _____
(cleft palate)

Root

Uvul
*(From a Latin word **uvula**, meaning grape. It refers to the central tag-like structure extending down from the soft palate, the uvula.)*

Combining forms **Uvul/o**

 WORD EXERCISE 11

Without using your Exercise Guide, build a word which means:

(a) removal of the uvula _____

Without using your Exercise Guide, build a word which means:

(b) incision into the uvula _____

Root

Phas
*(From a Greek word **phasis**, meaning speech.)*

Combining form **-phasia**

 WORD EXERCISE 12

Using your Exercise Guide, find the meaning of:

(a) a**phas**ia _____

(b) dys**phas**ia _____

There are many varieties and causes of aphasia. Common types are:

Motor aphasia
    due to an inability to move muscles involved in speech.

Sensory aphasia
    inability to recognize spoken (or written) words.
(Sometimes the word **aphonia** is used to refer to a loss of voice.)

Root

Odont
*(From a Greek word **odontos**, meaning tooth.)*

Combining forms **Odont/o**

 WORD EXERCISE 13

Without using your Exercise Guide, build words which mean:

(a) scientific study of teeth (dentistry) _____

(b) any disease of teeth _____

(c) condition of toothache (pain) _____

Using your Exercise Guide, find the meaning of:

(d) peri**odont**ics _____
    (includes all tissues supporting teeth)

(e) end**odonto**logy _____
    (includes pulp and roots)

(f) orth**odont**ics _____

(g) orth**odont**ist _____

(h) prosth**odont**ics _____

A prosthesis is any artificial replacement for a body part, in this case the replacement of lost teeth and associated structures.

 Root

Rhin
*(From a Greek word **rhinos**, meaning nose.)*

Combining forms **Rhin/o**

We have already used **rhin/o** when studying the nose and mouth. Here we include some more complex words.

 WORD EXERCISE 14

Using your Exercise Guide, find the meaning of:

(a) **rhino**phonia _____

(b) **rhino**manometry _____

(c) **rhino**phyma _____

Without using your Exercise Guide, write the meaning of:

(d) **rhino**rrhagia _____
(also known as epistaxis)

Root | **Sinus**
(A Latin word meaning hollow/cavity.)

Combining forms **Sin/o, sinus-**

WORD EXERCISE 15

Using your Exercise Guide, find the meaning of:

(a) **sin**us _____

(b) **sino**bronchitis _____

Without using your Exercise Guide, write the meaning of:

(c) **sinus**itis _____
(of the paranasal sinuses)

(d) **sino**gram _____

Root | **Antr**
(From a Greek word **antron**, meaning cave. Here it refers to the superior maxillary sinus, the antrum of Highmore.)

Combining forms **Antr/o**

WORD EXERCISE 16

Using your Exercise Guide, build words which mean:

(a) instrument to view the antrum _____

(b) inflammation of the tympanum and antrum _____

Without using your Exercise Guide, write the meaning of:

(c) **antro**tomy _____
(usually performed to drain out infected fluid)

(d) **antro**nasal _____

(e) **antro**cele _____

Using your Exercise Guide, find the meaning of:

(f) **antro**buccal _____

Root | **Faci**
(From a Latin word **facies**, meaning face.)

Combining forms **Faci/o**

WORD EXERCISE 17

Without using your Exercise Guide, write the meaning of:

(a) **faci**al _____

(b) **facio**plegia _____

(c) **facio**plasty _____

Medical equipment and clinical procedures

Revise the names of all instruments and examinations used in this unit before completing Exercise 18.

WORD EXERCISE 18

Match each term in Column A with a description from Column C by placing an appropriate number in Column B.

Column A	Column B	Column C
(a) antroscope	_____	1. instrument which measures force of jaws
(b) sialangiography	_____	2. technique of recording the tongue (movement in speech)
(c) gnathodyna-mometer	_____	3. instrument for viewing maxillary antrum

Column A	Column B	Column C
(d) rhinomanometer _____		4. an artificial part of the body, e.g. false tooth
(e) prosthesis _____		5. technique of making an X-ray of salivary ducts
(f) glossography _____		6. instrument which measures air pressure in nose

ANATOMY EXERCISE

Now complete the Anatomy Exercise on page 139.

Quick Reference

Medical roots relating to the nose and mouth:

Aden/o	gland
Antr/o	antrum/maxillary sinus
Bucc/o	cheek
Cheil/o	lip
Faci/o	face
Gingiv/o	gum
Gloss/o	tongue
Gnath/o	jaw
Labi/o	lip
Laryng/o	larynx
Lingu/o	tongue
Nas/o	nose
Odont/o	tooth
Or/o	mouth
Palat/o	palate
Phag/o	eating/consuming
Pharyng/o	pharynx
Ptyal/o	saliva
Rhin/o	nose
Sial/o	saliva/salivary glands
Sin/o	sinus
Sinus-	sinus
Stomat/o	mouth
Uvul/o	uvula

Abbreviations

You should learn common abbreviations related to the nose and mouth. Note, however, some are not standard and their meaning may vary from one hospital to another. There is a more extensive list for reference on page 259.

dmft	decayed missing filled teeth (deciduous)
DMFT	decayed missing filled teeth (permanent)
ging	gingiva (gums)
La	labial (lips)
LaG	labia and gingiva (lips and gums)
NAS	nasal
NP	nasopharynx
NPO	non per os/nothing by mouth
odont	odontology
Os	mouth
po/PO	per os/by mouth
Subling	sublingual/under the tongue

   ## NOW TRY THE WORD CHECK

WORD CHECK

This self-check exercise lists all the word components used in this unit. First write down the meaning of as many word components as you can. Then check your answers using the Exercise Guide and Quick Reference box or the Glossary of Word Components (pp. 269–279).

Prefixes

a- _____

dys- _____

endo- _____

macro- _____

ortho- _____

peri- _____

poly- _____

prostho- _____

sub- _____

Combining forms of word roots

aden/o _____

aer/o _____

angi/o _____

antr/o _____

bronch/o _____

bucc/o _____

cheil/o _____

dynam/o _____

faci/o _____

gingiv/o _____

gloss/o _____

gnath/o _____

labi/o _____

laryng/o _____

lingu/o _____

lith/o _____

man/o _____

myc/o _____

nas/o _____

odont/o _____

or/o _____

palat/o _____

phag/o _____

pharyng/o _____

ptyal/o _____

rhin/o _____

sial/o _____

sin/o, sinus- _____

stomat/o _____

trich/o _____

tympan/o _____

uvul/o _____

Suffixes

-agogue _____

-al _____

-algia _____

-cele _____

-dynia _____

-eal _____

-ectomy _____

-genic _____

-gram _____

-graphy _____

-ia _____

-ic _____

-ist _____

-itis _____

-lalia _____

-logy _____

-meter _____

-metry _____

-osis _____

-pathy _____

-phagia _____

-phasia _____

-phonia _____

-phyma _____

-plasty _____

-plegia _____

-rrhagia _____

-rrhaphy _____

-rrhoea
(Am. -rrhea) _____

-schisis _____

-scope _____

-tomy _____

-us _____

> NOW TRY THE SELF-ASSESSMENT

 SELF-ASSESSMENT

Test 12A

Below are some combining forms which refer to the anatomy of the nose and mouth. Indicate which part of the system they refer to by putting a number from the diagrams (Figs 66 and 67) next to each word.

(a) gloss/o _____

(b) stomat/o _____

(c) cheil/o _____

(d) gingiv/o _____

(e) palat/o _____

(f) rhin/o _____

(g) odont/o _____

(h) faci/o _____

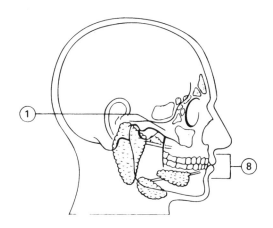

Figure 66 Sagittal section of the head showing sinuses and salivary glands

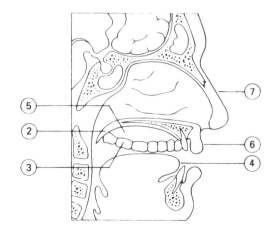

Figure 67 Sagittal section of the nasal cavity

Score

8

Test 12B
Prefixes and suffixes

Match the prefixes and suffixes in Column A with a meaning in Column C by inserting an appropriate number in Column B.

Column A	Column B	Column C
(a) -agogue	_____	1. condition of voice
(b) -cele	_____	2. split
(c) -dynia	_____	3. suturing/ stitching
(d) -ectomy	_____	4. inflammation
(e) endo-	_____	5. condition of speech
(f) -itis	_____	6. condition of paralysis
(g) -logy	_____	7. straight
(h) -metry	_____	8. measurement
(i) ortho-	_____	9. disease
(j) -pathy	_____	10. condition of excessive flow (of blood)
(k) peri-	_____	11. many
(l) -phasia	_____	12. surgical repair
(m) -phonia	_____	13. condition of pain

Column A	Column B		Column C
(n) -plasty	_____	14.	hernia/protrusion/ swelling
(o) -plegia	_____	15.	removal of
(p) poly-	_____	16.	inside/within
(q) prostho-	_____	17.	study of
(r) -rrhagia	_____	18.	around
(s) -rrhaphy	_____	19.	inducing/ stimulating
(t) -schisis	_____	20.	addition of artificial part

Score

20

Test 12C

Combining forms of word roots

Match each combining form in Column A with a meaning in Column C by inserting the appropriate number in Column B.

Column A	Column B		Column C
(a) antr/o	_____	1.	gum
(b) bucc/o	_____	2.	tooth
(c) cheil/o	_____	3.	sinus
(d) dynam/o	_____	4.	pressure (rare)
(e) faci/o	_____	5.	larynx
(f) gingiv/o	_____	6.	uvula
(g) gloss/o	_____	7.	tongue
(h) gnath/o	_____	8.	nose
(i) labi/o	_____	9.	maxillary sinus/antrum of Highmore
(j) laryng/o	_____	10.	hair
(k) man/o	_____	11.	mouth
(l) odont/o	_____	12.	jaw
(m) palat/o	_____	13.	cheek/inside mouth
(n) ptyal/o	_____	14.	palate
(o) rhin/o	_____	15.	lip (i)
(p) sial/o	_____	16.	lip (ii)
(q) sin/o	_____	17.	force

Column A	Column B		Column C
(r) stomat/o	_____	18.	face
(s) trich/o	_____	19.	saliva (i)
(t) uvul/o	_____	20.	saliva (ii)

Score

20

Test 12D

Write the meaning of:

(a) glossodynamometer _____

(b) sialometry _____

(c) stomatoglossitis _____

(d) gnathopalatoschisis _____

(e) odontogenic _____

Score

5

Test 12E

Build words which mean:

(a) incision into a salivary gland (use sial/o) _____

(b) suturing of the palate _____

(c) condition of fungi in nose _____

(d) pertaining to the lips _____

(e) surgical repair of the palate _____

Score

5

Check answers to Self-Assessment Tests on page 254.

13 The muscular system

Objectives

Once you have completed Unit 13 you should be able to:

- understand the meaning of medical words relating to the muscular system

- build medical words relating to the muscular system

- associate medical terms with their anatomical position

- understand medical abbreviations relating to the muscular system.

Exercise Guide

Use this list of word components and their meanings to complete the word exercises in this unit.

Prefixes

dys-	difficult/painful
electro-	electrical
hyper-	above normal/excessive

Roots/Combining forms

aesthesi/o	sensation
cardi/o	heart
esthesi/o (Am.)	sensation
fibr/o	fibre
neur/o	nerve
paed/o	child
ped/o (Am.)	child
phren/o	diaphragm

Suffixes

-al	pertaining to
-algia	condition of pain
-ar	pertaining to
-genic	pertaining to formation/ originating in
-globin	protein
-gram	X-ray/tracing/recording
-graph	usually an instrument that records
-graphy	technique of recording/making an X-ray
-ia	condition of
-ic	pertaining to
-itis	inflammation of
-kymia	condition of involuntary twitching of muscle
-logy	study of
-lysis	breakdown/disintegration
-malacia	condition of softening
-meter	measuring instrument
-oma	tumour/swelling
-osis	abnormal condition/disease/ abnormal increase
-paresis	slight paralysis
-pathy	disease of
-plasty	surgical repair/reconstruction
-rrhaphy	suture/stitch/suturing
-rrhexis	break/rupture
-sclerosis	abnormal condition of hardening
-spasm	involuntary muscle contraction
-tome	cutting instrument
-tomy	incision into
-tonia	condition of tension/tone
-trophy	nourishment/development
-tropic	pertaining to affinity for/ stimulating

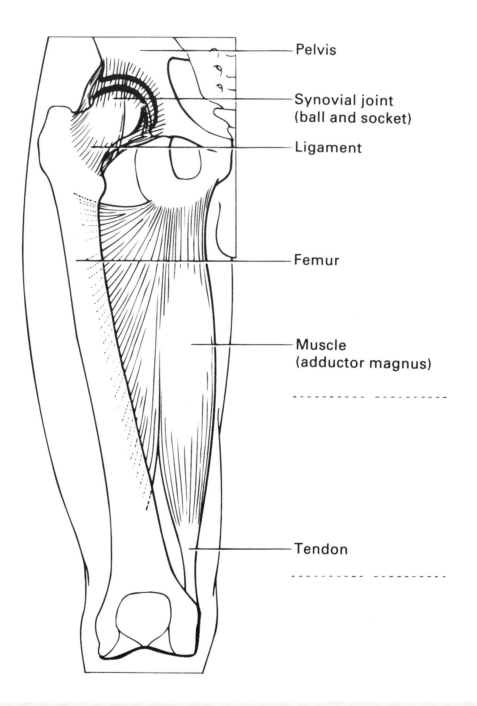

Pelvis

Synovial joint (ball and socket)

Ligament

Femur

Muscle (adductor magnus)

- - - - - - - - - - - - - - - - - -

Tendon

- - - - - - - - - - - - - - - - - -

Figure 68   Muscle arrangement in the thigh

ANATOMY EXERCISE

When you have finished Word Exercises 1–7, look at the word components listed below. Complete Figure 68 by writing the appropriate combining form on each dotted line – more than one component may relate to the same position. (You can check their meanings in the Quick Reference box on p. 153.)

Muscul/o   Tendin/o
My/o   Ten/o

The muscular system

Muscles compose 40–50% of the body's weight. The function of muscle is to effect the movement of the body as a whole and to move internal organs involved in the vital processes required to keep the body alive. There are three types of muscles tissue:

- Skeletal muscle – moves the vocal chords, diaphragm and limbs.
- Cardiac muscle – moves the heart.
- Smooth muscle – moves the internal organs, bringing about movement of food through the intestines and urine through the urinary tract. It is also found in the walls of blood vessels where it acts to maintain blood pressure.

Use the Exercise Guide at the beginning of this unit to complete Word Exercises 1–7 unless you are asked to work without it.

Root	my
	(From a Greek word **myos**, *meaning muscle.)*
Combining forms	**My/o, myos**

WORD EXERCISE 1

Using your Exercise Guide, find the meaning of:

(a) **myo**neural _____

(b) **myo**cardiopathy _____

(c) **myo**dystrophy _____

(d) **myos**itis _____

(e) **myo**fibrosis _____

Using your Exercise Guide, build words using my/o which mean:

(f) abnormal condition of hardening of a muscle _____

(g) tumour of a muscle _____

(h) muscle protein _____

(i) spasm of a muscle _____

The combining form **lei/o** (from Latin, meaning smooth) is added to myo to give **leiomy/o** which refers to smooth muscle. A **leiomy**oma is a tumour/swelling of smooth muscle.

Using your Exercise Guide, find the meaning of:

(j) **myo**kymia _____

(k) **myo**tonia _____

(l) **myo**paresis _____

(m) **myo**rrhexis _____

(n) **myo**malacia _____

The contraction of a muscle can be measured, using an instrument known as a **myo**graph.

Using your Exercise Guide, build words which mean:

(o) the technique of recording muscular contraction _____

(p) the technique of recording the electrical currents generated in muscular contraction _____

(q) trace/recording made by a myograph _____

Root	Rhabd
	(From a Greek word **rhabdos**, *meaning stripe. It is used with* **my/o** *when referring to striped/striated muscle.)*
Combining forms	**Rhabd/o**

WORD EXERCISE 2

Without using your Exercise Guide, write the meaning of:

(a) **rhabdo**myoma _____

Using your Exercise Guide, find the meaning of:

(b) **rhabdo**myolysis _____

Root	Muscul
	(From a Latin word **musculus**, *meaning muscle.)*
Combining forms	**Muscul/o**

WORD EXERCISE 3

Using your Exercise Guide, find the meaning of:

(a) **musculo**tropic _____

(b) **musculo**phrenic _____

Without using your Exercise Guide, write the meaning of:

(c) **muscul**ar dystrophy _____

Root	Kine
	*(From a Greek word **kinein**, meaning movement/motion.)*
Combining forms	**Kine**
	Also derived from this root: **kinesi/o, kines/o, kinet/o**

WORD EXERCISE 4

Using your Exercise Guide, find the meaning of:

(a) **kine**aesthesia _____
   (Am. kinesthesia)

(b) myo**kinesi**meter _____

(c) **kineto**genic _____

(d) hyper**kines**ia _____

Without using your Exercise Guide, build a word using kines/o which means:

(e) condition of difficult/ _____
   painful movement

A Greek word *taxis* is sometimes used when describing an ordered movement in response to a stimulus. **Ataxia** refers to a disordered movement which is irregular and jerky (a- meaning without, i.e. condition of without normal movement). There are many types of ataxia, e.g. motor ataxia – an inability to control muscles; Friedreich's ataxia – an inherited movement disorder.

Root	Ten
	*(From a Greek word **tenontos**, to stretch. It is used to mean tendon.)*
Combining forms	**Ten/o, tenont/o** *(Greek)* **Tend/o, tendon/o, tendin/o** *(Latin)*
	Note that the combining forms **tend/o, tendin/o** *are derived from Latin (**tendonis/tendines**, meaning tendon).*

WORD EXERCISE 5

Using your Exercise Guide, find the meaning of:

(a) **ten**algia _____

(b) **tendo**tome _____

Without using your Exercise Guide, write the meaning of:

(c) **tendin**itis _____

(d) **tenonto**logy _____

Using your Exercise Guide, build words which mean:

(e) repair of a muscle and _____
   tendon (use ten/o)

(f) incision of a muscle and _____
   tendon (use ten/o)

A tendon is a fibrous non-elastic cord of connective tissue which is continuous with the fibres of skeletal muscles. Its function is to attach muscle to bone. Tendons must be strong in tension because they are used to pull bones and thereby move the body. If a tendon is wide and thin it is known as an **aponeurosis**. This word is derived from:

apo-   Greek, meaning away from
neuro-   Greek, meaning tendon (but also used to mean nerve)
-osis   condition of

Several words are used with **aponeur/o**.

Using your Exercise Guide, find the meaning of:

(g) **aponeuro**rrhaphy _____

Without using your Exercise Guide, write the meaning of:

(h) **aponeur**itis   _____

_____

Root	**Orth**
	*(From a Greek word **orthos**, meaning straight.)*
Combining forms	**Orth/o**

WORD EXERCISE 6

Using your Exercise Guide, find the meaning of:

(a) **ortho**paedic   _____
(Am. orthopedic)
(Formerly this word just applied to the correction of deformities in children. It is now a branch of surgery dealing with all conditions affecting the locomotor system.)

Other common words related to this include:

> **Orthosis**
> structures/appliances used to correct deformities.
>
> **Orthotics**
> knowledge or use of orthoses.

Medical equipment and clinical procedures

Revise the names of all instruments and examinations in this unit before completing Exercise 7.

WORD EXERCISE 7

Match each term in Column A with a description in Column C by placing an appropriate number in Column B.

Column A	Column B	Column C
(a) myography	_____	1. appliance used to straighten deformities of the locomotor system
(b) electromyography	_____	2. recording/trace of muscular movement
(c) myogram	_____	3. a recording of the electrical activity of muscle
(d) myokinesiometer	_____	4. technique of recording electrical activity of muscle
(e) orthosis	_____	5. technique of making a recording of muscle (contraction)
(f) electromyogram	_____	6. instrument for measuring movement of muscle

ANATOMY EXERCISE

Now complete the Anatomy Exercise on page 150.

Quick Reference

Medical roots relating to the muscular system:

Aponeur/o	aponeurosis
Fibr/o	fibre
Kinesi/o	movement
Lei/o	smooth (muscle)
Muscul/o	muscle
My/o	muscle
Paed/o	child
Ped/o (Am.)	child
Rhabd/o	striated (muscle)
Tax/o	ordered movement
Tendin/o	tendon
Tend/o	tendon
Ten/o	tendon
Tenont/o	tendon

Abbreviations

You should learn common abbreviations related to the muscular system. Note, however, some are not standard and their meaning may vary from one hospital to another. There is a more extensive list for reference on page 259.

DTR	deep tendon reflex
EMG	electromyogram/electromyography
im	intramuscular
IMHP	intramuscular high potency
MAMC	mid-arm muscle circumference
MAP	muscle action potential
MD	muscular dystrophy
MFT	muscle function test
MNJ	myoneural junction
MS	muscle shortening/strength/ musculoskeletal
Ortho	orthopaedics (Am. orthopedics)
TJ	triceps jerk

NOW TRY THE WORD CHECK

WORD CHECK

This self-check exercise lists all the word components used in this unit. First write down the meaning of as many word components as you can. Then check your answers using the Exercise Guide and Quick Reference box or the Glossary of Word Components (pp. 269–279).

Prefixes

a- _____

dys- _____

electro- _____

hyper- _____

ortho- _____

Combining forms of word roots

aesthesi/o _____
(Am. esthesi/o)

aponeur/o _____

cardi/o _____

fibr/o _____

kinesi/o _____

lei/o _____

muscul/o _____

my/o _____

neur/o _____

paed/o _____
(Am. ped/o)

phren/o _____

rhabd/o _____

tax/o _____

tendin/o _____

tend/o _____

ten/o _____

tenont/o _____

Suffixes

-al _____

-algia _____

-genic _____

-globin _____

-gram _____

-graph _____

-graphy _____

-ic _____

-itis _____

-kymia _____

-logy _____

-lysis _____

-meter _____

-oma _____

-osis _____

-paresis _____

-pathy   _____

-rrhaphy   _____

-rrhexis   _____

-sclerosis _____

-spasm   _____

-taxia   _____

-tome   _____

-tonia   _____

-trophy   _____

-tropic   _____

Column A	Column B	Column C
(k) paed/o (Am. ped/o)	_____	11. condition of continuous slight contraction of muscle
(l) paresis	_____	12. nourishment
(m) phren/o	_____	13. fibre
(n) -rrhexis	_____	14. pertaining to affinity for/ acting on
(o) -sclerosis	_____	15. heart
(p) -spasm	_____	16. muscle (i)
(q) ten/o	_____	17. muscle (ii)
(r) -tonia	_____	18. sensation
(s) -trophy	_____	19. straight
(t) -tropic	_____	20. tendon

Score

20

> NOW TRY THE SELF-ASSESSMENT

SELF-ASSESSMENT

Test 13A

Prefixes, suffixes and combining forms of word roots

Match each word component from Column A with a meaning in Column C by inserting the appropriate number in Column B.

Column A	Column B	Column C
(a) aesthesi/o (Am. esthesi/o)	_____	1. child
(b) cardi/o	_____	2. movement
(c) electro-	_____	3. tumour/swelling
(d) fibr/o	_____	4. diaphragm
(e) -globin	_____	5. slight paralysis/ weakness
(f) kinesi/o	_____	6. rupture/break
(g) muscul/o	_____	7. hardening
(h) my/o	_____	8. electrical
(i) -oma	_____	9. protein
(j) ortho-	_____	10. involuntary contraction of muscle

Test 13B

Write the meaning of:

(a) electromyograph   _____

(b) kinesiology   _____

(c) myotenotomy   _____

(d) myoatrophy   _____

(e) musculoaponeurotic _____

Score

5

Test 13C

Build words which mean:

(a) condition of softening of muscle

(b) pertaining to originating in muscle

(c) disease of muscle

(d) suturing of a tendon (use ten/o)

(e) cutting of a tendon (use ten/o)

Score

5

Check answers to Self-Assessment Tests on page 255.

Objectives

Once you have completed Unit 14 you should be able to:

- understand the meaning of medical words relating to the skeletal system

- build medical words relating to the skeletal system

- associate medical terms with their anatomical position

- understand medical abbreviations relating to the skeletal system.

Exercise Guide

Use this list of word components and their meanings to complete the word exercises in this unit.

Prefixes

dys-	bad/difficult/painful
endo-	within/inside

Roots/Combining forms

calcin/o	calcium
cost/o	rib
fibr/o	fibre
lith/o	stone
petr/o	stone/rock (brittle)
por/o	pore
py/o	pus

Suffixes

-al	pertaining to
-algia	condition of pain
-blast	cell which forms .../immature germ cell
-centesis	puncture to remove fluid
-clasis	breaking
-clast	a cell which breaks
-desis	fixation/bind together by surgery
-ectomy	removal of
-genesis	capable of causing/forming
-genic	pertaining to formation/originating in
-gram	X-ray/tracing/recording
-graphy	technique of recording/making an X-ray
-ic	pertaining to
-itis	inflammation of
-lysis	breakdown/disintegration
-lytic	pertaining to breakdown/disintegration
-malacia	condition of softening
-oid	resembling
-olithesis	slipping
-oma	tumour/swelling
-osis	abnormal condition/disease/abnormal increase
-ous	pertaining to
-pathy	disease of
-phyte	plant/plant-like growth
-plasty	surgical repair/reconstruction
-scope	viewing instrument
-scopy	visual examination
-tome	cutting instrument
-trophy	nourishment/development

Details of synovial joint

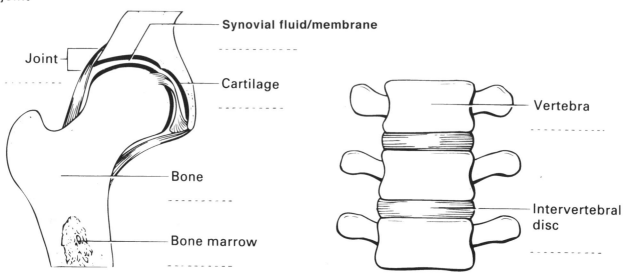

Figure 69 Joints

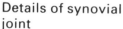

ANATOMY EXERCISE

When you have finished Word Exercises 1–9, look at the word components listed below. Complete Figure 69 by writing the appropriate combining form on each dotted line. (You can check their meanings in the Quick Reference box on p. 163.)

Arthr/o	Myel/o	Spondyl/o
Chondr/o	Oste/o	Synovi/o
Disc/o		

The skeletal system

The supporting structure of the body consisting of 206 bones is known as the skeletal system. This system has five main functions:

- it supports all tissues
- it protects vital organs and soft tissues
- it manufactures blood cells
- it stores minerals, which can be released into the blood
- it assists in movement.

Cartilage is found at the ends of bones and functions to form a smooth surface for the movement of one bone over another, e.g. in a joint. Bones in joints are held together by ligaments which are tough fibrous connective tissues.

Use the Exercise Guide at the beginning of this unit to complete Word Exercises 1–9 unless you are asked to work without it.

Root	**Oste**
	*(From a Greek word **osteon**, meaning bone.)*
Combining forms	**Oste/o**

WORD EXERCISE 1

Using your Exercise Guide, find the meaning of:

(a) **osteo**phyte _____
     (refers to a bony outgrowth at joint surface)

(b) **osteo**porosis _____
     (refers to loss of calcium/phosphorus/bone density)

(c) **osteo**petrosis _____
     (refers to spotty calcification of bone, which becomes brittle)

(d) **osteo**clasis _____

(e) **osteo**clast _____
     (a type of cell, compare with osteoblast)

(f) **osteo**dystrophy _____

Using your Exercise Guide, build words which mean:

(g) a cell which forms bone _____

(h) pertaining to breaking down of bone _____

(i) instrument to cut bone _____

(*Osseus* is a Latin word meaning of bone. It is used in **oss**eous, meaning pertaining to bone, and **oss**ification, meaning to form bone.)

Root	**Arthr**
	(From a Greek word **arthron**, meaning joint or articulation, i.e. the point where two or more bones meet.)
Combining forms	**Arthr/o**

WORD EXERCISE 2

Using your Exercise Guide, find the meaning of:

(a) **arthro**endoscope _____

(b) **arthro**pyosis _____

(c) **arthro**graphy _____

(d) **arthr**itis _____

Rheumatoid arthritis refers to a polyarthritis accompanied by general ill health and varying degrees of crippling joint deformities, pain and stiffness (ankylosis from Greek *agkylos* meaning bent/fusion).

(e) **arthro**desis _____
     (achieved by surgery; Fig. 70)

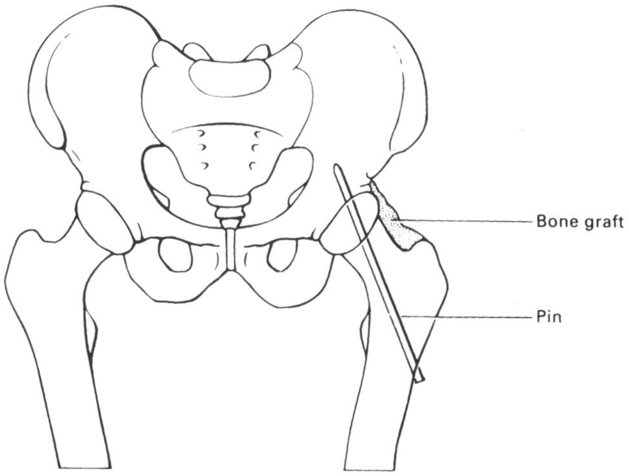

Bone graft

Pin

Figure 70 Arthrodesis of hip

Without using your Exercise Guide, write the meaning of:

(f) **arthro**clasis _____

Using your Exercise Guide, build words which mean:

(g) technique of viewing a joint _____

(h) puncture of a joint _____

(i) X-ray picture of a joint _____

(j) disease of a joint _____

(k) stony material in a joint _____

(l) surgical repair of a joint _____
     (This operation includes the formation of artificial joints, e.g. in a hip replacement where the natural joint is replaced with a metallic prosthesis; Fig. 71.)

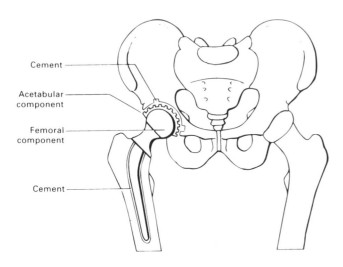

Cement

Acetabular
component

Femoral
component

Cement

Figure 71   Arthroplasty

Root   **Synovi**
*(From a New Latin word **synovia**,
meaning the fluid secreted by the
synovial membrane which lines the
cavity of a joint. Here the combining
form is used to mean synovial
membrane.)*

Combining forms   **Synovi/o**

WORD EXERCISE 3

Without using your Exercise Guide, write the meaning
of:

(a) arthro**synov**itis _____

Using your Exercise Guide, find the meaning of:

(b) **synov**ectomy _____

(c) **synovi**oma _____

Bursae are sacs of synovial fluid surrounded by a synovial membrane. They are found between tendons, ligaments and bones. Inflammation due to pressure, injury
or infection results in **burs**itis (from Latin *bursa*, meaning purse).

Root   **Chondr**
*(From a Greek word **chondros**,
meaning cartilage, the plastic-like
connective tissue found at the ends
of bones, e.g. in joints where it forms
a smooth surface for movement of a
joint.)*

Combining forms   **Chondr/o**

WORD EXERCISE 4

Without using your Exercise Guide, write the meaning
of:

(a) **chondr**ophyte _____
    (actually a cartilaginous growth)

(b) **chondr**osseous _____

(c) **chondr**oporosis _____

(d) **chondr**odystrophy _____

Using your Exercise Guide, find the meaning of:

(e) **Chondr**ocostal _____

(f) endo**chondr**al _____

Using your Exercise Guide, build words which mean:

(g) condition of pain in a _____
    cartilage

(h) condition of softening _____
    of cartilage

(i) formation of cartilage _____

(j) breakdown of cartilage _____

Using your Exercise Guide, find the meaning of:

(k) **chondr**ocalcinosis _____

A cartilage which is often damaged and may be
removed is the crescent-shaped cartilage in the knee
joint. The operation to remove this cartilage is known as
meniscectomy (from Latin *meniscus*, meaning crescent;
combining forms **menisc/o**).

Root   **Spondyl**
*(From Greek word **spondylos**,
meaning vertebra or vertebral
column.)*

Combining forms   **Spondyl/o**

WORD EXERCISE 5

Without using your Exercise Guide, write the meaning of:

(a) **spondyl**algia   _____

(b) **spondylo**pyosis   _____

Without using your Exercise Guide, build words which mean:

(c) breakdown/disintegration   _____
    of vertebrae

(d) any disease of vertebrae   _____

Using your Exercise Guide, find the meaning of:

(e) **spondyl**olithesis   _____
    (this applies to lumbar vertebrae)

Here we need to mention three other conditions of the vertebrae:

Kyphosis
  is an abnormally curved spine (as viewed from the side), commonly called hunch/humpback or dowager's hump. (**Kyph/o** is from Greek *kyphos*, meaning crooked/hump.) See Figure 72A.

Scoliosis
  is a lateral curvature of the vertebral column. (**Scoli/o** is from a Greek word *scoli*, meaning crooked/twisted.) See Figure 72B.

Lordosis
  is a forward curvature of the spine in the lumbar region (from a Greek word meaning to bend the body forward).

Two of these words can be combined as in:

Scoliokyphosis } both meaning lateral and
Kyphoscoliosis } posterior curvature of the spine.

Root   **Disc**
(*From a Latin word* **diskus**, *meaning disc. It refers to pads of connective tissue which act as shock absorbers between vertebrae, i.e. intervertebral discs.*)

Combining forms   **Disc/o. Disk/o** (*Am.*)

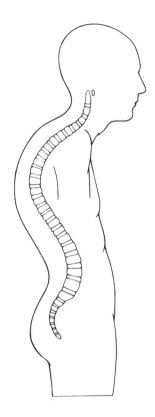

Figure 72   **(a) Kyphosis**

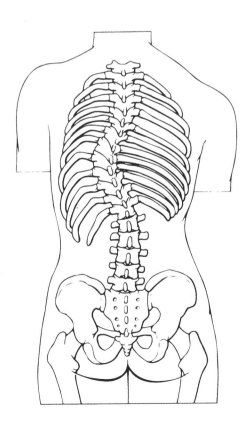

Figure 72   **(b) Scoliosis**

WORD EXERCISE 6

Using your Exercise Guide, find the meaning of:

(a) **disc**oid _____

(b) **disco**genic _____

Without using your Exercise Guide, build words which mean:

(c) technique of making an _____
X-ray of an intervertebral disc

(d) removal of an intervertebral disc _____

The excision of degenerated intervertebral discs requires the removal of a thin layer of bone from the vertebral arch. This operation is termed a **lamin**ectomy (from Latin *lamina*, meaning thin plate; combining forms **lamin/o**).

Root **Myel**
*(From a Greek word **myelos**, meaning marrow. Here we use it to mean the marrow of bones. Remember we have already used this root in reference to the spinal marrow and blood cells of the marrow cavities.)*

Combining forms **Myel/o**

 WORD EXERCISE 7

Without using your Exercise Guide, write the meaning of:

(a) osteo**myel**itis _____

(b) **myelo**fibrosis _____

Medical equipment and clinical procedures

Revise the names of all instruments and clinical procedures used in this unit and then try Exercise 8.

 WORD EXERCISE 8

Match each term in Column A with a description from Column C by placing an appropriate number in Column B.

Column A	Column B	Column C
(a) osteotome	_____	1. puncture of a joint to withdraw synovial fluid
(b) arthrodesis	_____	2. technique of making an X-ray of a joint
(c) replacement arthroplasty	_____	3. fixation of a joint by surgery
(d) arthrocentesis	_____	4. chisel-like instrument used to cut bone
(e) arthrography	_____	5. insertion of a metallic prothesis to replace a joint

The skeleton

There are many terms which refer to specific bones within the skeleton. Look at the diagram (Fig. 73) and then complete Exercise 9.

 WORD EXERCISE 9

Without using your Exercise Guide, build words which mean:

(a) surgical repair/reconstruction _____
of the collar bone

(b) condition of softening of _____
the cranium

(c) pertaining to between the ribs _____

(d) removal of a finger _____

(e) pertaining to the pelvis _____

(f) inflammation of an elbow joint _____

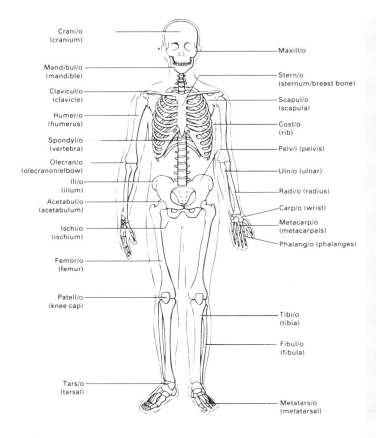

Crani/o (cranium)
Maxill/o
Mandibul/o (mandible)
Stern/o (sternum/breast bone)
Clavicul/o (clavicle)
Scapul/o (scapula)
Humer/o (humerus)
Cost/o (rib)
Spondyl/o (vertebra)
Pelv/i (pelvis)
Olecran/o (olecranon/elbow)
Uln/o (ulnar)
Ili/o (ilium)
Radi/o (radius)
Acetabul/o (acetabulum)
Carp/o (wrist)
Ischi/o (ischium)
Metacarp/o (metacarpals)
Phalang/o (phalanges)
Femor/o (femur)
Patell/o (knee cap)
Tibi/o (tibia)
Fibul/o (fibula)
Tars/o (tarsal)
Metatars/o (metatarsal)

Figure 73 The skeleton

(g) pertaining to the femur and tibia _____

(h) surgical fixation of the scapula   _____

(i) condition of pain in the   _____
     metatarsal region

(j) surgical operation to reconstruct _____
     the hip socket

ANATOMY EXERCISE

Now complete the Anatomy Exercise on page 158.

Quick Reference

Medical roots relating to the skeletal system:

Ankyl/o	fusion/adhesion/bent
Arthro	joint
Burs/o	bursa
Calcin/o	calcium
Chondr/o	cartilage
Cost/o	rib
Disc/o	intervertebral disc
Fibr/o	fibre
Kyph/o	crooked/humped
Lamin/o	lamina/part of vertebral arch
Lord/o	bend forward
Menisc/o	meniscus
Myel/o	bone marrow
Osse/o	bone
Oste/o	bone
Petr/o	stone/rock
Por/o	passage/pore
Scoli/o	crooked/twisted
Spondyl/o	vertebra
Synovi/o	synovial fluid/membrane

Abbreviations

You should learn common abbreviations related to the skeletal system. Note, however, some are not standard and their meaning may vary from one hospital to another. There is a more extensive list for reference on page 259.

BM(T)	bone marrow transplant
C 1–7	cervical vertebrae 1–7
CDH	congenital dislocation of the hip
Fx	fracture
L 1–5	lumbar vertebrae 1–5
OA	osteoarthritis
Osteo	osteomyelitis
PID	prolapsed intervertebral disc
RA	rheumatoid arthritis
RF (RhF)	rheumatoid factor
T 1–12	thoracic vertebrae 1–12
THR	total hip replacement

> ## NOW TRY THE WORD CHECK

WORD CHECK

This self-check exercise lists all the word components used in this unit. First write down the meaning of as many word components as you can. Then check your answers using the Exercise Guide and Quick Reference box or the Glossary of Word Components (pp. 269–279).

Prefixes

dys- _____

endo- _____

inter- _____

Combining forms of word roots

ankyl/o _____

arthro _____

burs/o _____

calcin/o _____

chondr/o _____

cost/o _____

disc/o _____

fibr/o _____

kyph/o _____

lamin/o _____

lith/o _____

lord/o _____

menisc/o _____

myel/o _____

osse/o _____

oste/o _____

petr/o _____

phyt/o _____

por/o _____

py/o _____

scoli/o _____

spondyl/o _____

synovi/o _____

Suffixes

-al _____

-algia _____

-blast _____

-centesis _____

-clasis _____

-clast _____

-desis _____

-ectomy _____

-genesis _____

-genic _____

-gram _____

-graphy _____

-ic _____

-itis _____

-lysis _____

-lytic _____

-malacia _____

-oid _____

-olithesis _____

-oma _____

-osis _____

-pathy _____

-plasty _____

-scope _____

-scopy _____

-tome _____

-trophy _____

Combining forms referring to specific parts of the skeleton

acetabul/o _____

carp/o _____

clavicul/o _____

cost/o _____

crani/o _____

femor/o _____

fibul/o _____

humer/o _____

ili/o _____

ischi/o _____

mandibul/o _____

maxill/o _____

metacarp/o _____

metatars/o _____

olecran/o _____

patell/o _____

pelv/i _____

phalang/o _____

radi/o _____

scapul/o _____

spondyl/o _____

stern/o _____

tars/o _____

tibi/o _____

uln/o _____

> **NOW TRY THE SELF-ASSESSMENT** ◁ |

SELF-ASSESSMENT

Test 14A

Below are some combining forms which refer to the anatomy of the skeletal system and its movement. Indicate which part of the system they refer to by putting a number from the diagram (Fig. 74) next to each word.

(a) synovi/o _____

(b) tendin/o _____

(c) my/o _____

(d) arthr/o _____

(e) oste/o _____

(f) chondr/o _____

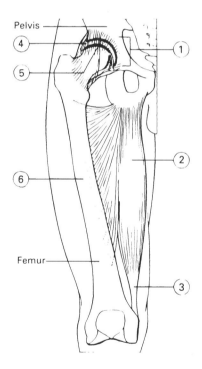

Figure 74 Muscle and skeletal arrangement in the thigh

Score

6

Test 14B
Prefixes and suffixes

Match each prefix or suffix in Column A with a meaning in Column C by inserting the appropriate number in Column B.

	Column A	Column B		Column C
(a)	-al		1.	resembling
(b)	-algia		2.	tumour/swelling
(c)	-blast		3.	slipping/dislocation
(d)	-centesis		4.	condition of pain
(e)	-clast		5.	technique of viewing
(f)	-desis		6.	surgical repair
(g)	dys-		7.	cell which breaks down a matrix
(h)	-genesis		8.	pertaining to destruction/breaking down
(i)	-ic		9.	condition of softening
(j)	inter-		10.	instrument to cut
(k)	-itis		11.	inflammation of
(l)	-lytic		12.	puncture to remove fluid
(m)	-malacia		13.	producing/forming
(n)	-oid		14.	pertaining to (i)
(o)	-olithesis		15.	pertaining to (ii)
(p)	-oma		16.	instrument to view
(q)	-plasty		17.	difficult/painful/bad
(r)	-scope		18.	germ cell
(s)	-scopy		19.	to bind together
(t)	-tome		20.	between

Score

20

Test 14C
Combining forms of word roots

Match each combining form in Column A with a meaning in Column C by inserting the appropriate number in Column B.

	Column A	Column B		Column C
(a)	arthr/o		1.	bone
(b)	burs/o		2.	marrow (of bone)
(c)	calcin/o		3.	synovia/synovial membrane
(d)	chondr/o		4.	pus
(e)	cost/o		5.	joint
(f)	disc/o		6.	vertebrae
(g)	fibr/o		7.	bursa/sac of fluid
(h)	kyph/o		8.	stone/rock
(i)	lamin/o		9.	calcium
(j)	lord/o		10.	meniscus/crescent-shaped
(k)	menisc/o		11.	bend forward
(l)	myel/o		12.	cartilage
(m)	oste/o		13.	crooked
(n)	petr/o		14.	fibre
(o)	phyt/o		15.	hunchback
(p)	por/o		16.	thin plate/lamina of vertebra
(q)	py/o		17.	rib
(r)	scoli/o		18.	passage/pore
(s)	spondyl/o		19.	plant-like growth
(t)	synovi/o		20.	intervertebral disc

Score

20

Test 14D

Write the meaning of:

(a) arthrochondritis   _____

(b) bursolith   _____

(c) spondylodesis   _____

(d) chondroclast   _____

(e) kyphotic   _____

Score

5

Test 14E

Build words which mean:

(a) condition of pain in a joint   _____

(b) inflammation of synovia
and adjacent bones   _____

(c) condition of softening of
vertebrae   _____

(d) disease of joints and bones   _____

(e) germ cell of the synovial
membrane   _____

Score

5

Check answers to Self-Assessment Tests on page 255.

15

The male reproductive system

Objectives

Once you have completed Unit 15 you should be able to:

- understand the meaning of medical words relating to the male reproductive system

- build medical words relating to the male reproductive system

- associate medical terms with their anatomical position

- understand medical abbreviations relating to the male reproductive system.

Exercise Guide

Use this list of word components and their meanings to complete the word exercises in this unit.

Prefixes

a-	without
crypt-	hidden
oligo-	deficiency/few

Roots/Combining forms

cyst/o	bladder
fer/o	to carry
posth/o	prepuce/foreskin

Suffixes

-algia	condition of pain
-cele	swelling/protrusion/hernia
-cide	something that kills/killing
-ectomy	removal of
-genesis	forming/capable of causing
-graphy	technique of recording/making an X-ray
-ia	condition of
-ic	pertaining to
-ism	process of
-itis	inflammation of
-lysis	breakdown/disintegration
-megaly	enlargement
-meter	measuring instrument
-oma	tumour/swelling
-ous	pertaining to
-pathia	condition of disease
-pathy	disease of
-pexy	surgical fixation/fix in place
-plasty	surgical repair/reconstruction
-rrhagia	condition of bursting forth/discharge of blood
-rrhaphy	suture/stitch/suturing
-rrhea (Am.)	excessive flow/discharge
-rrhoea	excessive flow/discharge
-sect(ion)	cut/cutting/excision
-stomy	opening into
-tomy	incision into
-uria	condition of urine

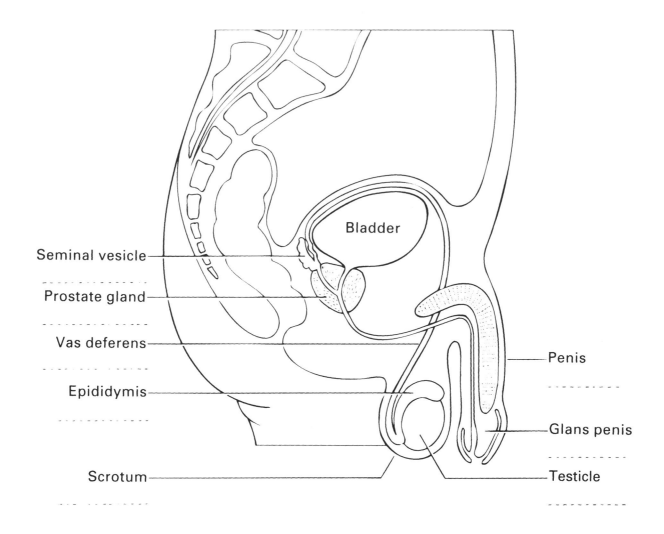

Figure 75 The male reproductive system

 ANATOMY EXERCISE

When you have finished Word Exercises 1–11, look at the word components listed below. Complete Figure 75 by writing the appropriate combining form on each dotted line. (You can check their meanings in the Quick Reference box on p. 175.)

Balan/o	Phall/o	Vas/o
Epididym/o	Prostat/o	Vesicul/o
Orchi/o	Scrot/o	

The male reproductive system

The male possesses paired reproductive organs known as the testes (synonymous with testicles). These are held in position outside the main cavities of the body by a sac known as the scrotum. Each testis produces millions of sperm cells (spermatozoa) which carry the male's genetic information. Once mature, sperms are mixed with glandular secretions to form a liquid known as semen. Semen containing active swimming sperms is ejaculated from the penis during sexual intercourse. Sperms swim along the reproductive tract of the female to the oviducts where they may fuse with an egg in the process of fertilization.

Use the Exercise Guide at the beginning of this unit to complete Word Exercises 1–11 unless you are asked to work without it.

Root	Orch
	(From a Greek word **orchi***, meaning testis (or testicle), i.e. the male reproductive organ which produces spermatozoa.)*
Combining forms	**Orchi/i, orchi/o, orchid/o**

WORD EXERCISE 1

Using your Exercise Guide, find the meaning of:

(a) **orchido**pathy _____

(b) **orchio**cele _____
(synonymous with scrotal hernia/scrotocele)

(c) crypt**orchi**sm _____
(The testes should descend from the abdominal cavity approximately 2 months prior to birth. Failure to do this produces an undescended testis.)

(d) **orchio**pexy (**orchido**pexy) _____

Using your Exercise Guide, build words (using either **orch/i/o** or **orchid/o**) which mean:

(e) incision into a testicle _____

(f) surgical repair of a testicle _____

(g) removal of a testicle _____

(h) condition of pain in a testicle _____

Without using your Exercise Guide, write the meaning of:

(i) crypt**orchido**pexy _____
(synonymous with **orchido**pexy)

Root	Scrot
	(From a Latin word **scrotum***, which refers to the pouch which contains the testicles.)*
Combining forms	**Scrot/o**

WORD EXERCISE 2

Without using your Exercise Guide, build words which mean:

(a) removal of the scrotum _____

(b) plastic surgery/repair of the scrotum _____

(c) hernia/protrusion of the scrotum _____
(synonymous with **orchiocele**)

Two other conditions can result in a swelling of the testis:

> **Hydrocele**
> a swelling/protrusion/hernia due to an accumulation of fluid within the testis.
>
> **Varicocele**
> a swelling/protrusion/hernia of veins of the spermatic cords within the testis (from Latin *varicosus*, meaning varicose vein). Varicoceles need to be removed as they lead to pain and infertility.

Root	Phall
	(From a Greek word **phallos***, meaning the penis or male copulatory organ. It is also the male organ of urination.)*
Combining forms	**Phall/o**

WORD EXERCISE 3

Using your Exercise Guide, build words which mean:

(a) inflammation of the penis _____

(b) pertaining to the penis _____

Without using your Exercise Guide, build a word which means:

(c) removal of the penis _____

Penis is a Latin word referring to the male organ of copulation. **Pen**itis and **pen**ile are synonymous with (a) and (b) above. An abnormally enlarged penis is known as megalo**pen**is or megalo**phall**us.

Several abnormalities of the penis have been noted at birth. The urethra sometimes opens on to the dorsal (upper) surface of the penis. This is known as an **epi-spadia** (*epi-* meaning above, and *-spadia* condition of drawing out). Sometimes the urethra opens on to the posterior (lower) surface. This is a **hypospadia** (condition of drawing out below).

The swelling of the penis during erotic stimulation is known as tumescence (from Latin *tumescere*, meaning to swell). The subsidence of the swelling is known as detumescence (*de* meaning lack of). Once erect the penis can be inserted into the vagina in the act of sex. Words used synonymously with sex include:

Coitus
from Latin *coire*, meaning to come together.

Intercourse
from Latin *intercurrere*, meaning to run between.

Copulation
from Latin *copulare*, meaning to bind together.

The failure to produce an erection and perform the sexual act is known as impotence (from Latin *impotentia*, meaning inability). This condition is often due to psychological problems, but it can arise from lesions within the reproductive tract or nervous system.

Root

Balan
*(From a Greek word **balanos**, meaning acorn. Here it refers to the sensitive, swollen end of the penis, known as the glans penis, which is covered with the prepuce or foreskin.)*

Combining forms **Balan/o**

WORD EXERCISE 4

Without using your Exercise Guide, build a word which means:

(a) inflammation of the glans penis _____

Using your Exercise Guide, find the meaning of:

(b) **balano**rrhagia _____

(c) **balano**posthitis _____

The **prepuce**, or covering foreskin of the glans penis, sometimes needs to be cut, a process known as **preputio**tomy. This is performed to relieve phimosis, a condition in which the foreskin is too tight and cannot retract.

The prepuce is removed in the process of circumcision (i.e. cutting around). This is often performed for religious rather than medical reasons.

Root

Epididym
*(Derived from Greek words **epi** – on, **didymos** – twins/testicles. It refers to a coiled tube, the epididymis, which forms the first part of the duct system of each testis. The epididymes store sperm.)*

Combining forms **Epididym/o**

WORD EXERCISE 5

Without using your Exercise Guide, build words which mean:

(a) inflammation of the epididymis _____

(b) removal of the epididymis _____

Without using your Exercise Guide, write the meaning of:

(c) **epididymo**-orchitis _____

Root

Vas
(A Latin word meaning vessel or duct. Here it is used to mean vas deferens, the main secretory duct of the testis along which mature sperms move towards the penis.)

Combining forms **Vas/o**

WORD EXERCISE 6

Without using your Exercise Guide, write the meaning of:

(a) **vas**ectomy _____

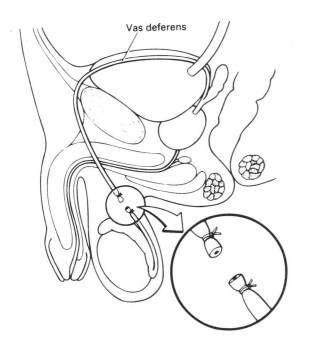

Vas deferens

Figure 76 **Vasectomy**

(This operation (Fig. 76) is performed to sterilize the male, i.e. to make him incapable of reproduction. The cut ends of a section of the vas are tied off. This is known as bilateral ligation (from Latin *ligare*, meaning to bind). Following vasectomy, a reduced volume of semen is produced which contains no sperm.)

Using your Exercise Guide, find the meaning of:

(b) **vaso**epididymostomy _____

(c) **vaso**epididymography _____

(d) **vaso**section _____

(e) **vaso**rrhaphy _____

Without using your Exercise Guide, write the meaning of:

(f) **vaso**-orchidostomy _____

(g) **vasovaso**stomy _____

(h) **vaso**tomy _____

Root **Vesicul**
*(From a Latin word **vesicula**, meaning vesicle/little bladder. Seminal vesicles are pouches lying near the base of the bladder which secrete a nutrient fluid which is a component of semen.)*

Combining forms **Vesicul/o**

WORD EXERCISE 7

Without using your Exercise Guide, build words which mean:

(a) technique of making an X-ray _____
     of the seminal vesicles

(b) incision into a seminal vesicle _____

Without using your Exercise Guide, write the meaning of:

(c) vaso**vesicul**ectomy _____

Root **Prostat**
*(From Greek **prostates**, meaning one who stands before. It is used to refer to the prostate gland surrounding the neck of the bladder and urethra in males. Secretions from the prostate gland are added to the semen during intercourse.)*

Combining forms **Prostat/o**

WORD EXERCISE 8

Using your Exercise Guide, find the meaning of:

(a) **prostato**cystotomy _____

(b) **prostato**megaly _____

Without using your Exercise Guide, write the meaning of:

(c) **prostat**ectomy _____
     (In elderly men there is a progressive enlargement of the prostate (prostatism) and this obstructs the urethra, interfering with the passage of urine. Part or all of the gland can be removed by transurethral resection (TUR) to alleviate this condition (*trans*, meaning across, *resection*, meaning removal/excision). TUR involves inserting an endoscope into the urethra and using it to view and cut out pieces of prostate gland.)

(d) **prostato**vesiculectomy _____

Root **Semin**
*(From a Latin word **seminis**, meaning seed. It now refers to semen, the liquid secretion of the testicles, or to glands associated with the reproductive system.)*

Combining forms **Semin/i**

WORD EXERCISE 9

Using your Exercise Guide, find the meaning of:

(a) **semini**ferous _____
(Spermatozoa flow along seminiferous tubules of the testis.)

(b) **semin**uria _____

(c) **semin**oma _____
(A malignancy of the testis. A change in size and shape of the testes are symptoms of this condition; their size can be measured with an **orchidometer**. When a testis is removed it can be replaced with a prosthesis.)

In**semina**tion refers to the deposition of semen in the female reproductive tract (from Latin *seminare*, meaning to sow).

Artificial insemination (AI) refers to the insertion of semen into the uterus via a cannula (tube) instead of by coitus. The sperm used in this procedure can be from two sources:

• AI by husband (AIH). In this procedure semen from the patient's husband is inseminated into the wife. It is used when there is difficulty in conceiving because of physical and/or psychological problems.
• AI by donor (AID). In this procedure semen from a male other than the female's partner is used. AID is used when the partner is sterile.

Root	**Sperm**
	*(From a Greek word **sperma**, meaning seed. It is used to mean sperm cells or spermatozoa (sing. spermatozoon). Sperm are ejaculated from the male during the peak of sexual excitement known as orgasm.)*
Combining forms	**Sperm/o, spermat/o** *Also* **sperm/i** *(from New Latin* **spermium**).

WORD EXERCISE 10

Using your Exercise Guide, find the meaning of:

(a) a**sperm**ia _____

(b) oligo**sperm**ia _____

(c) **spermi**cide _____
(often used in conjunction with condoms and other contraceptives)

Using your Exercise Guide, build words using spermat/o which mean:

(d) condition of disease/ _____
abnormality of sperms

(e) formation of sperms _____

(f) breakdown/disintegration _____
of sperms

(g) flow of sperm _____
(abnormal, without orgasm)

Sperm counts are performed to estimate the number of sperms, the percentage of abnormal sperms and their mobility. The actual number of sperms is important in determining the fertility of the male. A sperm count of less than 60 million sperms per cm^3 of semen results in decreased fertility, even though only one sperm is required to fertilize an egg!

Semen containing sperms can be preserved at very low temperatures in a cryostat. The frozen sperm remain capable of fertilizing eggs and they are used for artificial insemination.

Recently it has become possible to use sperm to fertilize eggs outside the body in laboratory glassware, a process known as in vitro fertilization (*vitro* meaning glass).

Medical equipment and clinical procedures

Revise the names of all instruments and procedures mentioned in this unit and then try Exercise 11.

WORD EXERCISE 11

Match each term in Column A with a description from Column C by placing an appropriate number in Column B.

Column A	Column B	Column C
(a) sperm count	_____	1. fusion of an egg and sperm in laboratory glassware

Column A	Column B	Column C
(b) transurethral resection	_____	2. material used to tie a cut vas
(c) vasectomy	_____	3. instrument to measure the size of a testicle
(d) orchidometer	_____	4. cutting of prostate through the urethra
(e) in vitro fertilization	_____	5. estimate of numbers of spermatozoa in 1 cm³ semen
(f) vasoligature	_____	6. the cutting and removal of a section of the sperm duct

ANATOMY EXERCISE

Now complete the Anatomy Exercise on page 170.

Abbreviations

You should learn common abbreviations related to the male reproductive system. Note, however, some are not standard and their meaning may vary from one hospital to another. There is a more extensive list for reference on page 259.

AI	artificial insemination
AID	artificial insemination by donor
ICSH	interstitial cell stimulating hormone
pros	prostate
PSA	prostate specific antigen
SPP	suprapubic prostatectomy
STD	sexually transmitted disease
Syph	syphilis
TUR	transurethral resection
TURP	transurethral resection of prostate
VD	venereal disease
WR	Wasserman reaction test for syphilis

> NOW TRY THE WORD CHECK

Quick Reference

Medical roots relating to the male reproductive system:

Balan/o	glans penis
Cyst/o	bladder
Epididym/o	epididymis
Orchi/o	testis
Phall/o	penis
Posth/o	prepuce/foreskin
Prostat/o	prostate
Scrot/o	scrotum
Semin/i	semen/testis
Sperm/i	spermatozoa/sperm
Varic/o	varicose vein
Vas/o	vas deferens/vessel
Vesicul/o	seminal vesicle

 ## WORD CHECK

This self-check exercise lists all the word components used in this unit. First write down the meaning of as many word components as you can. Then check your answers using the Exercise Guide and Quick Reference box or the Glossary of Word Components (pp. 269–279).

Prefixes

a-   _____

crypt-   _____

epi-   _____

hypo-   _____

oligo-   _____

trans-   _____

Combining forms of word roots

balan/o _____

cyst/o _____

epididym/o _____

fer/o _____

hydr/o _____

megal/o _____

orchi/o _____

phall/o _____

posth/o _____

prostat/o _____

scrot/o _____

semin/i _____

sperm/i _____

varic/o _____

vas/o _____

vesicul/o _____

Suffixes

-algia _____

-cele _____

-cide _____

-ectomy _____

-genesis _____

-graphy _____

-ia _____

-ic _____

-ism _____

-itis _____

-ligation _____

-lysis _____

-oma _____

-ous _____

-pathia _____

-pexy _____

-plasty _____

-rrhagia _____

-rrhaphy _____

-rrhoea
(Am. -rrhea) _____

-sect(ion) _____

-spadia _____

-stomy _____

-tomy _____

-uria _____

> **NOW TRY THE SELF-ASSESSMENT**

SELF-ASSESSMENT

Test 15A

Below are some combining forms which refer to the anatomy of the male reproductive system. Indicate which part of the system they refer to by putting a number from the diagram (Fig. 77) next to each word.

(a) scrot/o _____

(b) orchid/o _____

(c) phall/o _____

(d) balan/o _____

(e) vas/o _____

(f) prostat/o _____

(g) vesicul/o _____

(h) epididym/o _____

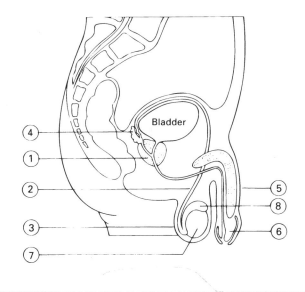

Bladder

Figure 77 The male reproductive system

Score

8

Test 15B
Prefixes and suffixes

Match each prefix or suffix in Column A with a meaning in Column C by inserting the appropriate number in Column B.

Column A	Column B	Column C
(a) -cele	_____	1. fixation
(b) -cide	_____	2. condition of drawing out
(c) crypt-	_____	3. hidden
(d) epi-	_____	4. condition of urine/urination
(e) -genesis	_____	5. opening into
(f) -ia	_____	6. across
(g) -ic	_____	7. back
(h) -ism	_____	8. suturing
(i) oligo-	_____	9. on/above/upon
(j) -ous	_____	10. bursting forth (of blood)
(k) -pexy	_____	11. pertaining to (i)
(l) re-	_____	12. pertaining to (ii)
(m) -rrhagia	_____	13. process of
(n) -rrhaphy	_____	14. excessive flow/discharge

Column A	Column B	Column C
(o) -rrhoea (Am. -rrhea)	_____	15. producing/ forming
(p) -sect	_____	16. hernia/ protrusion/ swelling
(q) -spadia	_____	17. condition of
(r) -stomy	_____	18. to kill
(s) trans-	_____	19. cut
(t) -uria	_____	20. little/scanty/few

Score

20

Test 15C
Combining forms of word roots

Match each combining form in Column A with a meaning in Column C by inserting the appropriate number in Column B.

Column A	Column B	Column C
(a) balan/o	_____	1. to carry
(b) cyst/o	_____	2. testis
(c) epididym/o	_____	3. penis
(d) fer/o	_____	4. glans penis
(e) hydr/o	_____	5. prostate gland
(f) megal/o	_____	6. prepuce
(g) orchid/o	_____	7. semen
(h) phall/o	_____	8. epididymis
(i) posth/o	_____	9. varicose vein
(j) prostat/o	_____	10. vessel
(k) scrot/o	_____	11. vesicle (seminal)
(l) semin/i	_____	12. water
(m) varic/o	_____	13. scrotum
(n) vas/o	_____	14. bladder
(o) vesicul/o	_____	15. abnormal enlargement

Score

15

Test 15D

Write the meaning of:

(a) orchidoepididymectomy   _____

(b) phallorrhoea   _____
    (Am. phallorrhea)

(c) epididymovasectomy   _____

(d) vasoligation   _____

(e) spermaturia   _____

Score

5

Test 15E

Build words which mean:

(a) stitching/suturing of the testis   _____

(b) condition of pain in the prostate   _____

(c) formation of an opening between   _____
    the vas and epididymis

(d) inflammation of the scrotum   _____

(e) excessive flow/discharge from   _____
    the prostate

Score

5

Check answers to Self-Assessment Tests on page 255.

16 The female reproductive system

Objectives

Once you have completed Unit 16 you should be able to:

- understand the meaning of medical words relating to the female reproductive system

- build medical words relating to the female reproductive system

- associate medical terms with their anatomical position

- understand medical abbreviations relating to the female reproductive system.

Exercise Guide

Use this list of word components and their meanings to complete the word exercises in this unit.

Prefixes

a-	without
ante-	before
dys-	difficult/painful
endo-	within/inside
eu-	good
micro-	small
multi-	many
neo-	new
nulli-	none
oligo-	deficiency/little/few
peri-	around
pre-	before/in front of
primi-	first
pro-	before
secundi-	second

Roots/ Combining forms

cyst/o	bladder (cyst)
cyt/e	cell
fer/o	to carry
haem/o	blood
hem/o (Am.)	blood
myc/o	fungus
perine/o	perineum
periton/e/o	peritoneum
phleb/o	vein
placent/o	placenta
rect/o	rectum
trachel/o	neck
vesic/o	bladder

Suffixes

-agogue	agent which induces/promotes
-al	pertaining to
-algia	condition of pain
-arche	beginning
-blast	cell which forms .../immature germ cell
-cele	swelling/protrusion/hernia
-centesis	puncture
-dynia	condition of pain
-ectomy	removal of
-fuge	agent that suppresses/removes
-genesis	formation of
-genic	pertaining to formation
-gram	X-ray/tracing/recording
-graphy	making an X-ray/technique of recording
-ia	condition of
-ic	pertaining to
-ischia	condition of reducing/holding back
-itis	inflammation of
-lithiasis	abnormal condition of stones
-logy	study of
-malacia	condition of softening
-meter	measuring instrument
-metry	process of measuring
-oma	tumour/swelling
-osis	abnormal condition/disease of
-ous	pertaining to
-pathia	condition of disease
-pathy	disease of
-pause	stopping
-pexy	surgical fixation/fix in place
-plasty	surgical repair/reconstruction
-poiesis	formation
-ptosis	falling/displacement/prolapse
-rrhagic	pertaining to bursting forth (of blood)
-rrhaphy	suturing/stitching
-rrhexis	breaking/rupturing
-rrhea (Am.)	excessive discharge/flow
-rrhoea	excessive discharge/flow
-sclerosis	abnormal condition of hardening
-scope	viewing instrument
-scopy	visual examination/technique of viewing
-staxis	dripping
-stenosis	abnormal condition of narrowing
-stomy	formation of an opening/an opening
-tome	cutting instrument
-tomy	incision into
-toxic	pertaining to poisoning
-trophin	hormone that stimulates/nourishes
-tropic	pertaining to stimulating/affinity for
-tubal	pertaining to a tube

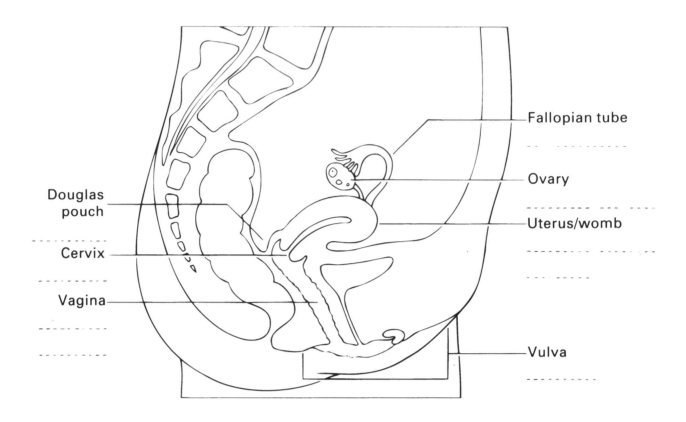

Figure 78 Section through female

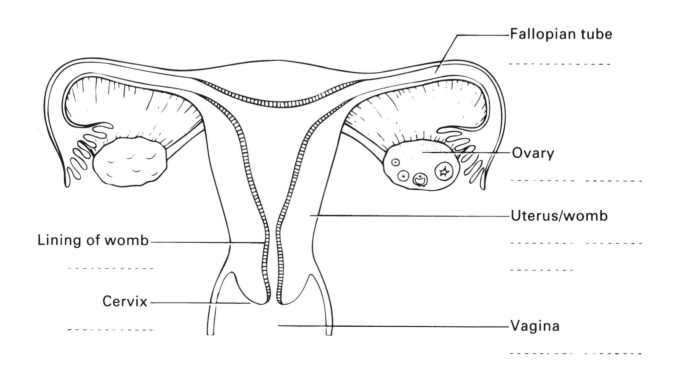

Figure 79 The female reproductive system

ANATOMY EXERCISE

When you have finished Word Exercises 1–14, look at the word components listed below. Complete Figures 78 and 79 by writing the appropriate combining form on each dotted line – more than one component may relate to the same position. (You can check their meanings in the Quick Reference box on p. 192.)

Cervic/o

Colp/o

Culd/o

Endometri/o

Hyster/o

Metr/o

Oophor/o

Ovari/o

Salping/o

Uter/o

Vagin/o

Vulv/o

The female reproductive system

The female possesses paired reproductive organs known as ovaries; these are located in the upper pelvic cavity on either side of the uterus. The function of the ovaries is to produce reproductive cells known as ova (eggs). The ovaries pass through a regular ovarian cycle in which one egg is released (ovulation) every 28 days. The egg passes into the oviduct where it may be fertilized by sperms ejaculated into the female reproductive tract by the male. Should an egg be fertilized, it will divide and grow into a new individual after implanting into the uterus. If the egg is not fertilized, it will disintegrate and may pass out of the body at menstruation.

Use the Exercise Guide at the beginning of this unit to complete Word Exercises 1–26 unless you are asked to work without it.

Root **Oo**
*(From a Greek word **oon** meaning egg.)*

Combining form **Oo-**

WORD EXERCISE 1

Using your Exercise Guide, find the meaning of:

(a) **oo**blast _____

(b) **oo**cyte _____

(c) **oo**genesis _____

Root **Oophor**
*(From a Greek word **oophoron**, derived from oion – egg, pherein – to bear. We use it to mean ovary, the egg-bearing gland.)*

Combining forms **Oophor/o**

WORD EXERCISE 2

Using your Exercise Guide, build words which mean:

(a) removal of an ovary _____

(b) fixation of an ovary _____

(c) incision of an ovary _____

Using your Exercise Guide, find the meaning of:

(d) **oophoro**cystectomy _____
(Cyst refers to an ovarian cyst, a bladder-like growth in the ovary.)

(e) **oophoro**stomy _____

Root **Ovari**
*(From a New Latin word **ovarium**, meaning ovary, derived from **ova**, meaning egg.)*

Combining forms **Ovari/o**

WORD EXERCISE 3

Without using your Exercise Guide, build words which mean:

(a) removal of an ovary   _____
(synonymous with oophorectomy)

(b) incision into an ovary   _____
(often used to mean the removal of an ovarian cyst)

Using your Exercise Guide, find the meaning of:

(c) **ovario**rrhexis   _____

(d) **ovario**tubal   _____
(The tube refers to an oviduct.)

(e) **ovario**centesis   _____

Approximately every 28 days an egg (or ovum) is released from one of the ovaries. This process is known as ovulation. Once released, the egg is picked up by the oviduct and it moves towards the uterus. An ovary which fails to release an egg is described as anovular (i.e. without eggs).

> **Root**
>
> **Salping**
> *(From Greek **salpingos**, meaning trumpet tube. Here it refers to the trumpet-shaped oviduct or Fallopian tube. This tube collects eggs ovulated from the ovary and passes them to the uterus.)*
>
> *Combining forms*   **Salping/o**

WORD EXERCISE 4

Without using your Exercise Guide, write the meaning of:

(a) **salpingo**-oophorectomy   _____

(b) ovario**salping**ectomy   _____

(c) **salpingo**pexy   _____

Using your Exercise Guide, find the meaning of:

(d) **salpingo**cele   _____

(e) **salpingo**-oophoritis   _____

Using your Exercise Guide, build words which mean:

(f) technique of making an   _____
X-ray of the oviduct
(follows an injection of
opaque dye)

(g) abnormal condition of   _____
calcareous stones/deposits
in oviduct

(h) surgical repair of the   _____
oviduct

> **Root**
>
> **Uter**
> *(From a Latin word **uterus**, meaning womb, the chamber in which a fertilized egg grows into a fetus and a baby.)*
>
> *Combining forms*   **Uter/o**

WORD EXERCISE 5

Using your Exercise Guide, build words which mean:

(a) condition of pain in the uterus   _____

(b) hardening of the uterus   _____

Without using your Exercise Guide, write the meaning of:

(c) **utero**tubal   _____

(d) **utero**salpingography   _____

Using your Exercise Guide, find the meaning of:

(e) **utero**vesical   _____

(f) **utero**rectal   _____

(g) **utero**placental   _____
(The placenta is a disc-shaped structure which attaches the fetus to the lining of the uterus.)

A common disorder of the uterus is the presence of uterine fibroids, which are benign tumours of dense fibrous tissue and muscle. They are removed by **fibroidectomy/myomectomy**. (**Myom** is from *myoma*, meaning muscle tumour.)

Root   **Hyster**
*(From Greek word **hystera**, meaning womb, i.e. uterus.)*

Combining forms   **Hyster/o**

WORD EXERCISE 6

Using your Exercise Guide, build words which mean:

(a) instrument to view the womb   _____

(b) abnormal condition of   _____
falling/displaced womb
(also known as a prolapse)

(c) X-ray picture of the womb   _____

Without using your Exercise Guide, write the meaning of:

(d) **hystero**salpingography   _____

(e) **hystero**salpingostomy   _____

(f) **hystero**salpingo-oophorectomy   _____

Using your Exercise Guide, find the meaning of:

(g) **hystero**trachelorrhaphy   _____

(h) **hystero**trachelotomy   _____

Root   **Metr**
*(From a Greek word **metra**, meaning womb.)*

Combining forms   **Metr/a, metr/o**

 ## WORD EXERCISE 7

Using your Exercise Guide, find the meaning of:

(a) **metro**staxis   _____

(b) **metro**pathia haemorrhagica   _____
(Am. metropathia
hemorrhagica)

(c) **metro**peritonitis   _____

(d) **metro**phlebitis   _____

(e) **metro**cystosis   _____

(f) **metro**ptosis   _____

Using your Exercise Guide, build words which mean:

(g) condition of narrowed womb   _____

(h) condition of softening of uterus   _____

The endometrium (meaning part within the womb) refers to the lining of the mucosa of the uterus. The endometrium grows during the 28-day menstrual cycle and disintegrates when it ends, producing the menstrual flow.

Using your Exercise Guide, find the meaning of:

(i) endo**metr**itis   _____

(j) endo**metr**ioma   _____

Without using your Exercise Guide, write the meaning of:

(k) endo**metr**iosis   _____
(refers to the endometrial tissue in abnormal locations)

 Root   **Men**
*(From a Latin word **mensis**, meaning month. It refers to menstruation, that is, monthly bleeding from the womb. The bleeding arises from the disintegration of the endometrium.)*

Combining forms   **Men/o**

WORD EXERCISE 8

Without using your Exercise Guide, write the meaning of:

(a) **men**ostaxis   _____

Using your Exercise Guide, find the meaning of:

(b) **men**arche   _____

(c) **men**opause   _____

(d) a**men**orrhoea   _____
(Am. amenorrhea)

(e) dys**menor**rhoea   _____
     (Am. dysmenorrhea)

(f) oligo**menor**rhoea   _____
     (Am. oligomenorrhea)

(g) pre**men**strual   _____

Curettage of the lining of the uterus

This is a surgical procedure in which the uterus is scraped with a curette, a surgical instrument with a curved spoon-like tip. The curette is designed for scraping tissue for diagnostic or therapeutic reasons. Dilatation and curettage first dilates the uterus and then scrapes it. It is often used to remove an incomplete abortion.

Root	**Cervic**
	*(From a Latin word **cervix**, meaning the neck of the uterus, the cervix uteri.)*
Combining forms	**Cervic/o**

WORD EXERCISE 9

Without using your Exercise Guide, build words which mean:

(a) inflammation of the cervix   _____

(b) removal of the cervix   _____

Adult women are advised to have periodic cervical smears. This procedure involves taking a sample of cells from the cervix and subjecting them to cytological examination (Pap test, named after cytologist G. Papanicolaou). Neoplastic cells can be removed in their early stages of growth, thereby preventing cervical cancer. The risk of developing cervical cancer is related to the number of sexual partners and may be the result of transmission of a virus.

Root	**Colp**
	*(From a Greek word **colpos**, meaning hollow. It is now used to mean vagina, a hollow chamber which receives the penis during copulation and through which a baby will pass at birth.)*
Combining forms	**Colp/o**

WORD EXERCISE 10

Using your Exercise Guide, find the meaning of:

(a) **colpo**scopy   _____

(b) **colpo**microscope   _____
     (used in situ, i.e. to examine the vagina directly)

Without using your Exercise Guide, write the meaning of:

(c) **colpo**gram   _____

(d) **colpo**perineorrhaphy   _____

The perineum is the region between the thighs bounded by the anus and vulva in the female. Perineotomy is used synonymously with episiotomy (*episi* – meaning pubic region). This incision is made during the birth of a child when the vaginal orifice does not stretch sufficiently to allow an easy birth.

(e) **colpo**hysterectomy   _____

(f) metro**colpo**cele   _____

(g) cervico**colp**itis   _____

Without using your Exercise Guide, build words which mean:

(h) surgical repair of the   _____
     perineum and vagina

(i) surgical fixation of the vagina   _____

Root	**Vagin**
	*(From a Latin word **vagina**, meaning sheath. It refers to the vagina, the musculo-membranous passage extending from the cervix uteri to the vulva. Synonymous with **colpos**.)*
Combining forms	**Vagin/o**

WORD EXERCISE 11

Without using your Exercise Guide, write the meaning of:

(a) **vagino**perineotomy   _____

(b) **vagino**perineorrhaphy   _____

(c) **vagino**vesical   _____

Using your Exercise Guide, build words which mean:

(d) abnormal condition of fungal   _____
infection of the vagina

(e) disease of the vagina   _____

Investigations of disorders of the vagina and cervix usually require the use of a vaginal speculum to hold the walls of the vagina apart. There are many types of vaginal specula, one of which is shown in Figure 80.

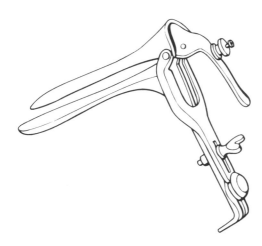

Figure 80   Vaginal speculum

Two small glands situated on either side of the external orifice of the vagina are known as **Bartholin's glands**. These produce mucus which lubricates the vagina. Sometimes these glands become inflamed, a condition known as **bartholin**itis (after C. Bartholin, a Danish anatomist).

Root	**Vulv**
	*(From a Latin word **vulva**, meaning womb. It is used to mean vulva, pudendum femina or external genitalia.)*

Combining forms   **Vulv/o**

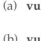

WORD EXERCISE 12

Without using your Exercise Guide, write the meaning of:

(a) **vulvo**vaginitis   _____

(b) **vulvo**vaginoplasty   _____

Root	**Culd**
	*(From a French word **cul-de-sac**, meaning bottom of the bag or sack. Here it is used to mean the blindly ending Douglas cavity or rectouterine pouch, which lies above the posterior vaginal fornix.)*

Combining forms   **Culd/o**

WORD EXERCISE 13

Without using your Exercise Guide, write the meaning of:

(a) **culdo**scope   _____
(This allows examination of the uterus, oviducts, ovaries and peritoneal cavity; Fig. 81)

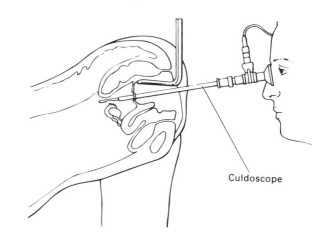

Culdoscope

Figure 81   Culdoscopy

(b) **culdo**scopy   _____

(c) **culdo**centesis   _____

Root | **Gynaec**
(From a Greek word **gyne***, meaning woman.)*

Combining forms **Gynaec/o**
Gynec/o *(Am.)*

WORD EXERCISE 14

Using your Exercise Guide, find the meaning of:

(a) **gynaeco**logy _____
(Am. gynecology; refers to diseases peculiar to women, i.e. of the female reproductive tract)

(b) **gynaeco**genic _____
(Am. gynecogenic)

ANATOMY EXERCISE

Now complete the Anatomy Exercise on page 181.

Abbreviations

You should learn common abbreviations related to the female reproductive system. Note, however, some are not standard and their meaning may vary from one hospital to another. There is a more extensive list for reference on page 259.

D & C	dilatation and curettage
DUB	dysfunctional uterine bleeding
Gyn	gynaecology (Am. gynecology)
in utero	within the uterus
IUCD	intrauterine contraceptive device
IUFB	intrauterine foreign body
LMP	last menstrual period
Pap	Papanicolaou smear test
PMB	post-menopausal bleeding
PMS	premenstrual syndrome
PV	per vagina
VE	vaginal examination

Terms relating to pregnancy, birth and lactation

After approximately 9 months (**the period of gestation**) a baby is expelled from the mother's body by muscular contractions of the uterus. The onset of uterine contractions is termed labour (or **parturition**). The period immediately following birth is known as the **puerperium**, at which time the reproductive organs tend to revert to their original state. The terms **antepartum** and **postpartum** are also used to indicate the periods before and after birth. **Ante** is usually used to mean up to 3 months before birth.

Occasionally, fertilized eggs can grow outside the uterus (extrauterine). These are known as **ectopic** pregnancies. The most common ectopic site is the Fallopian tube. Rupture of this by a pregnancy constitutes a surgical emergency.

The successful entry of a sperm into an egg at fertilization is known as **conception**. In this process a new individual is created. To complete its development, the conceptus must be implanted into the endometrium of the uterus. This event initiates **pregnancy**.

Following the implantation of the fertilized egg, a structure known as the **placenta** develops (from Latin meaning cake). This is a vascular structure, developed about the third month of pregnancy and attached to the wall of the uterus. Through the placenta the fetus is supplied with oxygen and nutrients and wastes are removed. The placenta is expelled as the afterbirth, usually within 1 hour of birth.

Root | **Gravida**
(A Latin word meaning heavy or pregnant. It is used to describe a woman in relation to her pregnancies.)

Combining form **-gravida**

WORD EXERCISE 15

Using your Exercise Guide, find the meaning of:

(a) primi**gravida** _____
(gravida I)

(b) secundi**gravida** _____
(gravida II)

(c) multi**gravida** _____
(more than twice)

(d) nulli**gravida** _____

Root | **Para**
(From a Latin word **parere**, meaning to bear/bring forth. It is used to refer to a woman and the number of her previous pregnancies.)

Combining form | **-para**

WORD EXERCISE 16

Without using your Exercise Guide, write the meaning of:

(a) primi**para** _____
(Primipara can be used synonymously with uni-para (_uni_ – one).)

(b) secundi**para** _____

(c) multi**para** _____

(d) nulli**para** _____

Another word which refers to pregnancy is **cyesis** (from Greek _kyesis_, meaning conception). **Pseudocyesis** refers to a false pregnancy, i.e. signs and symptoms of early pregnancy, a result of an overwhelming desire to have a child.

Root | **Fet**
(From a Latin word **fetus**, i.e. an unborn baby. A human embryo becomes a fetus 8 weeks after fertilization, i.e. when the organ systems have been laid down.)

Combining forms | **Fet/o**

Note. Foetus is an alternative spelling of fetus. Once the usual spelling in British English, it is becoming less common.

WORD EXERCISE 17

Without using your Exercise Guide, write the meaning of:

(a) **feto**logy _____

(b) **feto**scope _____

(c) **feto**placental _____

Using your Exercise Guide, build words which mean:

(d) pertaining to poisoning _____
of the fetus

(e) measurement of the fetus _____

The part of the fetus which lies in the lower part of the uterus is known as the presenting part. In a normal birth the vertex of the skull forms the presenting part and it enters the birth canal first. If other parts enter first, e.g. the buttocks, they are known as **malpresentations**.

Various manoeuvres can be made to turn or change the position of the fetus in the uterus. The term **version** (from Latin _vertere_, meaning to turn) is used for these manoeuvres. Many types have been described, e.g.:

Cephalic version
changes the position of the fetus from breech (buttocks first) to cephalic (head first) towards the birth canal.

External version
changes the position of the fetus by manipulation through the abdominal wall.

Internal version
changes the position of the fetus by hand within the uterus.

Root | **Amni**
(From a Greek word **amnia**, meaning the bowl in which blood was caught. It is now used to mean the fetal membrane which retains the amniotic fluid surrounding a developing fetus.)

Combining forms | **Amni/o**

WORD EXERCISE 18

Using your Exercise Guide, find the meaning of:

(a) **amnio**tome _____

Without using your Exercise Guide, build words which mean:

(b) technique of cutting the amnion _____

(c) an instrument to visually _____
    examine the amnion
    (see Fig. 82)

Without using your Exercise Guide, write the meaning of:

(d) **amnio**graphy _____

(e) **amnio**gram _____

(f) feto**amnio**tic _____

(g) **amnio**centesis _____

Figure 82 shows the developing amnion and Figure 83 the position of the needle used to withdraw amniotic fluid during amniocentesis.

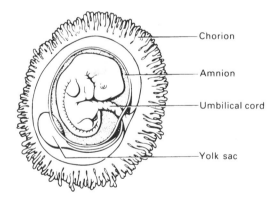

Figure 82 Amnion and related structures (showing 5-week embryo)

This procedure is used to remove amniotic fluid for analysis, to inject solutions that will induce abortion or infuse dyes for radiographic studies. Various fetal abnormalities can be detected by analysing the amniotic

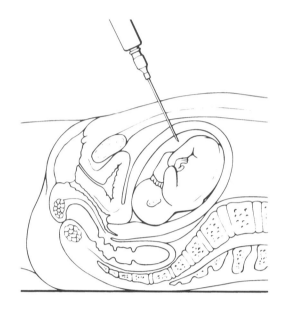

Figure 83 Amniocentesis (performed at 15 weeks)

fluid, e.g. spina bifida. This is a condition in which the vertebral arches fail to surround the spinal cord, exposing the cord and meninges which may protrude through the defective vertebrae. This disorder can be detected before birth by the presence of increased levels of alpha-fetoprotein (AFP) in the amniotic fluid. AFP is also raised when the fetus is anencephalic.

Genetic disorders can also be identified by analysing the chromosomes present in cells sloughed off the developing fetus into the amniotic fluid, e.g. Down syndrome (mongolism). In this condition 47 chromosomes are present instead of the normal 46. Parents can use the information from amniocentesis to decide to continue a pregnancy or abort a defective fetus.

The outermost of the fetal membranes is known as the **chorion** (from Greek, meaning afterbirth/outer membrane). It develops extensions, known as villi, which become part of the placenta. The combining form **chori/o** is used to mean chorion (see Fig. 82).

Without using your Exercise Guide, write the meaning of:

(h) chorio**amnion**ic _____

(i) chorio**amnion**itis _____

Root	**Obstetric** *(From a Latin word **obstetrix**, meaning midwife.)*
Combining form	**Obstetric**

Obstetrics
The science dealing with the care of the pregnant woman during all stages of pregnancy and the period following birth.

Obstetrician
A person who specializes in obstetrics. Often doctors specialize in obstetrics and gynaecology.

Obstetrical forceps
These consist of two flat blades connected to a handle. They are used to pull on a fetal head or rotate it to facilitate vaginal delivery (Figs 84 and 85).

Figure 84   Obstetrical forceps

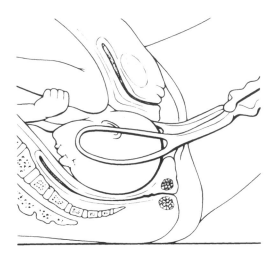

Figure 85   Obstetrical forceps in use

Another device which is used by obstetricians to assist delivery is the **vacuum extractor**. This suction device is attached to the head as it presents through the birth canal and is used to pull on the head.

Root   **Placent**
(From a Latin word **plakoenta**, meaning a flat cake.)

Combining forms   **Placent/o**

WORD EXERCISE 19

Without using your Exercise Guide, build words which mean:

(a) technique of making an   _____
X-ray of the placenta

(b) any disease of the placenta   _____

Many abnormalities of the placenta have been noted. Two common disorders are:

Adherent placenta
This is a placenta which is fused to the uterine wall so that separation is slow and delivery of the placenta is delayed. When the placenta is not expelled it is known as a **retained placenta**.

Placenta praevia (Am. placenta previa)
Here the placenta forms abnormally in the lower part of the uterus over the internal opening of the cervix. This condition gives rise to haemorrhage during pregnancy and threatens the life of the fetus.

Root   **Toc**
(From a Greek word **tokos**, meaning birth/labour.)

Combining forms   **Toc/o, -tocia** (also **tok/o**)

WORD EXERCISE 20

Without using your Exercise Guide, write the meaning of:

(a) dys**toc**ia   _____

(b) **toco**logy   _____
(synonymous with obstetrics)

Using your Exercise Guide, find the meaning of:

(c) eu**toc**ia   _____

The process of labour can be monitored by recording uterine contractions using a tocograph. The procedure is known as tocography.

If labour is late or slow, the uterus can be induced to produce forcible contractions by the administration of oxytocin, a hormone that is produced naturally by the pituitary gland. Various compounds with oxytocin-like activity are available for this purpose.

The 6–8 weeks following birth is known as the **puerperium**. It is the time when the reproductive system involutes (reverts) to its state before pregnancy. Puerperal sepsis is a serious infection of the genital tract occurring within 21 days of abortion or childbirth (from Latin *puerperus*, meaning childbearing).

Other problems can arise following birth, e.g.:

Postpartum haemorrhage
(Am. postpartum hemorrhage)
excessive bleeding from birth canal.

Eclampsia
sudden convulsion due to toxaemia of pregnancy. Usually there are signs of pre-eclampsia in pregnancy, e.g. albuminuria, hypertension and oedema.

Root

Nat
*(From a Latin word **natalis**, meaning birth.)*

Combining forms   **Nat/o, -natal**

WORD EXERCISE 21

Using your Exercise Guide, find the meaning of:

(a) neo**nat**al   _____

(b) ante**nat**al   _____

(c) peri**nat**al   _____

Without using your Exercise Guide, write the meaning of:

(d) pre**nat**al   .   _____

(e) neo**nat**ology   _____
     (A neonate is a newborn baby up to 1 month old.)

Root

Mamm
*(From a Latin word **mamma**, meaning breast. It refers to the mammary glands (breasts) which secrete milk during lactation which follows pregnancy.)*

Combining forms   **Mamm/o**

WORD EXERCISE 22

Without using your Exercise Guide, write the meaning of:

(a) **mammo**graphy   _____

(b) **mammo**plasty   _____
     (sometimes performed to increase or decrease the size of breasts)

Using your Exercise Guide, find the meaning of:

(c) **mammo**tropic   _____

Root

Mast
*(From a Greek word **mastos**, meaning breast.)*

Combining forms   **Mast/o**

WORD EXERCISE 23

Without using your Exercise Guide, build words which mean:

(a) technique of making   _____
     X-ray of breast

(b) surgical repair of breast   _____

(c) removal of breast   _____

There are two forms of this operation:

*   Simple mastectomy – removal of the breast and overlying skin
*   Radical mastectomy – removal of the breast, overlying skin, underlying muscle and lymphatic tissue.

Some patients opt for the removal of a breast cancer (mastadenoma) by a simpler procedure known as a lumpectomy, in which just the mass of abnormal cells is removed.

Without using your Exercise Guide, write the meaning of:

(d) **gynaeco**mastia   _____
     (Am. gynecomastia; seen in males)

Root **Lact**
*(From a Latin word **lactis**, meaning milk.)*

Combining forms   **Lact/o, lact/i**

WORD EXERCISE 24

Using your Exercise Guide, find the meaning of:

(a) **lact**agogue   _____

(b) **lacti**ferous   _____

(c) **lacto**meter   _____
(for specific gravity)

(d) **lacto**trophin   _____
(a hormone synonymous
with prolactin)

(e) pro**lact**in   _____
(hormone acts on breasts)

(f) **lacti**fuge   _____

Without using your Exercise Guide, write the meaning of:

(g) **lacto**genic   _____

Root **Galact**
*(From a Greek word **galaktos**, meaning milk.)*

Combining forms   **Galact/o**

WORD EXERCISE 25

Without using your Exercise Guide, write the meaning of:

(a) **galact**agogue   _____

(b) **galacto**rrhoea   _____
(Am. galactorrhea; an abnormal condition)

Using your Exercise Guide, find the meaning of:

(c) **galact**ischia   _____

(d) **galacto**poiesis   _____

Medical equipment and clinical procedures

Revise the names of all instruments and procedures introduced in this unit before completing Exercise 26.

WORD EXERCISE 26

Match each term in Column A with a description from Column C by placing the appropriate number in Column B.

Column A	Column B	Column C
(a) vaginal speculum	_____	1. technique of recording uterine contractions
(b) colposcope	_____	2. spoon-shaped device used for scraping tissue from uterus
(c) Pap test	_____	3. technique of examining peritoneal cavity via vaginal fornix and rectouterine pouch
(d) culdoscopy	_____	4. instrument used to cut amnion
(e) fetoscope	_____	5. instrument used to view the vagina and cervix
(f) curette	_____	6. instrument used to measure the specific gravity of milk
(g) amniotome	_____	7. technique of examining cells from a cervical smear
(h) lactometer	_____	8. instrument to assist passage of a baby through the birth canal
(i) obstetrical forceps	_____	9. instrument to hold walls of the vagina apart
(j) tocography	_____	10. instrument inserted into amniotic cavity to visually examine a fetus

Quick Reference

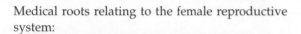

Medical roots relating to the female reproductive system:

Amni/o	amnion
Bartholin/o	Bartholin's glands of the vagina
Cervic/o	cervix
Chori/o	chorion/outer fetal membrane
Colp/o	vagina
Culd/o	Douglas cavity/rectouterine pouch
Fet/o (Am.)	fetus
Galact/o	milk
-gravida	pregnancy/pregnant woman
Gynaec/o	female
Gynec/o (Am.)	female
Hyster/o	uterus
Lact/o/i	milk
Mamm/o	breast
Mast/o	breast
Men/o	menses/menstruation/ monthly flow
Metr/o	uterus/womb
Nat/o	birth
Obstetric	pertaining to midwifery
Oo-	egg
Oophor/o	ovary
Ovari/o	ovary
-para	to bear/bring forth offspring
Perine/o	perineum
Placent/o	placenta
Salping/o	Fallopian tube
Toc/o	labour/birth
Trachel/o	neck
Uter/o	uterus
Vagin/o	vagina
Vulv/o	vulva

Abbreviations

You should learn common abbreviations related to obstetrics. Note, however, some are not standard and their meaning may vary from one hospital to another. There is a more extensive list for reference on page 259.

AB, ab, abor	abortion
AFP	alpha-fetoprotein
APH	antepartum haemorrhage (Am. hemorrhage)
BBA	born before arrival
C-Sect	caesarean section (Am. cesarean)
FDIU	fetal death in utero
GI and GII	gravida I and gravida II
IUD	intrauterine death
LCCS	low cervical caesarean section (Am. cesarean)
LGA	large for gestational age
NFTD	normal full-term delivery
Obs–Gyn	obstetrics and gynaecology (Am. gynecology)

> ## NOW TRY THE WORD CHECK

WORD CHECK

This self-check exercise lists all the word components used in this unit. First write down the meaning of as many word components as you can. Then check your answers using the Exercise Guide and Quick Reference box or the Glossary of Word Components (pp. 269–279).

Prefixes

a- _____

ante- _____

dys- _____

endo- _____

eu- _____

extra- _____

micro- _____

multi- _____

neo- _____

nulli- _____

oligo- _____

peri- _____

post- _____

pre- _____

primi- _____

pro- _____

pseudo- _____

secundi- _____

Combining forms of word roots

amni/o _____

bartholin/o _____

cervic/o _____

chori/o _____

colp/o _____

culd/o _____

cyst/o _____

cyt/o _____

fer/o _____

fet/o _____

fibr/o _____

galact/o _____

gravida _____

gynaec/o _____
(Am. gynec/o)

haem/o _____
(Am. hem/o)

hyster/o _____

lact/o _____

mamm/o _____

mast/o _____

men/o _____

metr/o _____

myc/o _____

nat/o _____

obstetric- _____

oo- _____

oophor/o _____

ovari/o _____

-para _____

perine/o _____

peritone/o _____

phleb/o _____

placent/o _____

rect/o _____

salping/o _____

sten/o _____

toc/o` _____

trachel/o _____

uter/o _____

vagin/o _____

vesic/o _____

vulv/o _____

Suffixes

-agogue _____

-al _____

-algia _____

-arche _____

-blast _____

-cele _____

-centesis _____

-dynia _____

-ectomy _____

-fuge _____

-genesis _____

-genic _____

-gram _____

-graphy _____

-ia _____

-ic _____

-ischia _____

-itis _____

-lithiasis _____

-logy _____

-malacia _____

-meter _____

-metry _____

-natal _____

-osis _____

-ous _____

-pathia _____

-pathy _____

-pause _____

-pexy _____

-plasty _____

-poiesis _____

-ptosis _____

-rrhagic _____

-rrhaphy _____

-rrhexis _____

-rrhoea _____
(Am. -rrhea)

-sclerosis _____

-scope _____

-scopy _____

-staxis _____

-stenosis _____

-stomy _____

-tome _____

-tomy _____

-toxic _____

-trophic _____

-tropic _____

-tubal _____

> **NOW TRY THE SELF-ASSESSMENT**

SELF-ASSESSMENT

Test 16A

Below are some combining forms which refer to the anatomy of the female reproductive system. Indicate which part of the system they refer to by putting a number from the diagrams (Figs 86 and 87) next to each word.

(a) oophor/o _____

(b) salping/o _____

(c) hyster/o _____

(d) endometr/o _____

(e) cervic/o _____

(f) colp/o _____

(g) vulv/o _____

(h) culd/o _____

Score

8

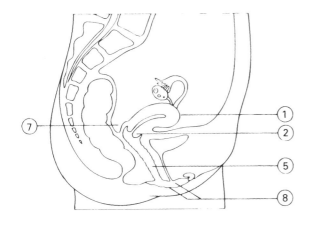

Figure 86 **Section through female**

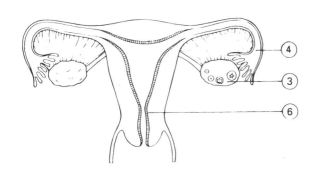

Figure 87 **The female reproductive system**

Column A	Column B	Column C
(i) oligo-	_____	9. pertaining to tube/oviduct
(j) -ous	_____	10. before (i)
(k) -pause	_____	11. before (ii)
(l) -pexy	_____	12. good
(m) post-	_____	13. fixation by surgery
(n) pre-	_____	14. pertaining to stimulating
(o) primi-	_____	15. pertaining to
(p) -rrhagia	_____	16. second
(q) secundi-	_____	17. none
(r) -staxis	_____	18. first
(s) -tropic	_____	19. condition of blocking/holding back
(t) -tubal	_____	20. many

Score

20

Test 16B
Prefixes and suffixes

Match each prefix and suffix in Column A with a meaning in Column C by inserting the appropriate number in Column B.

Column A	Column B	Column C
(a) -agogue	_____	1. to drip (blood)
(b) ante-	_____	2. pertaining to birth
(c) eu-	_____	3. stop/pause
(d) -ischia	_____	4. new
(e) multi-	_____	5. stimulate/induce
(f) -natal	_____	6. after
(g) neo-	_____	7. few/little
(h) nulli-	_____	8. condition of bursting forth (of blood)

Test 16C
Combining forms of word roots

Match each combining form in Column A with a meaning in Column C by inserting the appropriate number in Column B.

Column A	Column B	Column C
(a) cervic/o	_____	1. woman
(b) colp/o	_____	2. breast (i)
(c) culd/o	_____	3. breast (ii)
(d) gravida	_____	4. menstruation/monthly
(e) gynaec/o (Am. gynec/o)	_____	5. birth
(f) hyster/o	_____	6. vulva (external genitalia)
(g) lact/o	_____	7. placenta
(h) mamm/o	_____	8. pregnant heavy/pregnant woman

Column A	Column B	Column C
(i) mast/o	_____	9. perineum/area between anus and vulva
(j) men/o	_____	10. pertaining to midwifery and childbirth
(k) metr/o	_____	11. to bear/bring forth baby
(l) nat/o	_____	12. uterus (i)
(m) obstetric-	_____	13. uterus (ii)
(n) oo-	_____	14. uterus (iii)
(o) oophor/o	_____	15. neck (of womb)
(p) ovari/o	_____	16. Douglas pouch/ rectouterine cavity
(q) -para	_____	17. vagina (i)
(r) perine/o	_____	18. vagina (ii)
(s) placent/o	_____	19. egg
(t) salping/o	_____	20. ovary (i)
(u) trachel/o	_____	21. ovary (ii)
(v) uter/o	_____	22. cervix uteri
(w) vagin/o	_____	23. Fallopian tube/trumpet
(x) vesic/o	_____	24. milk
(y) vulv/o	_____	25. bladder

Score

25

Test 16D

Write the meaning of:

(a) tocometer _____

(b) oophorohysterectomy _____

(c) mastopexy _____

(d) hysterorrhexis _____

(e) metropathy _____

Score

5

Test 16E

Build words which mean:

(a) surgical repair of the Douglas pouch/rectouterine pouch _____

(b) formation of an opening into a Fallopian tube _____

(c) rupture of the amnion _____

(d) displacement/prolapse of the vagina (use colp/o) _____

(e) study of cells of the vagina (use colp/o) _____

Score

5

Check answers to Self-Assessment Tests on page 256.

17 The endocrine system

Objectives

Once you have completed Unit 17 you should be able to:

- understand the meaning of medical words relating to the endocrine system

- build medical words relating to the endocrine system

- associate medical terms with their anatomical position

- understand medical abbreviations relating to the endocrine system.

Exercise Guide

Use this list of word components and their meanings to complete the word exercises in this unit.

Prefixes

acro-	extremities/point
hyper-	above normal/excessive
hypo-	below normal/deficient
para-	beside/near

Roots/Combining forms

aden/o	gland
blast/o	germ cell/cell which forms ...
chondr/o	cartilage
gloss/o	tongue
-gyne	woman
kal/i	potassium
natr/i	sodium

Suffixes

-aemia	condition of blood
-al	pertaining to
-ectomy	removal of
-emia (Am.)	condition of blood
-genesis	formation of
-genic	pertaining to formation/ originating in
-globulin	protein
-ia	condition of
-ic	pertaining to
-ism	process of
-itis	inflammation of
-megaly	enlargement
-micria	condition of small size
-oma	tumour/swelling
-osis	abnormal condition/disease of
-plasia	condition of growth/formation of (cells)
-ptosis	falling/displacement/prolapse
-static	pertaining to stopping/ controlling
-tomy	incision into
-toxic	pertaining to poisoning
-trophic	pertaining to nourishment
-tropic	pertaining to affinity for/ stimulating
-uresis	excrete in urine/urinate
-uria	condition of urine

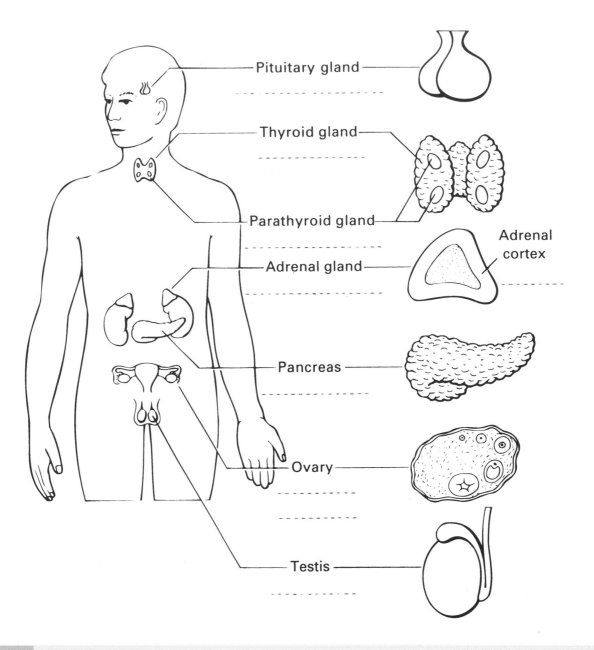

The endocrine system

ANATOMY EXERCISE

When you have finished Word Exercises 1–6, look at the word components listed below. Complete Figure 88 by writing the appropriate combining form on each dotted line – more than one component may relate to the same position. (You can check their meanings in the Quick Reference box on p. 203.)

Adren/o   Orchid/o   Parathyroid/o
Adrenocortic/o   Ovari/o   Pituitar-
Hypophys-   Pancreat/o   Thyr/o
Oophor/o

The endocrine system

The endocrine system is composed of a diverse group of glands which secrete hormones directly into the bloodstream. Once released, hormones travel in the blood to all parts of the body. Low concentrations of hormones in the blood stimulate specific target tissues and exert a regulatory effect on their cellular processes.

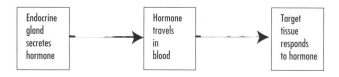

The concentration of hormones which circulate in the blood is precisely regulated by the brain and the endocrine glands. Many disorders of these glands affect the output of hormones. Abnormal levels of hormones produce symptoms which range from minor to severely disabling disease and death.

In this unit we will examine terms associated with each endocrine gland.

Use the Exercise Guide at the beginning of this unit to complete Word Exercises 1–6 unless you are asked to work without it.

The pituitary gland

Root	**Pituitar** *(From a Latin word **pituita**, meaning slime/phlegm. It refers to a small gland which grows at the base of the brain on a stalk. It is commonly called the 'master' gland of the endocrine system because it releases tropic hormones which regulate other endocrine glands.)*
Combining form	**-pituitar**ism *(This is used when referring to the process of pituitary secretion.)*

WORD EXERCISE 1

Using your Exercise Guide, find the meaning of:

(a) hypo**pituitar**ism _____

(b) hyper**pituitar**ism _____

One of the hormones produced by the pituitary gland is somatotrophin or human growth hormone.

Underproduction of this results in **acromicria** and **dwarfism**. Overproduction of growth hormone produces **acromegaly** and **giantism**.

(c) acromicria _____

(d) acromegaly _____

Once it was realized that the pituitary gland is not the source of spit and phlegm, scientists renamed the gland the **hypophysis** (*hypo* – below, *physis* – growth, i.e. growth below the brain). Pituitary and hypophysis are now used synonymously. The hypophysis consists of a down-growth from the brain, known as the neurohypophysis, and attached to it a glandular part, known as the adenohypophysis.

Removal of the hypophysis is known as **hypophys**ectomy.

The thyroid gland

Root	**Thyr** *(From a Greek word **thyreoidos**, meaning resembling a shield. It refers to the shield-shaped thyroid gland which lies above the trachea. It secretes the thyroid hormones tri-iodothyronine, T_3 and thyroxine, T_4, which control the metabolic rate of all cells.)*
Combining forms	**Thyr/o, -thyroid**

WORD EXERCISE 2

Using your Exercise Guide, find the meaning of:

(a) **thyr**oglossal _____

(b) **thyr**oadenitis _____

(c) **thyr**oglobulin _____

(d) **thyr**ochondrotomy _____

(e) **thyr**otoxicosis _____
(Graves' disease)

A symptom of this disorder is exophthalmos, protruding eyes. The extent of this can be measured using a technique known as exophthalmometry.

(f) para**thyr**oid _____

(This refers to another endocrine gland which lies beside the thyroid gland. The parathyroid consists of four small glands which secrete parathyroid hormone.)

(g) para**thyr**oidectomy _____

Without using your Exercise Guide, write the meaning of:

(h) hyperpara**thyr**oidism _____
(leads to excess calcium in blood, hypercalcaemia; Am. hypercalcemia)

(i) **thyro**megaly _____

Without using your Exercise Guide, build words which mean:

(j) process of secreting above _____
normal levels of thyroid
hormone

(k) process of secreting below _____
normal levels of thyroid
hormone

In infants this results in poor growth and mental retardation and is known as cretinism. In adults the condition is known as myxoedema (Am. myxedema) and it gives rise to dry skin which appears swollen.

Using your Exercise Guide, build words which mean:

(l) downward displacement of _____
the thyroid

(m) pertaining to affinity for _____
the thyroid gland

(n) pertaining to originating in _____
the thyroid gland

Enlargement of the thyroid gland is also known as goitre. It is a feature of many thyroid diseases, e.g.:

Simple goitre
can be due to deficiency of iodine in the diet. Iodine is part of the thyroid hormone, thyroxine.

Toxic goitre
hyperthyroiditis or exophthalmic goitre (Graves' disease).

Malignant goitre
due to carcinoma of the thyroid.

Thyroid goitres can be investigated by the administration of radioactive iodine. This is taken up by the thyroid gland which becomes slightly radioactive. The presence of radioactivity in the gland can be detected with a scanner which can outline the gland. We will look at this in more detail in Unit 18.

The pancreas

 Root | **Pancreat**
(Derived from Greek **pankreas***, pan – all, kreas – flesh.)*

Combining forms **Pancreat/o**

We have already used this root in our studies of the digestive system. The pancreas also has a role to play as an endocrine gland. Small patches of tissue within the pancreas called the Islets of Langerhans secrete the hormones insulin and glucagon directly into the blood. These hormones regulate the amount of glucose in the blood.

WORD EXERCISE 3

Without using your Exercise Guide, write the meaning of:

(a) **pancreato**tropic _____
(Some of the pituitary hormones have such an action.)

Insulin (named after Latin *insula*, meaning island) is produced by the Islets of Langerhans. It enters the blood and stimulates the uptake of sugar by tissue cells. Its overall effect is to lower blood sugar levels in the body following the intake of glucose in the diet. The combining forms derived from this are **insulin/o** (meaning insulin or Islets of Langerhans).

Using your Exercise Guide, find the meaning of:

(b) **insulino**genesis _____

(c) **insulin**oma _____

Without using your Exercise Guide, write the meaning of:

(d) **insulin**itis _____

(e) hyper**insulin**ism _____

If the body fails to produce insulin, blood sugar levels will rise and glucose will appear in the urine. This abnormal condition is known as **diabetes mellitus**.

There are several types of diabetes mellitus. Here are two common types:

Type 1
early onset diabetes, seen in young subjects, due to hereditary factors and/or autoimmune disease. It is also known as insulin-dependent diabetes mellitus (IDDM). These patients require insulin injections to remain alive.

Type 2
late onset diabetes mellitus. This is also known as non-insulin-dependent diabetes mellitus (NIDDM). Dietary factors are involved and it can be controlled by a change in diet and/or drugs which lower blood sugar levels.

Complications of diabetes mellitus include a tendency to develop cataracts, retinopathy and neuropathy. It is diagnosed by blood glucose estimation and glucose tolerance tests. The latter test involves administering a known quantity of glucose and measuring the amounts which appear in the blood and urine in a set time.

Below are terms which can be used to describe sugar levels in blood and urine. The combining form **glyc/o** is used to mean sugar (from Greek *glykys*, meaning sweet).

Using your Exercise Guide, find the meaning of:

(f) hypo**glyc**aemia _____
    (Am. hypoglycemia)

(g) hyper**glyc**aemia _____
    (Am. hyperglycemia)

(h) **glyco**suria _____
    (Patients can estimate the state of their own blood sugar level from the amount present in their urine. Glucose oxidase papers can be used to test for glucose in the urine. The papers change colour in the presence of glucose.)

(i) **glyco**static _____

Untreated diabetes results in the tissue cells using fatty acids as a source of energy instead of sugar. This leads to the release of chemicals known as ketones into the blood and urine. Ketones such as acetone have a toxic effect on the body which is known as **ketosis**.

The adrenal gland

Adren
*(From Latin ad – to/near, **renes** – kidneys. It refers to the adrenal gland, a small triangle-shaped gland which lies above each kidney. The inner part of the gland, the medulla, secretes adrenalin. The outer cortex secretes steroid hormones.)*

Combining forms **Adren/o**

WORD EXERCISE 4

Without using your Exercise Guide, build words which mean:

(a) enlarged adrenal gland _____

(b) pertaining to poisonous _____
    to the adrenal

(c) pertaining to stimulating/ _____
    acting on the adrenal

The adrenal cortex is the outer layer of the adrenal gland. It produces a variety of steroid hormones (steroidogenesis). There are three main types:

Androgens
types of male sex hormone.

Glucocorticoids
hormones which control glucose, protein and lipid metabolism.

Mineralocorticoids
which regulate fluid and electrolyte balance.

Aldosterone is an example of a mineralocorticoid. It enables the body to retain sodium and excrete potassium. Abnormal aldosterone production may result in the disturbances of sodium and potassium levels named in (d), (e) and (f) below.

Using your Exercise Guide, find the meaning of:

(d) hypernatraemia _____
    (Am. hypernatremia)

(e) hypokalaemia _____
    (Am. hypokalemia)

(f) natriuresis _____

The combining forms **adrenocortic/o** are used when referring to the adrenal cortex itself. Corticosteroid refers to the steroid hormones of the adrenal cortex.

(g) **adrenocortico**trophic _____
(Some of the hormones of the pituitary have this effect.)

(h) **adrenocortico**hyperplasia _____

Major disorders of hormone production by the adrenal cortex include:

Hyperfunction

Cushing's syndrome
Over-production of adrenocorticotrophic hormone (ACTH) by the pituitary stimulates the adrenal to release steroids, which results in raised blood pressure, hyperglycaemia and increased sodium retention.

Adrenogenital syndrome
Associated with over-production of male sex hormones. This results in virilization (masculinization) in women and precocity (premature sexual maturity) in boys.

Hypofunction

Addison's disease
A deficiency in glucocorticoids and mineralocorticoids results in loss of sodium and water, and a fall in blood pressure. Patients will die within 4–14 days unless treated with mineralocorticoids.

The ovary and testis

Both the ovary and the testis are reproductive organs, in that they produce the sex cells, i.e. eggs and sperm, but they are also endocrine glands producing the sex hormones. Note that we have already used the combining forms for the ovary (oophor/o and ovari/o) and testis (orchid/o).

First, let us examine the endocrine role of the testis. The main sex hormone produced by the testis is **testosterone**. It is also produced in small quantities in the adrenal gland. Testosterone and other similar hormones are known as **androgens**. In males they stimulate the development of the reproductive tract and secondary sexual characteristics, such as growth of the beard and

male musculature. Androgens are therefore masculinizing hormones.

 Root **Andr**
*(From a Greek word **andros**, meaning man/male.)*

Combining forms **Andr/o**

WORD EXERCISE 5

Using your Exercise Guide, find the meaning of:

(a) **andro**gyne _____
(actually a female hermaphrodite)

(b) **andro**blastoma _____

The ovary is also an endocrine hormone which secretes several sex hormones:

Oestrogens (Am. estrogens)
These are female sex hormones produced by the ovary which regulate the development of the female reproductive tract, menstrual cycle and secondary sexual characteristics, such as the growth of pubic hair and the female body form. Compounds which have oestrogen-like actions on the body are described as **oestrogenic** (Am. estrogenic).

Progesterones
These are steroid hormones concerned with maintaining the receptivity of the uterus to fertilized eggs and the growth of the uterus during pregnancy.

Medical equipment and clinical procedures

Revise the names of medical equipment and procedures mentioned in this unit and then try Exercise 6. Some imaging procedures used for examining the endocrine system will be studied in Unit 18 as the techniques involved are similar to those used for other systems.

WORD EXERCISE 6

Match each term in Column A with a description from Column C by placing an appropriate number in Column B.

Column A	Column B	Column C
(a) adrenal function test	_____	1. imaging of thyroid gland following administration of radioactive iodine
(b) glucose tolerance test	_____	2. test for hypothyroidism by measuring concentration of iodine in blood
(c) protein bound iodine test (PBI)	_____	3. a test used to diagnose diabetes mellitus
(d) glucose oxidase paper strip test (Clinistix)	_____	4. measurement of 24-h output of corticosteroids
(e) thyroid scan	_____	5. indicates the relative amount of glucose in urine

Abbreviations

You should learn common abbreviations related to the endocrine system. Note, however, some are not standard and their meaning may vary from one hospital to another. There is a more extensive list for reference on page 259.

ACTH	adrenocorticotrophic hormone
BSS	blood sugar series
FSH	follicle-stimulating hormone
HGH	human growth hormone
HRT	hormone replacement therapy
IDDM	Insulin-dependent diabetes mellitus
LH	luteinizing hormone
NIDDM	non-insulin-dependent diabetes mellitus
OGTT	oral glucose tolerance test
PRL	prolactin
T_3, T_4	tri-iodothyronine, tetraiodothyronine (thyroxine)
TSH	thyroid stimulating hormone

ANATOMY EXERCISE

Now complete the Anatomy Exercise on page 198.

> ## NOW TRY THE WORD CHECK

Quick Reference

Medical roots relating to the endocrine system:

Aden/o	gland
Adren/o	adrenal gland
Andr/o	male
Cortic/o	cortex
Estr/o (Am.)	estrogen
-globulin	protein
Glyc/o	sugar
Insulin/o	insulin
Kal/i	potassium
Ket/o	ketones
Natr/i	sodium
Oestr/o	oestrogen
Pancreat/o	pancreas
-physis	growth
Pituitar-	pituitary
Progest/o	progesterone
Thyr/o	thyroid gland

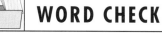

WORD CHECK

This self-check exercise lists all the word components used in this unit. First write down the meaning of as many word components as you can. Then check your answers using the Exercise Guide and Quick Reference box or the Glossary of Word Components (pp. 269–279).

Prefixes

acro-   _____

hyper-   _____

hypo-   _____

para-   _____

Combining forms of word roots

aden/o   _____

adren/o   _____

andr/o _____

blast/o _____

chondr/o _____

cortic/o _____

globulin _____

gloss/o _____

-gyne _____

insulin/o _____

kal/i _____

ket/o/n _____

natr/i _____

oestr/o
(Am. estr/o) _____

pancreat/o _____

physis _____

pituitar- _____

progest/o _____

thyr/o _____

Suffixes

-aemia
(Am. -emia) _____

-al _____

-ectomy _____

-genesis _____

-genic _____

-ia _____

-ic _____

-ism _____

-itis _____

-megaly _____

-micria _____

-oid _____

-oma _____

-osis _____

-plasia _____

-ptosis _____

-static _____

-tomy _____

-toxic _____

-trophic _____

-tropic _____

-uresis _____

-uria _____

> ## NOW TRY THE SELF-ASSESSMENT

SELF-ASSESSMENT

Test 17A

Below are some combining forms which refer to the anatomy of the endocrine system. Indicate which part of the system they refer to by putting a number from the diagram (Fig. 89) next to each word.

(a) adren/o _____

(b) parathyroid/o _____

(c) andr/o _____

(d) thyroid/o _____

(e) insulin/o _____

(f) oestr/o
(Am. estr/o) _____

(g) pituitar- _____

(h) adrenocortic/o _____

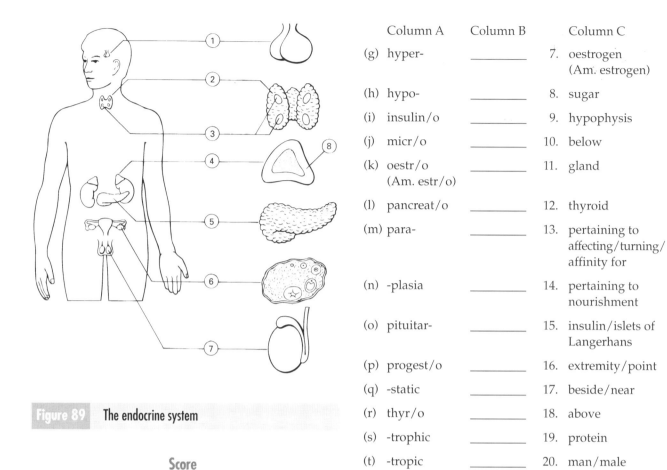

	Column A	Column B		Column C
(g)	hyper-	_____	7.	oestrogen (Am. estrogen)
(h)	hypo-	_____	8.	sugar
(i)	insulin/o	_____	9.	hypophysis
(j)	micr/o	_____	10.	below
(k)	oestr/o (Am. estr/o)	_____	11.	gland
(l)	pancreat/o	_____	12.	thyroid
(m)	para-	_____	13.	pertaining to affecting/turning/ affinity for
(n)	-plasia	_____	14.	pertaining to nourishment
(o)	pituitar-	_____	15.	insulin/islets of Langerhans
(p)	progest/o	_____	16.	extremity/point
(q)	-static	_____	17.	beside/near
(r)	thyr/o	_____	18.	above
(s)	-trophic	_____	19.	protein
(t)	-tropic	_____	20.	man/male

Score

8

Score

20

Test 17B

Prefixes, suffixes and combining forms of word roots

Match a word component from Column A with a meaning in Column C by inserting the appropriate number in Column B.

	Column A	Column B		Column C
(a)	acro-	_____	1.	germ cell
(b)	aden/o	_____	2.	small
(c)	andr/o	_____	3.	pancreas
(d)	blast/o	_____	4.	progesterone
(e)	-globin	_____	5.	pertaining to constant/ unchanging/ controlling
(f)	glyc/o	_____	6.	condition of growth (increase of cells)

Test 17C

Write the meaning of:

(a) thyroparathyroidectomy   _____

(b) pituicyte   _____

(c) adrenomegaly   _____

(d) glycotropic   _____

(e) hyperketonaemia (Am. hyperketonemia)   _____

Score

5

Test 17D

Build words which mean:

(a) process of producing too   _____
much insulin

(b) condition of too little sodium   _____
in the blood

(c) pertaining to nourishing the   _____
thyroid gland (use thyr/o)

(d) pertaining to acting on/   _____
stimulating the adrenal

(e) process of producing too   _____
little parathyroid hormone

Score

5

Check answers to Self-Assessment Tests on page 256.

18 Radiology and nuclear medicine

Objectives

Once you have completed Unit 18 you should be able to:

- understand the meaning of medical words relating to radiology and nuclear medicine

- build medical words relating to radiology and nuclear medicine

- understand medical abbreviations relating to radiology and nuclear medicine.

Exercise Guide

Use this list of word components and their meanings to complete the word exercises in this unit.

Prefixes

ultra-	beyond

Roots/Combining forms

angi/o	vessel
cardi/o	heart
encephal/o	brain
esophag/o (Am.)	esophagus/gullet
oesophag/o	oesophagus/gullet

Suffixes

-er	one who
-genic	pertaining to formation/ originating in
-gram	X-ray picture/tracing/recording
-graph	usually an instrument that records/an X-ray picture
-graphy	technique of recording/ making an X-ray
-ist	specialist
-logist	specialist who studies
-logy	study of
-scope	viewing instrument
-therapy	treatment

Radiology

Radiology is the study of the diagnosis of disease by the use of radiant energy (radiation). In the past this meant the use of X-rays to make an image of the internal components of the body. Today many other forms of radiation are used to aid both diagnosis and treatment of disease. Developments in physics and technology are bringing rapid changes to this branch of medicine.

Before completing the first exercise, review the terms below which are very relevant to this unit:

-gram
recording/picture/tracing/X-ray.

-graph
usually refers to an instrument which records by making a picture or tracing but it is also used here to mean a recording or X-ray picture.

-graphy
technique of making a recording, i.e. a picture, tracing or writing.

Use the Exercise Guide at the beginning of this unit to complete Word Exercises 1–10 unless you are asked to work without it.

Root   **Radi**
(From a Latin word **radius***, meaning a ray. Here it is used to mean the invisible rays produced by an X-ray machine. Also used for radiation/radioactivity.)*

Combining forms   **Radi/o**

WORD EXERCISE 1

Using your Exercise Guide, find the meaning of:

(a) **radio**logist _____
(a physician, i.e. medically qualified)

(b) **radio**graph _____
(refers to an X-ray picture)

(c) **radio**graphy _____

(d) **radio**grapher _____
(refers to a technician who is not medically qualified)

Some radiographic procedures require the use of a contrast medium or agent to improve the quality of the image. Contrast agents are required because there is little difference in the density of the soft parts of the body and X-rays pass through them without producing a distinct image of individual organs.

The contrast medium is administered to the patient and will fill cavities within the body which are then outlined on the radiograph.

Barium sulphate is a radio-opaque substance that absorbs X-rays. It will show up on X-ray film as a white area which has not allowed X-rays to pass. This property of barium sulphate makes it useful for outlining cavities, e.g. in the digestive tract where it is administered as:

A barium 'meal' (swallow)
To outline the upper parts of the digestive system the barium is given as a drink.

A barium enema
To outline the lower parts of the digestive system. Here the barium is injected via the anus into the rectum. Sometimes air is also injected with the barium to increase contrast. This is known as a **double contrast radiograph**.

Iodine is another contrast agent which can be added to make various fluids radio-opaque. It is often the contrast agent used in angiocardiography, arteriography and venography.

Root   **Roentgen**
(From the name of Wilhelm K. Roentgen, a German physicist who discovered X-rays. It is used to mean X-rays.)

Combining forms   **Roentgen/o**

WORD EXERCISE 2

Without using your Exercise Guide, write the meaning of:

(a) **roentgeno**graphy _____

(b) **roentgeno**logist _____
(synonymous with radiologist)

Using your Exercise Guide, find the meaning of:

(c) **roentgeno**gram   _____
(synonymous with radiograph, but as this German name is difficult to pronounce, radiograph is more commonly used)

(d) **roentgeno**cardiogram   _____

Sometimes it is important to observe an X-ray of the body moving directly by fluoroscopy. In this procedure X-rays pass through the body on to a phosphor screen (a fluorescent screen, i.e. one from which light flows). As the X-rays strike the screen, the phosphor emits light, producing an image. Thus the image is viewed as it is generated. It is useful for observing movement of the oesophagus (Am. esophagus), stomach and heart. If necessary, a recording/picture can be made of the light image from the screen. (**Fluor** is from Latin *fluere*, meaning to flow. It is used to mean something that is luminous, i.e. emitting light.)

Using your Exercise Guide, build a word which means:

(e) Instrument used for the direct   _____
X-ray examination of the body (fluoroscopy)

Without using your Exercise Guide, build a word which means:

(f) Technique of recording a   _____
radiographic image produced by fluoroscopy

	Cine
Root	*(From a Greek word* **kinein***, meaning movement. Here its combining forms are used to mean a moving film, i.e. a motion picture on film or video.)*

Combining forms   **Cine, cinemat/o**

WORD EXERCISE 3

Without using your Exercise Guide, write the meaning of:

(a) **cine**radiograph   _____

(b) roentgeno**cinemato**graphy   _____

Using your Exercise Guide, find the meaning of:

(c) **cine**angiocardiography   _____

(d) **cine**oesophagogram   _____
(Am. cine-esophagogram)

	Tom
Root	*(From a Greek word* **tomos***, meaning a slice or section.)*

Combining forms   **Tom/o**

A **tomograph** is an instrument which uses X-rays to obtain images of sections through the body. It uses a thin beam of X-rays which rotates around the patient. X-ray photons emitted from the patient are detected and converted into an image by a computer. The images produced by this device show more detail than a simple X-ray.

WORD EXERCISE 4

Without using your Exercise Guide, write the meaning of:

(a) **tomo**gram   _____

(b) **tomo**graphy   _____
(This procedure is also called computed tomography, computerized axial tomography, CT scanning and CAT scanning.)

Nuclear medicine

This is a branch of medicine which uses **radioisotopes** to diagnose and treat disease. In some texts it is referred to as nuclear radiology, nuclear imaging or radionuclide imaging.

Radioisotopes

These are elements which exhibit the property of spontaneous decay, emitting radiation in the process. The radiation is in the form of high-speed particles and energy-containing rays. Elements which emit alpha, beta or gamma radiation are used as diagnostic labels to trace the route and uptake of chemicals administered into the body. The radioisotope thus behaves like a transmitter, passing radiation from inside to the outside of the body. Ideally, radioisotopes should give off gamma radiation as alpha and beta particles can damage cells. Many different diagnostic techniques have been devised which use radioisotopes. One is described below.

First, a specific radioisotope known as a **tracer** is given to the patient. It is taken up or excluded by organs or tissues of interest to the investigation. The presence or absence of the tracer in a tissue can be detected by the fact that it emits gamma rays. These can be detected with a Geigy–Muller tube or gamma camera passed over the surface of the body, this is known as a **radioisotope scan**. Such techniques are used to image the heart, liver, biliary tract, bone, thyroid and kidney.

Here are examples of the use of specific radioisotopes:

$^{99\text{M}}$**Tc (technetium)**
$^{99\text{M}}$Tc is administered to the patient in trace quantities. It is excluded from normal brain tissue but it accumulates in some brain tumours. A tumour can be detected by locating the gamma rays emitted from it.

^{123}**I (iodine)**
^{123}I is administered to the patient and is rapidly taken up by the thyroid gland. A radioisotope scan of the gland will outline the now radioactive gland and information from this will aid the diagnosis of various thyroid disorders, e.g. thyrotoxicosis.

^{57}**Co (cobalt)**
^{57}Co is used to trace the uptake of vitamin B_{12} by the body and from this a diagnosis of megaloblastic anaemia can be made.

Root	**Scint** *(From a Latin word **scintilla**, meaning spark/emitting sparks/light.)*
Combining forms	**Scint/i, scintill/a**

In the process of **scintigraphy**, a radioisotope with an affinity for a particular organ or tissue is injected into the body. The distribution of the radioactivity can be followed using an instrument known as a **scintillation counter (scintiscanner)**. This device contains a **scintillator**, a substance that emits light when in contact with ionizing radiation. There is a flash of light for each ionizing event and the number of counts is therefore related to the amount of radioactivity present. Scintillation counters can be moved over the outer surface of the body to locate radioisotopes within particular organs and build an image (scintigram/scintiscan) of their distribution. The **gamma camera** mentioned earlier for scanning the body is a scintillation counter.

 WORD EXERCISE 5

Without using your Exercise Guide, write the meaning of:

(a) **scinti**gram _____

(b) **scinti**graphy _____

Another technique which traces the distribution of radioisotopes within the body is **positron emission tomography** (PET scanning). This procedure constructs a tomographic image of the location of radioactive isotopes that have been injected into the patient. These isotopes emit particles known as positrons which can be detected. An example is ^{18}F deoxyglucose which is taken up by active body cells for glucose metabolism. Differences in uptake by cells indicate variations in metabolism. Reduced cerebral uptake, for example, may indicate damage in a specific part of the brain.

Radiotherapy

Radiotherapy is the treatment of disease by X-rays and other forms of radiation. Radiotherapy is used to destroy malignant cancer cells by destroying them with a lethal dose of radiation.

^{60}Co (cobalt) emits highly penetrating gamma rays which can be aimed at tumours from a radiotherapy machine outside the body. Sometimes radioisotopes are administered into the body, for example ^{131}I (iodine) emits beta radiation which can destroy cells. Once administered into the body, it is preferentially absorbed by the thyroid gland which thus receives a dose of beta radiation sufficient to destroy thyroid cancer cells.

Other radioactive materials can be implanted in the body for a specific length of time, e.g. radon capsules (seeds). These contain radioactive radon gas and are left in place to destroy malignant cells. The capsules are removed after they have emitted a therapeutic dose of radiation.

 WORD EXERCISE 6

Without using your Exercise Guide, write the meaning of:

(a) **radio**therapy _____

(b) **radio**therapist _____
(a physician, medically qualified)

Ultrasonography

When high-frequency sound waves are directed at the body, internal organs and masses reflect the sound to a different extent. They are said to have different echo textures. These internal echoes are detected and converted into an image. The size and shape of easily recognized organs can be investigated using this technique and it is widely used for examining a fetus in utero.

Root	**Son** (From a Latin word **sonus**, meaning sound.)
Combining forms	**Son/o**

Note.   The next exercise refers to techniques using ultrasound, i.e. high-frequency sounds beyond human hearing.)

WORD EXERCISE 7

Using your Exercise Guide, find the meaning of:

(a) ultra**sono**gram _____
    (a picture/tracing)

Without using your Exercise Guide, write the meaning of:

(b) ultra**sono**graphy _____

(c) ultra**sono**graph _____
    (an instrument)

Root	**Echo** (A Greek word meaning the repetition of sounds owing to reflection by an obstacle. Here we are referring to the reflection of ultrasound, i.e. echoes.)
Combining form	**Echo-**

WORD EXERCISE 8

Using your Exercise Guide, find the meaning of:

(a) **echo**encephalogram _____

Using your Exercise Guide, build a word which means:

(b) pertaining to forming/ _____
    generating an echo

Without using your Exercise Guide, build words which mean:

(c) recording/picture of echo _____
    (synonymous with
    ultrasonogram)

(d) instrument which records _____
    echoes from the brain

(e) recording/picture of _____
    heart echoes

(f) technique of making a _____
    picture/tracing using echoes

Thermography

Thermography is the technique of recording temperature differences throughout the body on film.

Our bodies radiate a range of infrared waves at different frequencies. The frequency of the radiation depends on the temperature of the body. Thermography uses electronic equipment to convert infrared radiation into visible light which is then imaged. Thermography has proved of great benefit in the detection of breast and testicular tumours. Tumours contain abnormally active cells and so tend to be warmer than surrounding areas.

Root	**Therm** (From a Greek word **therme** meaning heat.)
Combining forms	**Therm/o**

WORD EXERCISE 9

Without using your Exercise Guide, write the meaning of:

(a) **thermo**gram _____

(b) scrotal **thermo**graphy _____

Medical equipment and clinical procedures

Revise the names of all instruments and techniques used in this unit before trying Exercise 10.

WORD EXERCISE 10

Match each term in Column A with a description in Column C by placing an appropriate number in Column B.

Column A	Column B	Column C
(a) radiography	_____	1. instrument which detects gamma rays from radioisotopes
(b) fluoroscopy	_____	2. technique of using ultrasound echoes to image the heart
(c) thermography	_____	3. chemical used to improve detail of an X-ray
(d) ultrasonograph	_____	4. technique of making an X-ray
(e) computerized tomograph	_____	5. instrument which makes tracing/ picture using reflected sound
(f) radiotherapy	_____	6. instrument which uses X-rays to image a slice through the body
(g) cineradiography	_____	7. direct observation of X-ray picture using a fluorescent screen
(h) gamma camera	_____	8. technique of recording body heat on film
(i) echocardiography	_____	9. treatment of disorders using radiation
(j) contrast medium	_____	10. technique of using X-rays to make a moving picture

Quick Reference

Medical roots relating to radiology and nuclear medicine:

Cine/o	movement/motion (picture)
Ech/o	reflected sound
Fluor/o	fluorescent/luminous/flow
Radi/o	radiation/X-ray
Roentgen/o	X-ray
Scint/i	spark/flash of light
Son/o	sound
Therm/o	heat
Tom/o	slice/section
Ultrason/o	ultrasound

Abbreviations

You should learn common abbreviations related to radiology and nuclear medicine. Note, however, some are not standard and their meaning may vary from one hospital to another. There is a more extensive list for reference on page 259.

AXR	abdominal X-ray
Ba	barium
CAT	computerized axial tomography
CXR	chest X-ray
DSA	digital subtraction angiography
DXT	deep X-ray therapy
EUA	examination under anaesthesia (Am. anesthesia)
MRI	magnetic resonance imaging
NMR	nuclear magnetic resonance
PET	positron emission tomography
US	ultrasound/ultrasonography
XR	X-ray

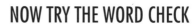

> **NOW TRY THE WORD CHECK**

WORD CHECK

This self-check exercise lists all the word components used in this unit. First write down the meaning of as many word components as you can. Then check your answers using the Exercise Guide and Quick Reference box or the Glossary of Word Components (pp. 269–279).

Prefixes

ultra- _____

Combining forms of word roots

angi/o _____

cardi/o _____

cine/o _____

ech/o _____

encephal/o _____

fluor/o _____

oesophag/o
(Am. esophag/o) _____

radi/o _____

roentgen/o _____

scint/o _____

son/o _____

therm/o _____

tom/o _____

Suffixes

-er _____

-genic _____

-gram _____

-graph _____

-graphy _____

-ist _____

-logy _____

-scope _____

-scopy _____

-therapy _____

> ## NOW TRY THE SELF-ASSESSMENT

SELF-ASSESSMENT

Test 18A

Prefixes, suffixes and combining forms of word roots

Match each word component in Column A with a meaning in Column C by inserting the appropriate number in Column B.

Column A	Column B	Column C
(a) angi/o	_____	1. X-ray/radiation
(b) cinemat/o	_____	2. X-rays
(c) ech/o	_____	3. specialist
(d) -er	_____	4. treatment
(e) fluor/o	_____	5. beyond/excess
(f) -genic	_____	6. slice/section/cut
(g) -gram	_____	7. sound
(h) -graph	_____	8. heat
(i) -graphy	_____	9. technique of recording/ making picture
(j) -ist	_____	10. technique of visual examination
(k) radi/o	_____	11. vessel
(l) roentgen/o	_____	12. picture/ tracing/X-ray picture
(m) scint/i	_____	13. movement/ motion picture
(n) -scope	_____	14. pertaining to formation/ originating in
(o) -scopy	_____	15. reflected sound
(p) son/o	_____	16. instrument to view
(q) -therapy	_____	17. luminous (to flow)
(r) -therm/o	_____	18. spark (flash or light)

	Column A	Column B		Column C
(s)	tom/o	_____	19.	instrument which records/tracing or picture, or the picture/ tracing/X-ray itself
(t)	ultra-	_____	20.	one who

Score

20

Test 18B

Write the meaning of:

(a) roentgenotherapy   _____

(b) sonologist   _____

(c) thermoradiotherapy   _____

(d) radiocinematograph   _____

(e) ultrasonotomography   _____

Score

5

Test 18C

Build words which mean:

(a) treatment using ultrasound   _____

(b) pertaining to examination by a fluoroscope   _____

(c) technique of making a picture of vessels using sparks/flashes of light   _____

(d) instrument used to detect and image heat from the body   _____

(e) technique of imaging the brain using echoes (use ech/o)   _____

Score

5

Check answers to Self-Assessment Tests on page 256.

19 Oncology

Objectives

Once you have completed Unit 19 you should be able to:

- understand the meaning of medical words relating to oncology
- build medical words relating to oncology
- understand medical abbreviations relating to oncology.

Exercise Guide

Use this list of word components and their meanings to complete the word exercises in this unit.

Roots/Combining forms

angi/o	vessel
chondr/o	cartilage
haem/o	blood
hem/o (Am.)	blood
leiomy/o	smooth muscle
mening/i	meninges (membranes of CNS)
rhabdomy/o	striated muscle

Suffixes

–genesis	formation of
–genic	pertaining to formation/ originating in
–ia	condition of
–ic	pertaining to
–ist	specialist
-logist	specialist who studies
–logy	study of
–lysis	breakdown/disintegration
–oma	tumour/swelling
–osis	abnormal condition/disease/ abnormal increase
–static	pertaining to stopping/ controlling
–tropic	pertaining to stimulating/ affinity for

Oncology

This is the branch of medicine which specializes in the study of malignant tumours commonly referred to as cancers. A tumour is a mass or swelling which consists of dividing cells that appear to be out of control. Benign tumours remain localized and do not threaten life. Malignant tumours spread and may lead to death. Tumours spread when they release cells into the blood and lymph; these cells multiply in new sites forming secondary growths or metastases (from Greek *meta* + *histanai*, *meta* meaning changed in form, *histanai* to place/set, i.e. a growth in a different position).

As the tumours grow they consume nutrients, depriving normal cells of essential metabolic components. A clinical feature called **cachexia** is seen in advanced stages of disease (from Greek *kakos* meaning bad and *hexis* meaning state). The body appears to suffer from malnutrition and becomes thin and 'wastes' away.

In this unit we will examine terms which relate to common types of tumour.

Use the Exercise Guide at the beginning of this unit to complete Word Exercises 1–3 unless you are asked to work without it.

Root	**Onc** *(From a Greek word **onkos**, meaning bulk. Here it is used to mean a tumour (Am. tumor).)*
Combining forms	**Onc/o**

WORD EXERCISE 1

Using your Exercise Guide, find the meaning of:

(a) **onc**osis _____

(b) **onco**genesis _____

(c) **onco**tropic _____

Using your Exercise Guide, build words which mean:

(d) pertaining to formation _____
of a tumour

(e) destruction/disintegration _____
of a tumour

(f) person who specializes in the _____
study and treatment of tumours

The process of tumour formation is also known as **neoplasia** and the tumour itself as a **neoplasm** (**neo** meaning new, **plasia**, from Greek *plassein*, meaning to form). Neoplastic, derived in the same way, is also used to mean pertaining to a new growth (synonymous with oncogenic).

Before we study the next word root, we need to examine the use of the suffix **-oma**. Used by itself in combination with a tissue type, it indicates a benign tumour, e.g. oste**oma** – a benign bone tumour.

Malignant tumours may also be designated by **-oma** but they are usually preceded by the word **malignant**, e.g. **malignant melanoma**, a malignant tumour of the pigment cells, **malignant lymphoma**, a tumour of lymphatic tissue.

(To confuse matters, -oma is occasionally used for a non-neoplastic condition such as haematoma (Am. hematoma), which refers to a swelling filled with blood and is not a new growth of cells.)

Two terms which are widely used when referring to malignant tumours are:

Carcinoma
a malignant tumour of epithelial origin. Remember epithelia cover organs and line cavities and may form membranes or glands.

Sarcoma
a malignant tumour of supporting tissues, i.e. connective tissues and muscle.

These terms are studied below.

Root	**Carcin** *(From a Greek word **karkinos**, meaning crab. It is used to mean a malignant tumour/cancer.)*
Combining forms	**Carcin/o**

A **carcin**oma is a tumour of an epithelium of which there are numerous types. They are usually named by using the word carcinoma preceded by the histological type and followed by the organ of origin, e.g.:

Squamous cell carcinoma of the lung
originates in non-glandular epithelium.

Adenocarcinoma of the breast
originates in a glandular epithelium within the breast.

Often carcinomas are more simply named, e.g. as carcinoma of the colon or carcinoma of the urinary bladder.

Note.   A substance which stimulates the formation of a malignant tumour is known as a carcinogen.

WORD EXERCISE 2

Without using your Exercise Guide, write the meaning of:

(a) **carcino**genic   _____

(b) **carcino**lysis   _____

Using your Exercise Guide, find the meaning of:

(c) **carcino**static   _____

Also from this root we have the word cancer, which is imprecisely used to mean carcinoma or cancer in situ. It is sometimes preceded by words which indicate the cause of a cancer, e.g.:

- radiologist's cancer
- smoker's cancer
- asbestos cancer.

Root	Sarc
	(From a Greek word **sarkoma**, *meaning a fleshy growth.)*
Combining forms	**Sarc/o**

Sarcomas are malignant tumours which are less common than carcinomas. They are derived from cells which have developed from the supporting tissues of the body, such as the connective tissues, i.e. bone, cartilage, blood and lymph, and from muscle tissue. The word sarcoma is preceded by the tissue type, e.g. osteo**sarc**oma, a malignant bone tumour.

Note.   **Sarcomat/o** are combining forms of sarcoma.

WORD EXERCISE 3

Using your Exercise Guide, find the meaning of:

(a) chondro**sarc**oma   _____

(b) leiomyo**sarc**oma   _____

(c) rhabdomyo**sarc**oma   _____

(d) meningeal **sarc**oma   _____

(e) haemangio**sarc**oma   _____
(Am. hemangiosarcoma)

Without using your Exercise Guide, write the meaning of:

(f) **sarcomat**osis   _____

Most malignant tumours arise from epithelial tissues. When a malignant tumour no longer resembles its tissue of origin and its cells are disordered, it is anaplastic (**ana** meaning backward, **plast** meaning growth).

Another form of malignant tumour is the mixed tissue tumour. These contain cells which resemble both epithelial and connective tissue cells.

Diagnosis of malignant tumours

Precise classification of malignant tumours is essential for determining their growth, tendency to metastasize and their prognosis (i.e. forecast of probable course of disease).

Attempts to develop an international language for describing the extent of malignant disease have been made. One of these is in widespread use and is known as the **TNM** system.

T – tumour
It categorizes the primary tumour and its size.

N – nodes
It defines the number of lymph nodes which have been invaded.

M – metastases
It indicates their presence or absence.

The extent of malignant disease defined by these categories is termed **staging**. Staging defines the size of tumour, its growth and progression at any one point.

Many different staging systems are in use for different cancers. It is not possible to study them here, but we have included a basic system which is outlined below.

T
- T_0 — no primary tumour
- T_1 — primary tumour limited to site of origin
- T_{2-4} — progressive increase in size of primary tumour
- T_x — primary tumour cannot be assessed
- T_{is} — primary tumour in situ

N
- N_0 — no evidence of spread to nodes
- N_1 — spread to nodes in immediate area
- N_{2-4} — increasing number of lymph nodes invaded
- N_x — lymph nodes cannot be assessed

M
- M_0 — no evidence of metastases
- M_{1-3} — ascending degrees of metastases

Using the above system, we can see the principle of how a cancer is staged:

$T_2\, N_1\, M_0$
This stage would indicate that the primary tumour is large and has spread to deeper structures (T_2). It has spread to one lymph node draining the area (N_1) and there is no evidence of a distant metastasis (M_0).

Staging is not an exact description of a tumour's progress but it is a useful way to estimate the course of the disease when planning treatment (therapy).

Medical equipment and clinical procedures

We have already described the main instruments and procedures which are used in the diagnosis and treatment of cancers in Unit 18. Tumours can be detected using radiography, CAT, thermography, MRI, etc., and radiotherapy is used to destroy them.

Other procedures used to destroy tumours include excision surgery and chemotherapy, i.e. treatment using cytotoxic drugs which poison tumour cells.

Quick Reference

Medical roots relating to oncology:

Aden/o	gland
Cancer/o	cancer
Carcin/o	cancerous/malignant
Melan/o	pigment
Onc/o	tumour
Sarc/o	fleshy/connective tissue

Abbreviations

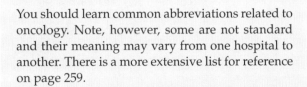

You should learn common abbreviations related to oncology. Note, however, some are not standard and their meaning may vary from one hospital to another. There is a more extensive list for reference on page 259.

BCC	basal cell carcinoma
BT	bone tumour
BX or Bx	biopsy
CA or Ca	cancer/carcinoma
CACX	cancer of the cervix
CF	cancer free
MEN	multiple endocrine neoplasia
Metas	metastasis
N & V	nausea & vomiting
SA	sarcoma
T	tumour
t	terminal

> ## NOW TRY THE WORD CHECK

WORD CHECK

This self-check exercise lists all the word components used in this unit. First write down the meaning of as many word components as you can. Then check your answers using the Exercise Guide and Quick Reference box or the Glossary of Word Components (pp. 269–279).

Prefixes

ana- _____

meta- _____

neo- _____

Combining forms of word roots

aden/o _____

angi/o _____

cancer/o _____

carcin/o _____

chem/o _____

chondr/o _____

cyt/o _____

haem/o _____
(Am. hem/o)

leiomy/o _____

melan/o _____

meningi/o _____

onc/o _____

rhabdomy/o _____

sarc/o _____

Suffixes

–genic _____

–genesis _____

–ia _____

–ic _____

–ist _____

–logy _____

–lysis _____

–oma _____

–osis _____

–plasia _____

–plastic _____

–static _____

–therapy _____

–toxic _____

–tropic _____

> **NOW TRY THE SELF-ASSESSMENT**

SELF-ASSESSMENT

Test 19A

Prefixes, suffixes and combining forms of word roots

Match each word component in Column A with a meaning in Column C by inserting the appropriate number in Column B.

Column A	Column B	Column C
(a) aden/o	_____	1. pertaining to
(b) ana-	_____	2. change position or form
(c) cancer/o	_____	3. pertaining to formation/ originating in
(d) carcinoma	_____	4. membranes of CNS
(e) chondr/o	_____	5. striated muscle
(f) -genic	_____	6. condition of growth (increase of cells)
(g) -ic	_____	7. pertaining to stopping/ controlling
(h) -ist	_____	8. pertaining to affinity for/ acting on
(i) leiomy/o	_____	9. gland
(j) melan/o	_____	10. cancer (general term)
(k) meningi/o	_____	11. cancer/tumour (medical term)
(l) meta-	_____	12. cartilage
(m) neo-	_____	13. benign tumour (when suffix is used alone)
(n) -oma	_____	14. malignant tumour of epithelium
(o) onc/o	_____	15. malignant tumour of supporting tissue

Column A	Column B	Column C
(p) -plasia	_____	16. specialist
(q) rhabdomy/o	_____	17. smooth muscle
(r) sarcomat/o	_____	18. pigment
(s) -static	_____	19. new
(t) -tropic	_____	20. backward

Score

20

Test 19B

Write the meaning of:

(a) fibrosarcoma   _____
(fibr/o – fibre/fibrous)

(b) gastric adenocarcinoma   _____
(gastr/o – stomach)

(c) hepatocellular carcinoma   _____
(hepat/o – liver)

(d) anaplastic thyroid carcinoma   _____
(thyr/o – thyroid)

(e) bronchogenic carcinoma   _____
(bronch/o – bronchus)

Score

5

Test 19C

Build words which mean:

(a) malignant tumour of lymph   _____
(use sarc/o)

(b) benign tumour of cartilage   _____

(c) a malignant tumour originating   _____
in bone (use sarc/o)

(d) condition of a new growth   _____
of cells

(e) the treatment of tumours   _____

Score

5

Check answers to Self-Assessment Tests on page 256.

Anatomical position

Objectives

Once you have completed Unit 20 you should be able to:

- understand the meaning of medical words relating to the anatomical position

- build medical words relating to regions and positions in the body

- associate medical terms with their anatomical position

- understand medical abbreviations relating to anatomical positions.

Exercise Guide

Use this list of word components and their meanings to complete the word exercises in this unit.

Prefixes

epi-	above/upon/on
hypo-	below/under

Roots/Combining forms

bucc/o	cheek
cardi/o	heart
cephal/o	head
chondr/o	cartilage
cost/o	rib
crani/o	cranium/skull
derm/o	skin
faci/o	face
-ganglion	ganglion
gastr/o	stomach
hepat/o	liver
ili/o	hip/ilium/flank
mamm/o	breast/mammary gland
nas/o	nose
or/o	mouth
ot/o	ear
stern/o	sternum
ven/o	vein
-version	turn
vertebr/o	vertebra/spine

Suffixes

–al	pertaining to
–ary	pertaining to
–iac	pertaining to
–ic	pertaining to

Anatomical position

In this unit we will examine a selection of terms which refer to the position of organs and tissues within the body. Many of these terms are also used to indicate the position of injuries, pain, disease and surgical operations.

The **anatomical position** of the body (Fig. 90) is a reference system which all doctors and medical texts use when describing body components. Note that the right and left sides refer to the sides of the patient not the observer. We always refer to position in the patient's body as if he/she were standing upright with arms at the sides and palms of the hands facing forward, head erect and eyes looking forward.

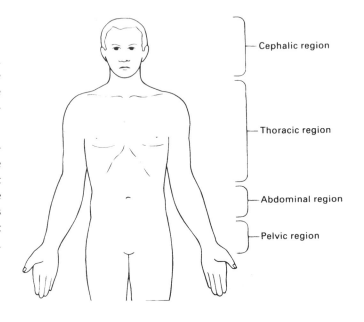

Figure 91 Regions of the trunk and head

Each of these regions can be subdivided (Fig. 92). The simplest example is perhaps the division of the abdominopelvic region into quadrants.

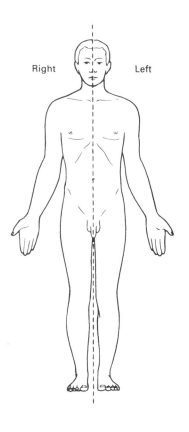

Figure 90 The anatomical position

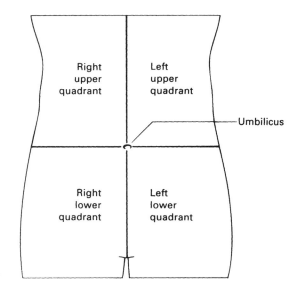

Figure 92 Abdominopelvic region (quadrants)

With the body in this position, it can be divided into regions, e.g. the trunk can be divided into thoracic, abdominal and pelvic regions (Fig. 91).

Doctors and health personnel often use this simple system to describe the position of abdominopelvic pain. The quadrants are formed by imaginary vertical and horizontal lines through the umbilicus. A more complex method is to divide the abdominopelvic region into nine regions (Fig. 93).

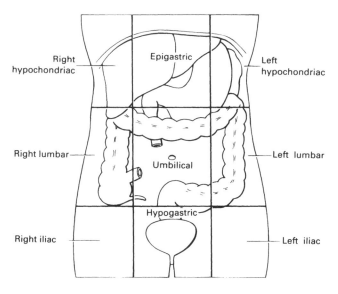

Right hypochondriac

Epigastric

Left hypochondriac

Right lumbar

Umbilical

Left lumbar

Right iliac

Hypogastric

Left iliac

Figure 93   Abdominopelvic region (nine regions)

Use the Exercise Guide at the beginning of this unit to complete Word Exercises 1–7 unless you are asked to work without it.

WORD EXERCISE 1

Using your Exercise Guide, find the meaning of:

(a) hypochondriac _____

Without using your Exercise Guide, write the meaning of:

(b) epigastric _____

(c) iliac _____

Note. The cartilage referred to in (a) is the cartilage of the rib-cage.

The cephalic regions and the upper and lower extremities can also be subdivided into regions. These are examined in the next two exercises.

WORD EXERCISE 2

Examine Figure 94 and match the regions listed in Column A with a number from the diagram:

Column A	Number
(a) cephalic region	_____
(b) cranial region	_____
(c) facial region	_____
(d) otic region	_____
(e) oral region	_____
(f) mammary region	_____
(g) nasal region	_____
(h) buccal region	_____

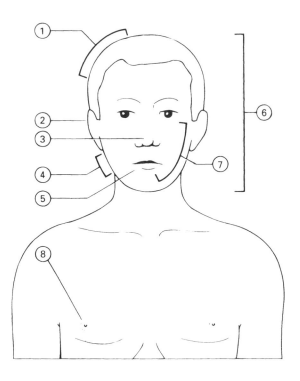

Figure 94   Regions of the head and thorax

WORD EXERCISE 3

Look at Figures 95 and 96 and label the regions of each limb by selecting an appropriate region from the list below. The first region has been labelled for you.

hallux region	great toe
crural region	leg
pedal region	foot
digital/phalangeal region	toes
patellar region	knee
femoral region	thigh
tarsal region	ankle
axillary region	armpit
palmar/volar region	palm
antebrachial region	forearm
digital/phalangeal region	fingers
brachial region	arm
pollex region	thumb
carpal region	wrist

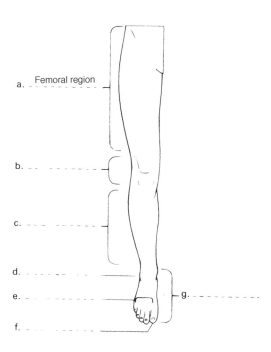

Figure 95   Leg regions

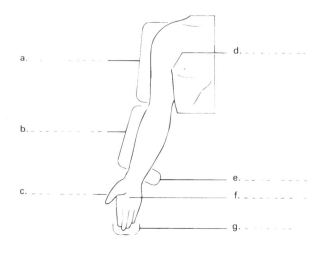

Figure 96   Arm regions

Now let us return to the anatomical position and draw an imaginary line along the middle of the body (Fig. 97). This is known as the **median line**.

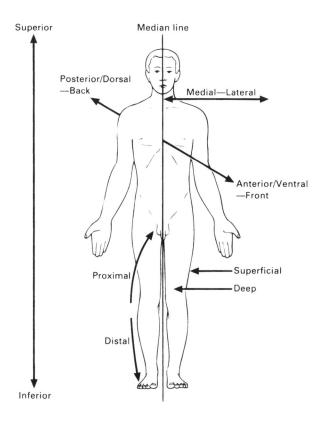

Figure 97   Anatomical directions

Parts of the body which lie nearer to the median line of the body than another are described as **medial** to that part. Any part which lies further away is said to be **lateral** to the first part. To summarize:

| **Medial** towards the median line |
| **Lateral** away from the median line |

Figure 97 also shows the use of:

| **Superior** towards the head, upper |
| **Inferior** away from the head, lower |
| **Anterior (ventral)** front |
| **Posterior (dorsal)** back |
| **Proximal** near point of attachment or point of origin |
| **Distal** further from point of attachment or origin |
| **Superficial** near the surface of the body |
| **Deep** away from the surface of the body |

 WORD EXERCISE 4

Using the information in Figure 97, complete the following sentences by deleting the incorrect word:

(a) The eyes are superior/inferior to the mouth.

(b) The mouth is superior/inferior to the nose.

(c) The ear is medial/lateral to the eye.

(d) The nostril is medial/lateral to the eye.

(e) The umbilicus lies on the anterior/posterior surface of the abdomen.

(f) The vertebrae lie close to the dorsal/ventral surface of the body.

(g) The wrist is proximal/distal to the elbow.

(h) The ankles are proximal/distal to the toes.

(i) The ribs are superficial/deep to the lungs.

These terms can also be applied to organ systems and tissues within the body. They too are described as if they are in the anatomical position, e.g. the digestive system (Fig. 98).

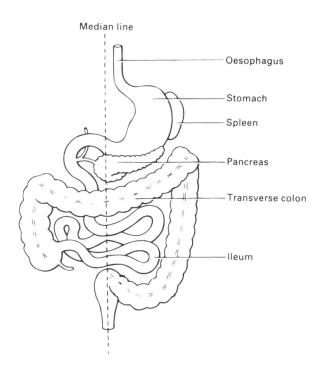

Figure 98 Digestive system position

 WORD EXERCISE 5

Using information from Figure 98, complete the following sentences by deleting the incorrect word:

(a) The pancreas is superior/inferior to the stomach.

(b) The oesophagus is superior/inferior to the stomach.

(c) The stomach is medial/lateral to the spleen.

(d) The oesophagus is proximal/distal to the stomach.

(e) The transverse colon is anterior/posterior to the ileum.

(f) The ileum is dorsal/ventral to the transverse colon.

Locating parts of the body

There are a large number of locative prefixes which act as prepositions when placed in front of word roots. These tell us about the position of structures within the body. Use the list of locative prefixes below to complete the next two exercises.

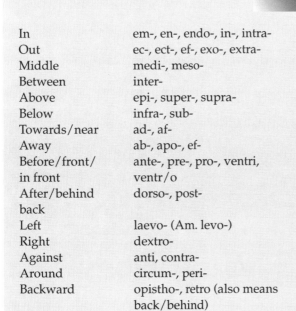

Locative prefixes

In	em-, en-, endo-, in-, intra-
Out	ec-, ect-, ef-, exo-, extra-
Middle	medi-, meso-
Between	inter-
Above	epi-, super-, supra-
Below	infra-, sub-
Towards/near	ad-, af-
Away	ab-, apo-, ef-
Before/front/ in front	ante-, pre-, pro-, ventri, ventr/o
After/behind back	dorso-, post-
Left	laevo- (Am. levo-)
Right	dextro-
Against	anti, contra-
Around	circum-, peri-
Backward	opistho-, retro (also means back/behind)
Beside	para-
Side	later-
Through	dia-, per-,
Upon	epi-
Across	trans-

WORD EXERCISE 6

Use the list above to fill in each blank with an appropriate locative prefix:

(a) The region beside the nose _____ nasal region

(b) Disc between vertebrae _____ vertebral disc

(c) Region upon the stomach _____ gastric region

(d) Pertaining to after a ganglion _____ ganglionic

(e) Condition of right displacement of heart _____ cardia

(f) Nerve below orbit of eye _____ orbital nerve

WORD EXERCISE 7

Use your Exercise Guide and the locative prefix list to find the meaning of:

(a) pericardial _____

(b) intravenous _____

(c) intercostal _____

(d) retroverted uterus _____

(e) suprahepatic _____

(f) infrasternal _____

(g) preganglionic _____

(h) extracellular _____

(i) subepidermal _____

Quick Reference

Medical roots relating to anatomical parts and positions of the body:

Anter/o	front/anterior
Axill/o	armpit
Brachi/o	arm
Bucc/o	cheek
Carp/o	carpal/wrist bones
Cephal/o	head
Crani/o	cranium
Crur/o	leg
Digit/o	finger/toe
Faci/o	face
Femor/o	femur/thigh
Hallux	great toe
Ili/o	ilium/flank
Infer/o	towards the feet/inferior
Later/o	side

Quick Reference (contd)

Medical roots relating to anatomical parts and positions of the body:

Mamm/o	breast/mammary gland
Nas/o	nose
Or/o	mouth
Ot/o	ear
Palm/o	palm
Patell/o	patella/knee cap
Ped/o	foot
Phalang/o	phalange/finger/toe
Pollex	thumb
Poster/o	back/posterior
Super/o	towards the head/superior
Tars/o	tarsus/ankle
Vol/o	palm

Abbreviations

You should learn common abbreviations related to anatomical position. Note, however, some are not standard and their meaning may vary from one hospital to another. There is a more extensive list for reference on page 259.

ant	anterior
inf	inferior
lat	lateral
LLQ	left lower quadrant
LUQ	left upper quadrant
med	medial
pos	position
post	posterior
prox	proximal
RLQ	right lower quadant
RUQ	right upper quadrant
sup	superior

NOW TRY THE WORD CHECK

WORD CHECK

This self-check exercise lists all the word components used in this unit. First write down the meaning of as many word components as you can. Then check your answers using the Exercise Guide and Quick Reference box or the Glossary of Word Components (pp. 269–279).

Prefixes

ab- _____

ad- _____

af- _____

ante _____

anti- _____

apo- _____

circum- _____

contra- _____

dextro- _____

dia- _____

dorso- _____

ec- _____

ect- _____

ef- _____

em- _____

en- _____

endo- _____

exo- _____

extra- _____

in- _____

infra- _____

inter- _____

intra- _____

laevo-
(Am. levo-) _____

medi- _____

meso- _____

opistho- _____

para- _____

per- _____

peri- _____

pre- _____

pro- _____

retro- _____

super- _____

supra- _____

trans- _____

ventro- _____

Combining forms of word roots

anter/o _____

axill/o _____

brachi/o _____

bucc/o _____

carp/o _____

cephal/o _____

crani/o _____

crur/o _____

derm/o _____

digit/o _____

faci/o _____

femor/o _____

hallux _____

ili/o _____

infer/o _____

later/o _____

mamm/o _____

nas/o _____

or/o _____

ot/o _____

palm/o _____

patell/o _____

ped/o _____

phalang/o _____

pollex _____

poster/o _____

super/o _____

tars/o _____

vol/o _____

Suffixes

-al _____

-ary _____

-ia _____

-ic _____

> **NOW TRY THE SELF-ASSESSMENT** ◁

SELF-ASSESSMENT

Test 20A
Combining forms relating to parts of body

Match each combining form in Column A with a meaning in Column C by inserting the appropriate number in Column B.

	Column A	Column B	Column C
(a)	abdomin/o	_____	1. head
(b)	axill/o	_____	2. leg
(c)	brachi/o	_____	3. great toe
(d)	carp/o	_____	4. ankle
(e)	cephal/o	_____	5. palm (i)
(f)	crani/o	_____	6. palm (ii)

Column A	Column B	Column C
(g) crur/o	_____	7. knee
(h) digit/o	_____	8. finger/toe (i)
(i) femor/o	_____	9. finger/toe (ii)
(j) hallux	_____	10. pelvis
(k) ili/o	_____	11. thumb
(l) palm/o	_____	12. thigh/femur
(m) patell/o	_____	13. abdomen
(n) ped/o	_____	14. skull/cranium
(o) pelv/i	_____	15. thorax
(p) phalang/o	_____	16. foot
(q) pollex	_____	17. arm
(r) tars/o	_____	18. armpit
(s) thorac/o	_____	19. ilium/flank
(t) vol/o	_____	20. wrist

Score

20

Test 20B

Locative prefixes

Match each locative prefix from Column A with a meaning in Column C by inserting the appropriate number in Column B.

Column A	Column B	Column C
(a) ab-	_____	1. through (i)
(b) ad-	_____	2. through (ii)
(c) circum-	_____	3. backward/behind
(d) dextro-	_____	4. across
(e) dia-	_____	5. between
(f) ec-	_____	6. side
(g) en-	_____	7. around (i)
(h) epi-	_____	8. around (ii)
(i) infra-	_____	9. away
(j) inter-	_____	10. before/in front of
(k) laevo- (Am. levo-)	_____	11. beside
(l) later-	_____	12. towards

Column A	Column B	Column C
(m) para-	_____	13. after/behind
(n) per-	_____	14. right
(o) peri-	_____	15. upon
(p) post-	_____	16. in
(q) pre-	_____	17. above
(r) retro-	_____	18. left
(s) supra-	_____	19. below
(t) trans-	_____	20. out

Score

20

Test 20C

Write the meaning of:

(a) interphalangeal _____

(b) dextroversion _____

(c) retrobuccal _____

(d) supracostal _____

(e) intracellular _____

Score

5

Test 20D

Build words which mean:

(a) pertaining to the side _____

(b) a turning towards the left _____

(c) pertaining to after a ganglion _____

(d) pertaining to below the liver _____

(e) pertaining to across the skin _____

Score

5

Check answers to Self-Assessment Tests on page 257.

Answers to word exercises

Unit 1 Levels of organization

Word Exercise 1

(a) Cyt – word root meaning cell, o – combining vowel, pathy – suffix meaning disease
(b) Disease of cells
(c) Study of disease
(d) Study of disease of cells
(e) Breakdown/disintegration of cells
(f) Pertaining to poisonous to cells
(g) Specialist who studies cells

Word Exercise 2

(a) Erythr – word root meaning red, o – combining vowel, cyte – word root meaning cell
(b) Red cell

Word Exercise 3

(a) Melanocyte
(b) Fibrocyte
(c) Lympho/lymphocyte (lymph cell)
Spermato/spermatocyte (sperm cell)
Oo/oocyte (egg cell)
Granulo/granulocyte (granular cell)
Chondro/chondrocyte (cartilage cell)

Word Exercise 4

(a) Bone-forming cell/immature bone cell
(b) Fibre-forming cell/immature fibre cell
(c) Immature blood cell/cell which forms blood cells

Word Exercise 5

(a) The chemistry of tissues (refers to study of)
(b) Study of diseased tissues
(c) Person who specializes in study of tissues
(d) Breakdown/disintegration of tissues

Word Exercise 6

(a) Small
(b) Instrument to view small objects
(c) Technique of viewing very small objects with a microscope
(d) Person who specializes in microscopy

Word Exercise 7

(a) The formation of organs
(b) Pertaining to nourishing/stimulating organs

Unit 2 The digestive system

Word Exercise 1

(a) Instrument to view the oesophagus
(b) Removal of oesophagus
(c) Incision into the oesophagus
(d) Inflammation of the oesophagus

Word Exercise 2

(a) Instrument to view the stomach
(b) Removal of part or all of stomach
(c) Incision into stomach
(d) Inflammation of the stomach, especially the lining
(e) Gastropathy
(f) Gastrology

Word Exercise 3

(a) Inflammation of the intestines
(b) Disease of the intestines
(c) Incision into the intestines
(d) Opening into the intestine (often to connect to stomach, ileum, jejunum or abdominal wall)
(e) Intestinal stone (compacted material in intestine)
(f) Enterology
(g) Enterologist
(h) Study of intestines and stomach (+ associated structures, e.g. liver and pancreas)
(i) Disease of intestines and stomach
(j) Inflammation of the intestines and stomach (often due to infection)
(k) Technique of viewing the intestines and stomach

Word Exercise 4

(a) Removal of stomach and pylorus
(b) Technique of viewing pylorus (with an endoscope)

Word Exercise 5

(a) Formation of an opening (anastomosis) between the intestine and duodenum
(b) Formation of an opening (anastomosis) between one part of the jejunum and another part of the jejunum
(c) Pertaining to the jejunum and duodenum
(d) Ileostomy
(e) Ileitis

Word Exercise 6

(a)   Large colon

(b)   Inflammation of the appendix

(c)   Removal of the colon

(d)   Opening into the colon (usually a connection between the colon and the abdominal wall; it acts as an artificial anus)

(e)   Caecostomy (Am. cecostomy)

(f)   Appendicectomy (Am. Appendectomy)

(g)   Gastrocolostomy

Word Exercise 7

(a)   Technique of viewing the sigmoid colon

(b)   Pertaining to beside the rectum

(c)   Inflammation around anus/rectum

(d)   Administration of fluid into anus/rectum (enema)

(e)   Condition of pain in the anus/rectum

(f)   Proctoscope

(g)   Proctocaecostomy (Am. proctocecostomy)

(h)   Caecosigmoidostomy (Am. cecosigmoidostomy)

Word Exercise 8

(a)   Inflammation of the peritoneum

(b)   Infusion/injection into peritoneum

Word Exercise 9

(a)   Breaking down of the pancreas

(b)   Enlargement of the liver

(c)   Liver tumour

(d)   Pertaining to poisonous to the liver

(e)   Formation of an opening between the stomach and hepatic duct

(f)   Pertaining to the duodenum and pancreatic duct

Word Exercise 10

(a)   Condition of absence of bile

(b)   Bile stone

(c)   Abnormal condition of stones in bile duct (or gall bladder)

(d)   Condition of bile in blood

(e)   Condition of bile in urine

(f)   Incision into gall bladder

(g)   Removal of gall bladder

(h)   Abnormal condition of stones in gall bladder

(i)   X-ray film demonstrating bile ducts (vessels)

(j)   Technique or process of making a cholangiogram

(k)   Abnormal condition of stones in common bile duct

(l)   Incision into common bile duct to remove stones

Word Exercise 11

(a)   Visual examination of the abdomen (i.e. abdominal cavity) with a laparoscope

(b)   Incision into the abdomen

Word Exercise 12

(a)   Enteroscope (4)

(b)   Endoscope (6)

(c)   Enteroscopy (7)

(d)   Endoscopy (9)

(e)   Endoscopist (8)

(f)   Colonoscopy (3)

(g)   Proctoscope (1)

(h)   Sigmoidoscopy (10)

(i)   Panendoscopy (5)

(j)   Photoendoscopy (2)

Unit 3 The breathing system

Word Exercise 1

(a)   Technique of viewing the nose

(b)   Disease of the nose

(c)   Condition of pain in the nose

(d)   Inflammation of the nose

(e)   Excessive flow/discharge from the nose

(f)   Surgical repair of the nose

Word Exercise 2

(a)   A tube which passes from nose to stomach (for suction or feeding)

(b)   A tube which passes from nose to oesophagus (for suction or feeding)

Word Exercise 3

(a)   Condition of pain in pharynx

(b)   Excessive flow/discharge from the pharynx

(c)   Pharyngoplasty

(d)   Pharyngorhinitis

Word Exercise 4

(a)   Study of the larynx

(b)   Removal of the pharynx and larynx

(c)   Laryngoscopy

(d)   Laryngorhinology

Word Exercise 5

(a)   Incision into the trachea

(b)   Formation of an opening into the trachea (to establish a safe airway) or the opening itself

Word Exercise 6

(a)   Bronchorrhoea (Am. bronchorrhea)

(b)   Bronchogram

(c)   Bronchography

(d)   Bronchoscope

(e)   The windpipe itself – bronchus

(f)   Condition of paralysis of the bronchi

(g)   Suturing of the bronchi

(h)   Dilatation of the bronchi

(i)   Abnormal condition of fungi in bronchi

(j)   Originating in the bronchi/pertaining to formation of bronchi

(k)   Pertaining to the bronchi and trachea

(l)   Inflammation of bronchi, trachea and larynx
(m)   Formation of an opening between the oesophagus and bronchus

Word Exercise 7

(a)   Incision into the lung
(b)   Suturing of the lung
(c)   Disease/abnormal condition of lung
(d)   Pneumonectomy
(e)   Pneumonopathy
(f)   Puncture of the lung (by surgery)
(g)   Fixation of a lung by surgery (to thoracic wall)

Word Exercise 8

(a)   Blood and air in thorax (pleural cavity)
(b)   Technique of making an X-ray after injection of air
(c)   Without breathing (temporary, due to low levels of carbon dioxide in blood)
(d)   Difficult/painful breathing
(e)   Above normal breathing (higher rate and depth)
(f)   Below normal breathing (low rate and depth)
(g)   Fast breathing

Word Exercise 9

(a)   Lobotomy
(b)   Lobectomy

Word Exercise 10

(a)   Pertaining to the lungs
(b)   Pertaining to the lungs

Word Exercise 11

(a)   Inflammation of the pleura
(b)   Puncture of the pleura
(c)   Pleurography
(d)   Condition of pain in the pleura
(e)   Adhesion/fixation of pleura

Word Exercise 12

(a)   Pertaining to the stomach and diaphragm
(b)   Pertaining to the liver and diaphragm
(c)   Condition of paralysis of the diaphragm

Word Exercise 13

(a)   Thoracopathy
(b)   Thoracotomy
(c)   Puncture of the thorax (by surgery)
(d)   Instrument to view the thorax
(e)   Abnormal condition of narrowing of the thorax

Word Exercise 14

(a)   Pertaining to between the ribs
(b)   Pertaining to originating in the ribs/pertaining to forming ribs
(c)   Inflammation of cartilage of the ribs

Word Exercise 15

(a)   Bronchoscope (3)
(b)   Laryngoscopy (4)
(c)   Rhinoscope (8)
(d)   Pharyngoscope (6)
(e)   Bronchoscopy (7)
(f)   Rhinologist (1)
(g)   Tracheostomy tube (5)
(h)   Laryngoscope (2)

Word Exercise 16

(a)   Thoracoscope (5)
(b)   Stethoscope (7)
(c)   Spirometer (6)
(d)   Spirography (3)
(e)   Nasal speculum (1)
(f)   Nasogastric tube (8)
(g)   Pleurography (2)
(h)   Spirometry (4)

Unit 4 The cardiovascular system

Word Exercise 1

(a)   Condition of pain in the heart
(b)   Instrument to view the heart
(c)   Instrument which records the heart beat (force and form)
(d)   Tracing/recording made by a cardiograph
(e)   Condition of fast heart rate
(f)   Cardiomegaly
(g)   Cardioplasty
(h)   Cardiopathy
(i)   Cardiology
(j)   The heart muscle
(k)   Disease of heart muscle
(l)   Stitching/suturing of heart
(m)   Instrument which records electrical activity of heart
(n)   Inflammation inside heart (lining)
(o)   Inflammation of all of heart
(p)   Condition of slow heart beat
(q)   Condition of right heart (heart displaced to right)
(r)   Technique of recording heart sounds
(s)   Technique of recording (ultrasound) echoes of heart
(t)   Tracing of electrical activity of heart

Word Exercise 2

(a)   Pericarditis
(b)   Fixation of the pericardium to the heart
(c)   Puncture of the pericardium (by surgery)
(d)   Removal of the pericardium

Word Exercise 3

(a)   Valvoplasty

(b)   Valvectomy

(c)   Instrument for cutting a heart valve

(d)   Pertaining to a valve

(e)   Incision into a valve

Word Exercise 4

(a)   Sudden contraction of a blood vessel

(b)   Pertaining to without blood vessels

(c)   Vasculitis

(d)   Vasculopathy

Word Exercise 5

(a)   X-ray picture of blood vessels (usually arteries)

(b)   X-ray picture of heart and major vessels

(c)   Technique of making an angiocardiogram

(d)   Angiology

(e)   Angioplasty

(f)   Tumour formed from blood vessels (non-malignant)

(g)   Dilatation of blood vessels

(h)   Formation of blood vessels

(i)   Hardening of blood vessels

Word Exercise 6

(a)   Aortopathy

(b)   Aortography

Word Exercise 7

(a)   Arteriorrhaphy

(b)   Arteriosclerosis

(c)   Removal of lining of artery

(d)   Abnormal condition of decay of arteries

(e)   Abnormal condition of narrowing of arteries

Word Exercise 8

(a)   X-ray picture of a vena cava

(b)   Technique of making an X-ray/tracing of the venae cavae

Word Exercise 9

(a)   Dilatation of a vein (varicosity or varicose vein)

(b)   Injection or infusion into a vein (of nutrients or medicines)

(c)   Venogram

(d)   Venography

Word Exercise 10

(a)   General dilatation of arteries and veins

(b)   Injection/infusion into a vein

(c)   Incision into vein

(d)   Cessation of movement of blood in a vein

(e)   Instrument to measure pressure within a vein

(f)   Concretion or stone within a vein

Word Exercise 11

(a)   Formation of a clot

(b)   Inflammation of a vein associated with a thrombus

(c)   Removal of the lining of an artery and a thrombus

(d)   Thrombosis

(e)   Thrombectomy

(f)   Formation of clots

(g)   Disintegration/breakdown of clots

Word Exercise 12

(a)   Formation of atheroma

(b)   Blockage caused by atheroma and embolus

Word Exercise 13

(a)   Surgical repair of an aneurysm

(b)   Suturing/stitching of an aneurysm

Word Exercise 14

(a)   Instrument which measures the force of the pulse (pressure and volume)

(b)   Instrument which measures pressure of the pulse (arterial blood pressure)

(c)   Technique of measuring the pulse

(d)   Instrument which records the pulse

(e)   Tracing/picture/recording of the pulse

(f)   Instrument which records the heart beat and pulse

Word Exercise 15

(a)   Cardioscope (6)

(b)   Cardiograph (4)

(c)   Electrocardiograph (5)

(d)   Cardiovalvotome (2)

(e)   Angiocardiography (3)

(f)   Sphygmomanometer (1)

Word Exercise 16

(a)   Echocardiography (6)

(b)   Sphygmocardiograph (5)

(c)   Stethoscope (2)

(d)   Phonocardiogram (1)

(e)   Electrocardiogram (3)

(f)   Phlebomanometer (4)

Unit 5 The blood

Word Exercise 1

(a)   The study of blood

(b)   Study of diseases of the blood

(c)   Pertaining to the force and movement of the blood (study of)

(d)   Formation of the blood

(e)   Cessation of blood flow/stopping of bleeding by clotting

(f)   Blood in the pericardial sac (around heart)

(g)   haematoma (Am. hematoma)

(h)   haemolysis (Am. hemolysis)

(i)   haematuria (Am. hematuria)

(j)   haemorrhage (Am. hemorrhage)

(k)   Too many blood cells (refers to conditions in which there is an increase in the number of circulating red blood cells)

(l)   Without blood (refers to condition of reduced number of red cells and/or quantity of haemoglobin)

(m)   Condition of decay of blood (due to infection)

(n)   Instrument which measures haemoglobin

(o)   Blood protein

(p)   Condition of haemoglobin in the urine

(q)   Condition of abnormal decrease of haemoglobin (colour)

(r)   Condition of abnormal increase of haemoglobin (colour)

Word Exercise 2

(a)   Condition of reduction in number of red blood cells

(b)   Formation of red blood cells

(c)   Immature germ cell which gives rise to red blood cells

(d)   Formation of red blood cells

(e)   Breakdown of red blood cells

(f)   Condition of erythrocyte blood, i.e. too many red blood cells

(g)   Abnormal condition of too many small cells (small erythrocytes)

(h)   Abnormal condition of too many large cells (large erythrocytes)

(i)   Abnormal condition of too many elliptical cells (elliptical erythrocytes)

(j)   Abnormal condition of too many unequal cells (unequally sized erythrocytes)

(k)   Abnormal condition of too many irregular/varied cells (variably shaped erythrocytes)

Word Exercise 3

(a)   Reticuloblast

(b)   Reticulocytosis

(c)   Reticulopenia

Word Exercise 4

(a)   Leucopenia

(b)   Leucopoiesis

(c)   Formation of white blood cells

(d)   Condition of white blood (synonymous with leukocythaemia, a malignant cancer of white blood cells)

(e)   Abnormal condition of white cells (an increase in white blood cells, usually transient in response to infection)

(f)   Tumour of leucocytes

(g)   Immature germ cell which gives rise to leucocytes

(h)   Abnormal condition of too many white germ cells (results in proliferation of leucocytes)

(i)   Pertaining to poisonous to white cells

Word Exercise 5

(a)   Marrow cell

(b)   Condition of fibres in marrow

(c)   Myeloblast

(d)   Myeloma

Word Exercise 6

(a)   Condition of reduction in the number of platelets

(b)   Formation of platelets

(c)   Breakdown of platelets

(d)   Disease of platelets

(e)   Instrument which measures the volume of thrombocytes in a sample of blood, or the actual value of the measured volume of thrombocytes in a sample

(f)   Withdrawal of blood, removal of red cells and retransfusion of remainder

(g)   Withdrawal of blood, removal of thrombocytes and retransfusion of remainder

(h)   Withdrawal of blood, removal of leucocytes and retransfusion of remainder

Word Exercise 7

(a)   Plasmapheresis (4)

(b)   Differential count (3)

(c)   Haematocrit (2)

(d)   Haemoglobinometer (5)

(e)   Blood count (1)

Unit 6 The lymphatic system

Word Exercise 1

(a)   Abnormal condition of lymph cells (too many cells)

(b)   Condition of bursting forth of lymph (from lymph vessels)

(c)   Technique of making an X-ray/tracing of lymphatic vessels

(d)   X-ray picture/tracing of a lymph vessel

(e)   Dilatation of a lymph vessel

(f)   Tumour of a lymph gland

(g)   Removal of a lymph gland

(h)   Disease of a lymph gland

(i)   Inflammation of a lymph gland

Word Exercise 2

(a)   Enlargement of the spleen

(b)   Enlargement of the liver and spleen

(c)   Surgical fixation of the spleen

(d)   Hernia/protrusion of the spleen

(e)   Condition of softening of spleen

(f)   Breakdown/disintegration of spleen

(g)   X-ray picture of the spleen

(h)   X-ray picture of portal vein and spleen

Word Exercise 3

(a) Tonsillitis

(b) Tonsillectomy

(c) Pertaining to the pharynx and tonsils

(d) Instrument to cut the tonsils

Word Exercise 4

(a) Thymocyte

(b) Thymopathy

(c) Thymocele

(d) Abnormal condition of ulceration of thymus

(e) Pertaining to lymphatics and thymus

Word Exercise 5

(a) Immunology

(b) Immunopathology

(c) Formation of immunity

(d) Self-immunity (immune system acts against self, producing an autoimmune disease)

(e) Protein of immune system (antibody)

Word Exercise 6

(a) Serology

Word Exercise 7

(a) Condition of pus in blood (infection in blood)

(b) Pertaining to generating pus

(c) Flow of pus (usually referring to pus flowing from teeth sockets)

(d) Formation of pus

Word Exercise 8

(a) Lymphography (5)

(b) Lymphangiography (4)

(c) Lymphadenography (6)

(d) Lymphogram (2)

(e) Splenoportogram (1)

(f) Tonsillotome (3)

Unit 7 The urinary system

Word Exercise 1

(a) Pertaining to the stomach and kidney

(b) X-ray/tracing of the kidney

(c) Technique of making an X-ray/tracing of kidney

Word Exercise 2

(a) Falling kidney (downward displacement)

(b) Abnormal condition of water in kidney (swelling)

(c) Swelling/hernia of a kidney

(d) Condition of pain in a kidney

(e) Nephropexy

(f) Nephroplasty

(g) Nephrotomy

(h) Nephrolithiasis

(i) Nephrectomy

(j) Inflammation of glomeruli (producing pus)

(k) Disease of glomeruli

(l) Abnormal condition of hardening of glomeruli

Word Exercise 3

(a) Inflammation of kidney and renal pelvis

(b) Incision to remove stone from renal pelvis

(c) Disease/abnormal condition of the kidney and renal pelvis

(d) Pyeloplasty

(e) Pyelogram

Word Exercise 4

(a) Hernia/protrusion of the ureter

(b) Removal of a ureterocele

(c) Condition of excessive flow of blood from the ureter

(d) Suturing of the ureter

(e) Dilatation of a ureter

(f) Visual examination of the kidney and ureters

(g) Formation of an opening into the ureter

(h) Ureteroenterostomy

(i) Ureterocolostomy

Word Exercise 5

(a) Inflammation of the bladder

(b) Removal of stones from bladder

(c) Inflammation of renal pelvis and bladder

(d) Falling/displacement of bladder

(e) Instrument to view the bladder

(f) Formation of an opening between rectum/anus and bladder

(g) Cystometer

(h) Cystometry

(i) Cystometrogram

Word Exercise 6

(a) Vesicostomy

(b) Vesicotomy

(c) Infusion/injection into the bladder

(d) Pertaining to the bladder

(e) Opening between sigmoid colon and bladder (to drain urine)

(f) Pertaining to the ureter and bladder

Word Exercise 7

(a) Process of measuring the urethra

(b) Inflammation of trigone and urethra

(c) Fixation (by surgery) of the urethra

(d) Urethralgia

(e) Urethrorrhagia

(f) Urethroscopy

(g) Tumour/boil in urethra

(h) Instrument for cutting urethra

(i) Abnormal condition of narrowing of urethra

(j) Condition of pain in the urethra

Word Exercise 8

(a) Pertaining to carrying urine
(b) Urine splitting/separating for analysis
(c) Instrument to measure urine

Word Exercise 9

(a) Technique of recording the urinary tract (X-ray)
(b) Person specializing in the study of the urinary tract
(c) Formation of urine
(d) Condition of little urine (diminished secretion of)
(e) Condition of albumin in urine
(f) Condition of urea (too much) in urine
(g) Condition of much urine
(h) Condition of painful/difficult (flow) of urine
(i) Condition of blood in urine
(j) Condition of pus in urine

Word Exercise 10

(a) Inflammation of kidney due to stones
(b) Condition of calculus or stones in urine
(c) Formation of stones
(d) Instrument to crush stones
(e) Washing of stones from bladder following crushing
(f) Instrument which uses shock waves to destroy stones
(g) The procedure of breaking stones using shock waves
(h) Excretion of stones in the urine

Word Exercise 11

(a) Diathermy (8)
(b) Cystoscope (10)
(c) Lithotriptor (7)
(d) Urinometer (9)
(e) Haemodialyser (2)
(f) Ureteroscopy (4)
(g) Urethrotome (3)
(h) Cystometer (5)
(i) Urethroscope (6)
(j) Lithotrite (1)

Unit 8 The nervous system

Word Exercise 1

(a) Study of nerves/nervous system
(b) Disease of the nervous system
(c) Condition of pain in nerves
(d) Nerve fibre tumour (arises from connective tissue around nerves)
(e) Inflammation of many nerves
(f) Pertaining to formation of nerves/originating in nerves
(g) Neurosclerosis
(h) Neuromalacia
(i) Neurologist
(j) Wasting/decay of nerves
(k) Pertaining to affinity for/stimulating nervous tissue
(l) Injury to nerve
(m) Nerve glue cell
(n) Tumour of nerve glue cells (gliocytes)

Word Exercise 2

(a) Disease of a plexus
(b) Pertaining to the formation of a plexus/originating in a plexus

Word Exercise 3

(a) Hernia/protrusion from head
(b) Pertaining to without a head
(c) A tumour of blood within the head (actually a collection of blood in sub-periosteal tissue, the result of an injury)
(d) Thing (baby) with water in head
(e) Microcephalic
(f) Cephalogram
(g) Cephalometry
(h) Thing (baby) with large head
(i) Pertaining to turning motion of head

Word Exercise 4

(a) Tumour of brain
(b) Abnormal condition of pus (infection) of brain
(c) Pertaining to without a brain
(d) Instrument which records electrical activity of the brain
(e) Encephalography
(f) Pneumoencephalography
(g) Electroencephalography
(h) Encephalopathy
(i) Encephalocele
(j) Tracing/picture of brain made using reflected ultrasound (echoes)
(k) Middle brain
(l) Inflammation of grey matter of brain

Word Exercise 5

(a) Cerebrosclerosis
(b) Cerebromalacia
(c) Cerebrosis

Word Exercise 6

(a) Ventriculoscopy
(b) Ventriculotomy
(c) Technique of making X-ray of brain ventricles
(d) Opening between the cistern (subarachnoid space) and ventricles

Word Exercise 7

(a) Craniotomy
(b) Craniometry

Word Exercise 8

(a) Ganglioma

(b) Pertaining to before a ganglion

(c) Pertaining to after a ganglion

(d) Removal of a ganglion

Word Exercise 9

(a) Meningitis

(b) Meningocele

(c) Meningorrhagia

(d) Hernia/protrusion of brain through meninges

(e) Inflammation of brain and meninges

(f) Disease of brain and meninges

(g) Tumour of the meninges

(h) Pertaining to above/upon the dura

(i) Swelling/tumour of blood beneath the dura

Word Exercise 10

(a) Inflammation of the ganglia and spinal roots

(b) Inflammation of nerves and spinal nerve roots

(c) Incision into a spinal root

Word Exercise 11

(a) Inflammation of the meninges and spinal cord

(b) Hernia/protrusion of the spinal cord through the meninges

(c) Inflammation of spinal nerve roots and spinal cord

(d) Inflammation of brain and spinal cord

(e) Wasting of the spinal cord

(f) Inflammation of grey matter of spinal cord

(g) Myelosclerosis

(h) Myelomalacia

(i) Myelography

(j) Condition of abnormal/difficult development/growth (of cells) of the spinal cord

(k) Without nourishment of the spinal cord (wasting away/poor growth)

(l) Abnormal condition of a tube (cavity) in spinal cord

Word Exercise 12

(a) Instrument to measure spine (curvature)

(b) Puncture of spine

(c) Splitting of spine

Word Exercise 13

(a) Condition of paralysis of all four limbs

(b) Condition of paralysis of half body, right or left side

(c) Condition of near/beside paralysis (lower limbs)

(d) Condition of two parts paralysed (similar parts on either side of body)

(e) Condition of paralysis of four limbs (synonymous with quadriplegia)

Word Exercise 14

(a) Condition of without sensation/state of being anaesthetized

(b) Pertaining to a drug which reduces sensation

(c) Study of anaesthesia

(d) Person who administers anaesthesia/specialist in anaesthesia

(e) Condition of anaesthesia of half the body (one side)

(f) Condition of decreased sensation

(g) Condition of increased sensation

(h) Post-anaesthesic/anaesthetic/anaesthesia

(i) Pre-anaesthesic/anaesthetic/anaesthesia

Word Exercise 15

(a) Abnormal condition of stupor/deep sleep (drug induced)

(b) Treatment with narcotics

Word Exercise 16

(a) Condition of sensing pain

(b) Condition of without sensation of pain

(c) Condition of excessive/above normal sensation of pain

(d) Pertaining to a loss of pain/drug which reduces pain

Word Exercise 17

(a) Study of the mind (behaviour)

(b) Pertaining to the mind

(c) Disease of the mind

(d) Abnormal condition/disease of the mind

(e) Drug which acts on/has an affinity for the mind

(f) Pertaining to body and mind (actually body symptoms of mental origin)

(g) (Study of) treatment of mind; a psychiatrist is a doctor who treats the mind

Word Exercise 18

(a) Condition of fear of heights (peaks, extremities)

(b) Condition of fear of open spaces

(c) Condition of fear of water

(d) Condition of fear of cancer

(e) Condition of fear of death/dead bodies

Word Exercise 19

(a) Pertaining to forming/causing epileptic fit

(b) Pertaining to following/after an epileptic fit

(c) Having form of epilepsy

Word Exercise 20

(a) Encephalography (5)

(b) Pneumoencephalography (4)

(c) Ventriculoscopy (6)

(d) Tendon hammer (1)

(e) Tomograph (2)

(f) Craniometry (3)

Word Exercise 21

(a) MRI (3)

(b)   Lumbar puncture (6)
(c)   Myelography (5)
(d)   CAT (1)
(e)   Electroencephalography (2)
(f)   Ventriculography (4)

Unit 9 The eye

Word Exercise 1

(a)   Ophthalmoscope
(b)   Ophthalmologist
(c)   Ophthalmoplegia
(d)   Ophthalmitis
(e)   Ophthalmomycosis
(f)   Pertaining to circular movement of eye
(g)   Inflammation of optic nerve
(h)   Inflammation of all eye
(i)   Instrument to measure tension (pressure) within the eye
(j)   Condition of inflammation of eye with mucus discharge
(k)   Condition of inflammation due to dryness of eye
(l)   In eye (displacement of eyes into sockets)
(m)   Out eye (bulging eyes)

Word Exercise 2

(a)   Pertaining to one eye
(b)   Pertaining to one eye
(c)   Pertaining to two eyes
(d)   Nerve which stimulates eye movement/action
(e)   Pertaining to nose and eye
(f)   Picture/tracing of electrical activity of eye
(g)   Pertaining to circular movement of eye

Word Exercise 3

(a)   Instrument to measure sight
(b)   Technique of measuring sight
(c)   Person who measures sight (specializes in optometry)
(d)   Instrument for measuring the muscles of sight (power of ocular muscles)
(e)   Condition of sensation of sight (ability to perceive visual stimuli)

Word Exercise 4

(a)   Condition of double vision
(b)   Condition of old man's vision
(c)   Condition of dim vision
(d)   Condition of half colour vision (faulty colour vision in half field of view)
(e)   Condition of painful/difficult/bad vision
(f)   Condition of without half vision (blindness in one half of visual field in one or both eyes)

Word Exercise 5

(a)   Blepharoplegia

(b)   Blepharospasm
(c)   Blepharoptosis
(d)   Blepharorrhaphy
(e)   Flow of pus from eyelid
(f)   Inflammation of eyelid glands (meibomian glands)
(g)   Condition of sticking together of eyelids
(h)   Slack, loose eyelids (causes drooping)

Word Exercise 6

(a)   Incision into sclera
(b)   Dilatation of sclera
(c)   Instrument to cut sclera

Word Exercise 7

(a)   Inflammation of cornea and sclera
(b)   Measurement of cornea (actually curvature of cornea)
(c)   Instrument to cut cornea
(d)   Surgical repair of cornea (corneal graft)
(e)   Puncture of the cornea
(f)   Abnormal condition of ulceration of cornea
(g)   Puncture of the cornea
(h)   To carve the cornea
(i)   Cone-like protrusion of the cornea

Word Exercise 8

(a)   Iridoptosis
(b)   Iridokeratitis
(c)   Motion/movement of iris (contraction and expansion)
(d)   Separation of iris
(e)   Hernia/protrusion of iris (through cornea)
(f)   Separation of iris and sclera
(g)   Incision into iris and sclera
(h)   Inflammation of iris and cornea

Word Exercise 9

(a)   Inflammation of ciliary body and iris
(b)   Condition of paralysis of ciliary body
(c)   Destruction through heat of ciliary body

Word Exercise 10

(a)   Goniometer
(b)   Gonioscope
(c)   Goniotomy

Word Exercise 11

(a)   Condition of paralysis of pupil
(b)   Measurement of pupil (diameter)

Word Exercise 12

(a)   Condition of unequal pupils
(b)   Surgical fixation of pupil into new position
(c)   Condition of equal pupils
(d)   Surgical repair of pupil

Word Exercise 13

(a) Inflammation of ciliary body and choroid
(b) Inflammation of choroid and sclera

Word Exercise 14

(a) Tumour of germ cells of retina
(b) Condition of softening of retina
(c) Splitting (separation of retina)
(d) Disease of the retina
(e) Technique of viewing the retina
(f) Electroretinogram
(g) Retinochoroiditis
(h) Choroidoretinitis

Word Exercise 15

(a) Swelling of the optic disc
(b) Retinopapillitis

Word Exercise 16

(a) Phacomalacia
(b) Phacoscope
(c) Phacosclerosis
(d) Aphakia
(e) Removal of lens bladder (capsule)
(f) Sucking out of lens

Word Exercise 17

(a) Instrument to measure scotomas
(b) Technique of measuring scotomas
(c) Instrument to record scotomas

Word Exercise 18

(a) Lacrimotomy
(b) Nasolacrimal

Word Exercise 19

(a) Tear bladder (lacrimal sac)
(b) Technique of making an X-ray of the lacrimal sac
(c) Formation of an opening between the nose and lacrimal sac
(d) Tear stone
(e) Abnormal condition of narowing lacrimal duct (apparatus)
(f) Pertaining to stimulation of tears
(g) Flow of mucus from lacrimal sac
(h) Condition of pus in lacrimal sac

Word Exercise 20

(a) Ophthalmoscope (4)
(b) Dacrycystogram (1)
(c) Keratome (5)
(d) Pupillometry (8)
(e) Optometry (7)
(f) Scotometry (2)
(g) Ophthalmotonometer (3)
(h) Optomyometer (6)

Word Exercise 21

(a) Sclerotome (5)
(b) Optometer (4)
(c) Keratometry (6)
(d) Pupillometer (8)
(e) Phacoscope (7)
(f) Retinoscopy (1)
(g) Tonography (2)
(h) Dacryocystography (3)

Unit 10 The ear

Word Exercise 1

(a) Otology
(b) Otoscope
(c) Otosclerosis
(d) Otopyosis
(e) Study of the larynx, nose and ear
(f) Abnormal condition of fungi in the ear
(g) Excessive flow of pus from the ear
(h) Condition of small ears
(i) Condition of large ears

Word Exercise 2

(a) Auriscope
(b) Pertaining to two ears
(c) Pertaining to within the ear
(d) Pertaining to having two ear flaps (pinnae)

Word Exercise 3

(a) Myringotomy
(b) Myringotome
(c) Myringomycosis

Word Exercise 4

(a) Tympanoplasty
(b) Tympanocentesis
(c) Inflammation of the middle ear/ear drum
(d) Incision into the middle ear/ear drum

Word Exercise 5

(a) Blocking up of Eustachian tube
(b) Pertaining to pharynx and Eustachian tube

Word Exercise 6

(a) Stapedectomy
(b) Cutting of tendon of stapes

Word Exercise 7

(a) Incision into the malleus

Word Exercise 8

(a) Pertaining to malleus and incus
(b) Pertaining to stapes and incus
(c) Pertaining to the incus and malleus

Word Exercise 9

(a) Cochleostomy

(b) Electrocochleography

Word Exercise 10

(a) Labyrinthitis

(b) Labyrinthectomy

Word Exercise 11

(a) Incision into the vestibule

(b) Pertaining to originating in the vestibule

Word Exercise 12

(a) Mastoidalgia

(b) Mastoidotomy

(c) Mastoidectomy

(d) Tympanomastoiditis

Word Exercise 13

(a) Audiology

(b) Instrument which measures hearing

(c) Tracing/recording made by an audiometer

(d) Technique of measuring hearing/using an audiometer

Word Exercise 14

(a) Audiometer (6)

(b) Audiometry (1)

(c) Aural speculum (7)

(d) Auriscope (2)

(e) Otoscopy (3)

(f) Aural syringe (4)

(g) Grommet (5)

Unit 11 The skin

Word Exercise 1

(a) Abnormal condition of the skin

(b) Outer skin (layer above/upon skin)

(c) Skin plant (fungus which infects skin)

(d) Thick skin

(e) Yellow skin

(f) Self surgical repair of skin (using one's own skin for a graft)

(g) Condition of dry skin

(h) Dermatomycosis

(i) Dermatome

(j) Hypodermic/subdermal

(k) Intradermal

Word Exercise 2

(a) Abnormal condition of the epidermis caused by excessive exposure to sun

(b) Abnormal condition of the epidermis (above normal thickening)

(c) Tumour of the epidermis

(d) Breakdown/disintegration of the epidermis

Word Exercise 3

(a) Nerve which performs an action to move hair (erects hair)

Word Exercise 4

(a) Abnormal condition of hair plants (fungal infection)

(b) Abnormal condition of hair

(c) Condition of sensitive hairs

(d) Condition of split hairs

(e) Broken/ruptured hairs

Word Exercise 5

(a) Excessive flow of sebum

(b) Sebaceous stone (actually hardened sebum)

(c) Pertaining to stimulating the sebaceous glands

Word Exercise 6

(a) Abnormal condition of sweating (excess)

(b) Condition of increased/above normal sweating

(c) Formation of sweat

(d) Abnormal condition of without sweating

(e) Inflammation of sweat glands

Word Exercise 7

(a) Abnormal condition of hidden nail (ingrowing)

(b) Condition of increased growth of nails

(c) Difficult/poor growth of nails (malformation)

(d) Without nourishment/wasting away of nails

(e) Condition beside a nail (inflammation)

(f) Splitting/parting of nails

(g) Condition of nail eating (actually biting)

(h) Onycholysis

(i) Onychomycosis

(j) Onychitis

(k) Rupture/breaking of nails

(l) Condition of without nails

(m) Condition of thickened nails

Word Exercise 8

(a) Melanocyte

(b) Melanosis

(c) Tumour of melanin (melanocytes), highly malignant

Word Exercise 9

(a) Excision biopsy (4)

(b) Dermatome (5)

(c) Medical laser (2)

(d) PUVA (6)

(e)   Epilation (1)

(f)   Electrolysis (3)

Unit 12 The nose and mouth

Word Exercise 1

(a)   Study of mouth

(b)   Condition of excessive flow (of blood) from mouth

(c)   Disease of mouth

(d)   Stomatodynia/stomatalgia

(e)   Stomatomycosis

Word Exercise 2

(a)   Pertaining to the mouth

(b)   Pertaining to the pharynx and mouth

(c)   Pertaining to the nose and mouth

Word Exercise 3

(a)   Glossology

(b)   Glossodynia/glossalgia

(c)   Glossopharyngeal (e.g. glossopharyngeal nerve IX)

(d)   Condition of paralysis of the tongue

(e)   Condition of hairy tongue

(f)   Protrusion/swelling of tongue

(g)   Condition of large tongue

(h)   Surgical repair of the tongue

Word Exercise 4

(a)   Removal of salivary gland

(b)   Technique of making X-ray/tracing of salivary vessels/ducts

(c)   Condition of much saliva (excess secretion)

(d)   X-ray of salivary glands and ducts

(e)   Sialolith

(f)   A drug which stimulates saliva (production)

(g)   Condition of eating air and saliva (excessive swallowing)

Word Exercise 5

(a)   Pertaining to formation of saliva/originating in saliva

(b)   Excessive flow of saliva

(c)   Stone in the saliva

Word Exercise 6

(a)   Gnathalgia/gnathodynia

(b)   Gnathoplasty

(c)   Gnathology

(d)   Stomatognathic

(e)   Instrument which measures force of jaw (closing force)

(f)   Split or cleft jaw

(g)   Inflammation of the jaw

Word Exercise 7

(a)   Surgical repair of mouth and lip

(b)   Split/cleft lip

(c)   Suturing of lips

(d)   Cheilitis

Word Exercise 8

(a)   Pertaining to larynx, tongue and lips

(b)   Labioglossopharyngeal

Word Exercise 9

(a)   Gingivitis

(b)   Gingivectomy

(c)   Pertaining to gums and lips

Word Exercise 10

(a)   Palatoplegia

(b)   Palatognathic

(c)   Palatoschisis

Word Exercise 11

(a)   Uvulectomy

(b)   Uvulotomy

Word Exercise 12

(a)   Condition of without speech/loss of voice

(b)   Condition of difficult speech

Word Exercise 13

(a)   Odontology

(b)   Odontopathy

(c)   Odontalgia

(d)   Pertaining to around the teeth (study of tissues that support the teeth)

(e)   Study of inside of teeth (pulp, dentine, etc.)

(f)   Pertaining to straight teeth (branch of dentistry dealing with the straightening of teeth and associated facial abnormalities)

(g)   Person who specializes in orthodontics

(h)   Pertaining to adding teeth (branch of dentistry dealing with the construction of artificial teeth and other oral components)

Word Exercise 14

(a)   Condition of nasal voice (speech through nose)

(b)   Technique of measuring pressure (air flow) in nose

(c)   Tumour/swelling/boil of nose

(d)   Condition of excessive flow of blood (from nose)

Word Exercise 15

(a)   Hollow/cavity in bone/anatomical part

(b)   Inflammation of bronchi and sinuses

(c)   Inflammation of a sinus

(d)   X-ray/tracing of sinus

Word Exercise 16

(a) Antroscope
(b) Antrotympanitis
(c) Incision into the antrum
(d) Pertaining to the nose and antrum
(e) Swelling/protrusion of antrum
(f) Pertaining to the cheek and antrum

Word Exercise 17

(a) Pertaining to the face
(b) Condition of paralysis of the face
(c) Surgical repair of the face

Word Exercise 18

(a) Antroscope (3)
(b) Sialangiography (5)
(c) Gnathodynamometer (1)
(d) Rhinomanometer (6)
(e) Prosthesis (4)
(f) Glossography (2)

Unit 13 The muscular system

Word Exercise 1

(a) Pertaining to nerve and muscle
(b) Disease of heart muscle
(c) Poor nourishment (growth) of muscle
(d) Inflammation of a muscle
(e) Abnormal condition of fibres in muscle
(f) Myosclerosis
(g) Myoma
(h) Myoglobin
(i) Myospasm
(j) Condition of involuntary twitching of muscle
(k) Condition of muscle tone (abnormal increased tone)
(l) Slight paralysis of muscle
(m) Rupture of a muscle
(n) Condition of softening of a muscle
(o) Myography
(p) Electromyography
(q) Myogram

Word Exercise 2

(a) Tumour of striated muscle
(b) Breakdown of striated muscle

Word Exercise 3

(a) Pertaining to affinity for/stimulating muscle
(b) Pertaining to the diaphragm muscles
(c) Poor nourishment (growth) of muscle. An inherited disease

Word Exercise 4

(a) Condition of sensation of movement
(b) Instrument which measures muscular movement
(c) Pertaining to forming movements
(d) Condition of above normal movement
(e) Dyskinesia

Word Exercise 5

(a) Condition of pain in a tendon
(b) Instrument to cut tendons
(c) Inflammation of tendons
(d) Study of tendons
(e) Tenomyoplasty
(f) Tenomyotomy
(g) Suturing of an aponeurosis
(h) Inflammation of an aponeurosis

Word Exercise 6

(a) Pertaining to straight child, a branch of surgery which deals with the restoration of function in the musculoskeletal system

Word Exercise 7

(a) Myography (5)
(b) Electromyography (4)
(c) Myogram (2)
(d) Myokinesiometer (6)
(e) Orthosis (1)
(f) Electromyogram (3)

Unit 14 The skeletal system

Word Exercise 1

(a) Bone plant (plant-like growth of bone)
(b) Abnormal condition of passages (pores) in bone
(c) Abnormal condition of stone-like bones
(d) Breaking down of bone
(e) Cell which breaks down bone
(f) Bad nourishment of bone (poor growth)
(g) Osteoblast
(h) Osteolytic
(i) Osteotome

Word Exercise 2

(a) Instrument to view within a joint
(b) Abnormal condition of pus in joint
(c) Technique of making an X-ray of joints
(d) Inflammation of a joint
(e) Fixation of a joint by surgery
(f) Breaking of a joint (actually breaking adhesions within a joint to improve mobility)
(g) Arthroscopy
(h) Arthrocentesis
(i) Arthrogram
(j) Arthropathy
(k) Arthrolith
(l) Arthroplasty

Word Exercise 3

(a) Inflammation of a synovial joint
(b) Removal of the synovial membranes/synovia
(c) Tumour/swelling of a synovial membrane

Word Exercise 4

(a) Plant-like growth of cartilage
(b) Pertaining to bone and cartilage
(c) Abnormal condition of passages (pores) in cartilage
(d) Bad nourishment of cartilage (poor growth)
(e) Pertaining to rib cartilage
(f) Pertaining to within cartilage
(g) Chondralgia
(h) Chondromalacia
(i) Chondrogenesis
(j) Chondrolysis
(k) Abnormal condition of calcified cartilage/abnormal increase in calcium in cartilage

Word Exercise 5

(a) Condition of pain in the vertebrae
(b) Abnormal condition of pus in vertebrae
(c) Spondylolysis
(d) Spondylopathy
(e) Slipping/dislocation of vertebrae

Word Exercise 6

(a) Resembling a disc
(b) Pertaining to forming a disc/originating in a disc
(c) Discography
(d) Discectomy

Word Exercise 7

(a) Inflammation of bone marrow
(b) Abnormal condition of fibres in marrow

Word Exercise 8

(a) Osteotome (4)
(b) Arthrodesis (3)
(c) Replacement arthroplasty (5)
(d) Arthrocentesis (1)
(e) Arthrography (2)

Word Exercise 9

(a) Claviculoplasty
(b) Craniomalacia
(c) Intercostal
(d) Phalangectomy
(e) Pelvic
(f) Olecranarthritis
(g) Tibiofemoral
(h) Scapulodesis
(i) Metatarsalgia
(j) Acetabuloplasty

Unit 15 The male reproductive system

Word Exercise 1

(a) Disease of the testes
(b) Hernia/protrusion/swelling of testes (through scrotum)
(c) Process of hidden testes, i.e. undescended
(d) Surgical fixation of the testes, i.e. into their normal position
(e) Orchiotomy/orchidotomy
(f) Orchioplasty/orchidoplasty
(g) Orchidectomy/orchiectomy
(h) Orchialgia/orchidalgia
(i) Surgical fixation of hidden testes, i.e. into their normal position

Word Exercise 2

(a) Scrotectomy
(b) Scrotoplasty
(c) Scrotocele

Word Exercise 3

(a) Phallitis
(b) Phallic
(c) Phallectomy

Word Exercise 4

(a) Balanitis
(b) Condition of bursting forth (of blood) from the glans penis
(c) Inflammation of the prepuce and glans penis

Word Exercise 5

(a) Epididymitis
(b) Epididymectomy
(c) Inflammation of the testes and epididymis

Word Exercise 6

(a) Removal of the vas deferens (a section of it to prevent transfer of sperm)
(b) Formation of an opening between the epididymis and the vas deferens
(c) Technique of making an X-ray of the epididymis and vas
(d) Cutting/excision of the vas deferens
(e) Suturing of the vas deferens
(f) Formation of an opening between the testes and the vas deferens
(g) Formation of an opening between the vas deferens and another part of the vas deferens
(h) Incision into the vas deferens

Word Exercise 7

(a) Vesiculography

(b)   Vesiculotomy
(c)   Removal of the seminal vesicles and vas deferens

Word Exercise 8

(a)   Incision into the bladder and prostate gland
(b)   Enlargement of the prostate gland
(c)   Removal of the prostate gland
(d)   Removal of the seminal vesicles and prostate gland

Word Exercise 9

(a)   Pertaining to carrying semen
(b)   Condition of semen in the urine
(c)   Tumour of semen (actually the germ cells of the testis)

Word Exercise 10

(a)   Condition of being without sperm
(b)   Condition of few sperm (low sperm count)
(c)   Killing of sperms (actually an agent which is used as a contraceptive by killing sperm)
(d)   Spermatopathia
(e)   Spermatogenesis
(f)   Spermatolysis
(g)   Spermatorrhoea (Am. spermatorrhea)

Word Exercise 11

(a)   Sperm count (5)
(b)   Transurethral resection (4)
(c)   Vasectomy (6)
(d)   Orchidometer (3)
(e)   In vitro fertilization (1)
(f)   Vasoligature (2)

Unit 16 The female reproductive system

Word Exercise 1

(a)   Germ cell which produces eggs
(b)   Egg cell (ovum)
(c)   Formation of eggs

Word Exercise 2

(a)   Oophorectomy
(b)   Oophoropexy
(c)   Oophorotomy
(d)   Removal of bladder (cyst) of ovary (an ovarian cyst)
(e)   Opening into an ovary/formation of an opening into an ovary

Word Exercise 3

(a)   Ovariectomy
(b)   Ovariotomy

(c)   Rupture/breaking of ovary
(d)   Pertaining to the oviduct and ovary
(e)   Puncture of an ovary

Word Exercise 4

(a)   Removal of an ovary and oviduct
(b)   Removal of an oviduct and ovary
(c)   Fixation of a Fallopian tube (by surgery)
(d)   Hernia/protrusion/swelling of oviduct
(e)   Inflammation of ovary and oviduct
(f)   Salpingography
(g)   Salpingolithiasis
(h)   Salpingoplasty

Word Exercise 5

(a)   Uteralgia/uterodynia
(b)   Uterosclerosis
(c)   Pertaining to the tubes (Fallopian) and uterus
(d)   Technique of making an X-ray of the oviduct and uterus
(e)   Pertaining to the bladder and uterus
(f)   Pertaining to the rectum and uterus
(g)   Pertaining to the placenta and uterus

Word Exercise 6

(a)   Hysteroscope
(b)   Hysteroptosis
(c)   Hysterogram
(d)   Technique of making an X-ray of the oviduct and uterus
(e)   Formation of an opening between the oviduct and uterus
(f)   Removal of ovary, oviduct and uterus
(g)   Suturing of the neck of the womb
(h)   Incision into the neck of the womb

Word Exercise 7

(a)   Excessive dripping/bleeding from womb
(b)   Condition of disease of womb with excessive loss of blood
(c)   Inflammation of the peritoneum around the womb
(d)   Inflammation of veins of womb
(e)   Abnormal condition of cysts in the womb
(f)   Abnormal condition of falling/prolapsed womb
(g)   Metrostenosis
(h)   Metromalacia
(i)   Inflammation within the lining of the womb (endometrium)
(j)   Tumour of the endometrium
(k)   Abnormal condition of the endometrium

Word Exercise 8

(a)   Excessive dripping of menses/prolonged menstruation
(b)   Beginning of menstruation
(c)   Stopping of menstruation (occurs in women aged 45–50 years approximately)

(d) Without menstrual flow (menstruation), e.g. as in pregnancy

(e) Difficult/painful/bad menstruation

(f) Reduced flow of menses/infrequent menstruation

(g) Before menstruation

Word Exercise 9

(a) Cervicitis

(b) Cervicectomy

Word Exercise 10

(a) Visual examination of the vagina

(b) Microscope used to view the lining of the vagina in situ

(c) Picture (in this case a differential list) of vaginal cells

(d) Suturing of the perineum and vagina

(e) Removal of the uterus through the vagina

(f) Hernia/protrusion/swelling of the uterus into vagina

(g) Inflammation of the vagina and cervix

(h) Colpoperineoplasty

(i) Colpopexy

Word Exercise 11

(a) Incision into the perineum and vagina

(b) Suturing of the perineum and vagina

(c) Pertaining to the bladder and vagina

(d) Vaginomycosis

(e) Vaginopathy

Word Exercise 12

(a) Inflammation of the vagina and vulva

(b) Surgical repair of the vagina and vulva

Word Exercise 13

(a) Instrument to view the rectouterine pouch

(b) Technique of viewing the rectouterine pouch

(c) Puncture of the rectouterine pouch

Word Exercise 14

(a) Study of women (particularly diseases of the female reproductive tract)

(b) Pertaining to woman-forming (feminizing)

Word Exercise 15

(a) A woman's first pregnancy

(b) A woman's second pregnancy

(c) A woman who is pregnant and has been pregnant more than twice before

(d) A woman who has never been pregnant

Word Exercise 16

(a) A woman who has had one pregnancy which resulted in a viable offspring

(b) A woman who has had two pregnancies which resulted in a viable offspring

(c) A woman who has had more than two pregnancies which resulted in a viable offspring

(d) A woman who has never borne a viable child

Word Exercise 17

(a) Study of the fetus

(b) Instrument to view the fetus

(c) Pertaining to the placenta and fetus

(d) Fetotoxic

(e) Fetometry

Word Exercise 18

(a) Instrument to cut the amnion

(b) Amniotomy

(c) Amnioscope

(d) Technique of making an X-ray of the amnion

(e) An X-ray picture of the amnion

(f) Pertaining to the amnion and fetus

(g) Puncture of the amnion to remove amniotic fluid

(h) Pertaining to the amnion and chorion (fetal membranes)

(i) Inflammation of the amnion and chorion

Word Exercise 19

(a) Placentography

(b) Placentopathy

Word Exercise 20

(a) Condition of difficult/painful/bad birth

(b) Study of labour/birth

(c) Condition of good (normal) birth

Word Exercise 21

(a) Pertaining to new birth

(b) Pertaining to before birth

(c) Pertaining to around/near birth

(d) Pertaining to before birth

(e) Study of neonates (new births)

Word Exercise 22

(a) Technique of making a breast X-ray

(b) Surgical reconstruction/repair of the breast

(c) Pertaining to affinity for/affecting the breast

Word Exercise 23

(a) Mastography

(b) Mastoplasty

(c) Mastectomy

(d) Condition of women's breasts (abnormal condition seen in males)

Word Exercise 24

(a) Agent stimulating/promoting milk production

(b) Pertaining to carrying milk

(c) Instrument to measure milk (specific gravity)

(d) Hormone which nourishes (develops/stimulates) milk

(e) Hormone which acts before milk, i.e. on breast to stimulate lactation
(f) Agent which stops milk
(g) Pertaining to forming milk/originating in milk

Word Exercise 25
(a) Agent which stimulates milk production
(b) Excessive flow of milk
(c) Condition of holding back/stopping milk
(d) Formation of milk

Word Exercise 26
(a) Vaginal speculum (9)
(b) Colposcope (5)
(c) Pap test (7)
(d) Culdoscopy (3)
(e) Fetoscope (10)
(f) Curette (2)
(g) Amniotome (4)
(h) Lactometer (6)
(i) Obstetrical forceps (8)
(j) Tocography (1)

Unit 17 The endocrine system

Word Exercise 1
(a) Process of secreting below normal level of pituitary secretion
(b) Process of secreting above normal level of pituitary secretion
(c) Condition of small extremities, i.e. hands and feet (owing to deficiency of growth hormone)
(d) Large extremities, i.e. hands and feet (owing to excess production of growth hormone in adults)

Word Exercise 2
(a) Pertaining to the tongue and thyroid gland
(b) Inflammation of the thyroid gland
(c) Thyroid protein
(d) Incision into thyroid cartilage
(e) Condition of poisoning by thyroid (owing to overstimulation of thyroid gland)
(f) Near/beside the thyroid/the parathyroid gland
(g) Removal of the parathyroid gland
(h) Process of secreting above normal levels of parathyroid hormones
(i) Enlargement of the thyroid gland
(j) Hyperthyroidism
(k) Hypothyroidism
(l) Thyroptosis
(m) Thyrotropic
(n) Thyrogenic

Word Exercise 3
(a) Pertaining to affinity for/acting on pancreas
(b) Formation of insulin (from Islets of Langerhans)
(c) Tumour of Islets of Langerhans

(d) Inflammation of Islets of Langerhans
(e) Process of secreting above normal level of insulin
(f) Condition of below normal levels of sugar in blood
(g) Condition of above normal levels of sugar in blood
(h) Condition of sugar in urine
(i) Pertaining to a constant glucose level (controlled level)

Word Exercise 4
(a) Adrenomegaly
(b) Adrenotoxic
(c) Adrenotropic
(d) Condition of above normal levels of sodium in blood
(e) Condition of below normal levels of potassium in blood
(f) Secretion of excess sodium in urine
(g) Pertaining to nourishing the adrenal cortex
(h) Condition of above normal growth of cells of adrenal cortex

Word Exercise 5
(a) Pertaining to male and female
(b) Tumour of germ cells of male, i.e. testis

Word Exercise 6
(a) Adrenal function test (4)
(b) Glucose tolerance test (3)
(c) PBI test (2)
(d) Glucose oxidase paper strip test (5)
(e) Thyroid scan (1)

Unit 18 Radiology and nuclear medicine

Word Exercise 1
(a) Specialist who studies radiology (medically qualified)
(b) An X-ray picture
(c) Technique of making an X-ray
(d) One who makes an X-ray (technician, not medically qualified)

Word Exercise 2
(a) Technique of making an X-ray/roentgenogram
(b) Specialist who studies roentgenology/X-rays (medically qualified)
(c) An X-ray picture
(d) X-ray picture of the heart
(e) Fluoroscope
(f) Fluorography

Word Exercise 3
(a) Moving X-ray picture
(b) Technique of making a moving X-ray

(c)   Technique of making a moving X-ray of the heart and vessels

(d)   Moving X-ray picture of the oesophagus (Am. esophagus)

Word Exercise 4

(a)   X-ray picture of a slice/section through body

(b)   Technique of making an X-ray of a slice/section through the body

Word Exercise 5

(a)   Picture of sparks, i.e. distribution of radioactivity within body (synonymous with scintiscan)

(b)   Technique of making a scintigram

Word Exercise 6

(a)   Treatment by radiation

(b)   Specialist who treats disease with radiation (medically qualified)

Word Exercise 7

(a)   Picture/tracing produced using ultrasound

(b)   Technique of making a picture/tracing using ultrasound

(c)   An instrument which uses ultrasound to make a picture/tracing

Word Exercise 8

(a)   Picture/tracing of the brain made using ultrasound echoes

(b)   Echogenic

(c)   Echogram

(d)   Echoencephalograph

(e)   Echocardiogram

(f)   Echography

Word Exercise 9

(a)   Picture/tracing of infrared heat within body

(b)   Technique of making a thermogram of infrared heat from the scrotum (used to detect testicular cancer)

Word Exercise 10

(a)   Radiography (4)

(b)   Fluoroscopy (7)

(c)   Thermography (8)

(d)   Ultrasonograph (5)

(e)   Computerized tomograph (6)

(f)   Radiotherapy (9)

(g)   Cineradiography (10)

(h)   Gamma camera (1)

(i)   Echocardiography (2)

(j)   Contrast medium (3)

Unit 19 Oncology

Word Exercise 1

(a)   Abnormal condition of tumours

(b)   Formation of tumours

(c)   Pertaining to affinity for a tumour

(d)   Oncogenic

(e)   Oncolysis

(f)   Oncologist

Word Exercise 2

(a)   Pertaining to the formation of a carcinoma (malignant tumour of an epithelium)

(b)   Destruction/disintegration of a carcinoma

(c)   Pertaining to stopping growth of a carcinoma

Word Exercise 3

(a)   Malignant tumour of cartilage

(b)   Malignant tumour of smooth muscle

(c)   Malignant tumour of striated muscle

(d)   Malignant tumour of meninges

(e)   Malignant tumour of blood vessels

(f)   Abnormal condition of sarcomas

Unit 20 Anatomical position

Word Exercise 1

(a)   Pertaining to below cartilage (of rib cage)

(b)   Pertaining to upon/above the stomach

(c)   Pertaining to the flank/hip

Word Exercise 2

(a)   6

(b)   1

(c)   7

(d)   2

(e)   5

(f)   8

(g)   3

(h)   4

Word Exercise 3

Leg regions

(a)   femoral region

(b)   patella region

(c)   crural region

(d)   tarsal region

(e)   digital/phalangeal region

(f)   hallux region

(g)   pedal region

Arm regions

(a)   brachial region

(b)   antebrachial region

(c)   pollex region

(d)   axillary region

(e)   carpal region

(f)   palmar/volar region

(g)   digital/phalangeal region

Word Exercise 4

(a)   Superior

(b)   Inferior
(c)   Lateral
(d)   Medial
(e)   Anterior
(f)   Dorsal
(g)   Distal
(h)   Proximal
(i)   Superficial

Word Exercise 5

(a)   Inferior
(b)   Superior
(c)   Medial
(d)   Proximal
(e)   Anterior
(f)   Dorsal

Word Exercise 6

(a)   Paranasal

(b)   Intervertebral
(c)   Epigastric
(d)   Postganglionic
(e)   Dextrocardia
(f)   Infraorbital

Word Exercise 7

(a)   Pertaining to around the heart
(b)   Pertaining to within a vein
(c)   Pertaining to between the ribs
(d)   Uterus turned backwards
(e)   Pertaining to above the liver
(f)   Pertaining to below the sternum
(g)   Pertaining to before/in front of a ganglion
(h)   Pertaining to outside cells
(i)   Under the epidermis

Answers to self-assessment tests

Levels of organization

Test 1A

(a)	7	(h)	4	(o)	16
(b)	14	(i)	17	(p)	20
(c)	18	(j)	12	(q)	11
(d)	19	(k)	5	(r)	15
(e)	8	(l)	10	(s)	6
(f)	3	(m)	1	(t)	13
(g)	9	(n)	2		

Test 1B

(a) Breakdown of cartilage
(b) Breakdown of white cells
(c) Pertaining to poisonous to tissues
(d) Disease of bone
(e) Immature lymph cell/cell which forms lymphocytes

Test 1C

(a) Microcyte
(b) Pathologist
(c) Cytopathologist
(d) Chondrology
(e) Cytopathic

The digestive system

Test 2A

(a)	15	(f)	4	(k)	3
(b)	14	(g)	13/12	(l)	7
(c)	10/11	(h)	5	(m)	8
(d)	2	(i)	12	(n)	6
(e)	9	(j)	1	(o)	11

Test 2B

(a)	14	(h)	17	(o)	11
(b)	20	(i)	15	(p)	13
(c)	2	(j)	7	(q)	10
(d)	5	(k)	12	(r)	4
(e)	19	(l)	3	(s)	18
(f)	9	(m)	16	(t)	8
(g)	6	(n)	1		

Test 2C

(a)	6	(h)	7	(o)	18
(b)	20	(i)	5	(p)	3
(c)	17	(j)	12	(q)	10
(d)	14	(k)	19	(r)	1
(e)	16	(l)	4	(s)	9

(f)	8	(m)	15	(t)	2
(g)	11	(n)	13		

Test 2D

(a) Inflammation of colon, intestine and stomach
(b) Technique of making an X-ray/recording of liver
(c) Pertaining to the rectum and ileum
(d) Instrument to view the sigmoid colon and rectum
(e) Enlargement of the pancreas

Test 2E

(a) Duodenitis
(b) Gastralgia
(c) Hepatotomy
(d) Proctology
(e) Ileoproctostomy

The breathing system

Test 3A

(a)	3	(e)	4	(i)	9
(b)	10	(f)	7/6	(j)	1
(c)	5	(g)	2		
(d)	6/7	(h)	8		

Test 3B

(a)	14	(h)	18	(o)	15
(b)	16	(i)	4	(p)	20
(c)	7	(j)	1	(q)	9
(d)	12	(k)	19	(r)	3
(e)	8	(l)	5	(s)	10
(f)	2	(m)	6	(t)	17
(g)	11	(n)	13		

Test 3C

(a)	3	(h)	13	(o)	17
(b)	19	(i)	12	(p)	9
(c)	5	(j)	10/11	(q)	11/10
(d)	18	(k)	14	(r)	20
(e)	7	(l)	2	(s)	4
(f)	15	(m)	6	(t)	8
(g)	1	(n)	16		

Test 3D

(a) Originating in bronchi/pertaining to formation of bronchi
(b) Abnormal condition of narrowing of trachea
(c) Specialist who studies lungs
(d) Instrument which records diaphragm (movement)

(e)   Condition of paralysis of larynx

Test 3E

(a)   Bronchoplasty
(b)   Bronchoscopy
(c)   Tracheorrhaphy
(d)   Rhinology
(e)   Costophrenic

The cardiovascular system

Test 4A

(a)	6	(c)	4	(e)	2
(b)	1	(d)	5	(f)	3

Test 4B

(a)	8	(h)	20	(o)	3/2
(b)	5	(i)	2/3	(p)	14
(c)	15	(j)	1	(q)	13
(d)	4	(k)	19	(r)	6
(e)	10	(l)	18	(s)	17
(f)	7	(m)	11	(t)	16
(g)	12	(n)	9		

Test 4C

(a)	12	(h)	1	(o)	18
(b)	9/10	(i)	13	(p)	20
(c)	6	(j)	14	(q)	17
(d)	2	(k)	3	(r)	5
(e)	7	(l)	15/16	(s)	10/9
(f)	8	(m)	4	(t)	16/15
(g)	11	(n)	19		

Test 4D

(a)   Inflammation of heart valves
(b)   Suturing of the aorta
(c)   Instrument to view vessels
(d)   Abnormal condition of narrowing of veins
(e)   Inflammation of lining of artery due to a clot

Test 4E

(a)   Thromboarteritis
(b)   Cardiocentesis
(c)   Arteriopathy
(d)   Phlebectomy
(e)   Angiocardiology

The blood

Test 5A

(a)	5	(c)	3/1	(e)	4
(b)	1/3	(d)	2		

Test 5B

(a)	10	(i)	3	(q)	5
(b)	17	(j)	12	(r)	11
(c)	9	(k)	7	(s)	16
(d)	6	(l)	2	(t)	15
(e)	13	(m)	21	(u)	24
(f)	19	(n)	4	(v)	14
(g)	20	(o)	18	(w)	8
(h)	22	(p)	23	(x)	1

Test 5C

(a)   Condition of white blood cells/leucocytes in urine
(b)   Abnormal condition of marrow cells (too many)
(c)   Condition of erythrocytes in urine
(d)   Condition of blood with thrombocytes (too many platelets)
(e)   Breakdown of phagocytes

Test 5D

(a)   Haemopathy (Am. hemopathy)
(b)   Erythrocytopenia
(c)   Haematologist (Am. hematologist)
(d)   Haemotoxic/haematotoxic (Am. hemotoxic/hematotoxic)
(e)   Neutropenia

The lymphatic system

Test 6A

(a)	5	(c)	2	(e)	4
(b)	3	(d)	1		

Test 6B

(a)	14	(h)	10	(o)	15
(b)	5	(i)	3	(p)	11
(c)	8	(j)	13	(q)	9
(d)	4	(k)	18	(r)	20
(e)	2	(l)	17	(s)	7
(f)	1	(m)	19	(t)	12
(g)	16	(n)	6		

Test 6C

(a)   Excessive flow of lymph
(b)   Pertaining to the spleen
(c)   Dilatation of a lymph gland
(d)   Breakdown of thymus
(e)   Specialist who studies sera

Test 6D

(a)   Lymphoma
(b)   Lymphography
(c)   Splenectomy
(d)   Splenorrhagia
(e)   Lymphangioma

The urinary system

Test 7A

(a)	4	(d)	3	(g)	5

(b) 2   (e) 7   (h) 8
(c) 1   (f) 6

Test 7B

(a) 9   (h) 17   (o) 10
(b) 7   (i) 18   (p) 6
(c) 15   (j) 2   (q) 20
(d) 16   (k) 5   (r) 1
(e) 14   (l) 13   (s) 3
(f) 11   (m) 8   (t) 4
(g) 12   (n) 19

Test 7C

(a) 17   (h) 18   (o) 16
(b) 8/9   (i) 12   (p) 7
(c) 11   (j) 5   (q) 13
(d) 15   (k) 3/2   (r) 14
(e) 1   (l) 4   (s) 10
(f) 19   (m) 20   (t) 9/8
(g) 2/3   (n) 6

Test 7D

(a) Incision to remove stones from the renal pelvis and kidney
(b) Abnormal condition of narrowing of the ureter
(c) Technique of recording/making an X-ray of urethra and bladder
(d) Hernia/protrusion of the bladder
(e) Dilatation of the pelvis

Test 7E

(a) Ureterectasis
(b) Sigmoidoureterostomy
(c) Cystography
(d) Urogram
(e) Nephrosclerosis

The nervous system

Test 8A

(a) 3   (e) 6   (h) 8
(b) 1   (f) 4   (i) 7
(c) 9   (g) 2   (j) 5
(d) 10

Test 8B

(a) 7/8   (h) 13   (o) 20
(b) 19   (i) 4/3   (p) 12
(c) 15   (j) 14   (q) 1
(d) 8/7   (k) 6   (r) 11
(e) 3/4   (l) 2   (s) 9/10
(f) 18   (m) 17   (t) 10/9
(g) 16   (n) 5

Test 8C

(a) 20   (h) 7   (o) 3

(b) 10   (i) 18   (p) 2
(c) 13   (j) 6   (q) 1
(d) 8   (k) 17   (r) 14
(e) 11   (l) 16   (s) 5
(f) 19   (m) 4   (t) 9
(g) 12   (n) 15

Test 8D

(a) 14   (h) 2   (o) 4
(b) 7   (i) 17   (p) 6
(c) 19   (j) 11   (q) 15
(d) 13   (k) 8   (r) 20
(e) 3   (l) 1   (s) 9
(f) 18   (m) 16   (t) 5
(g) 12   (n) 10

Test 8E

(a) Inflammation of the spinal cord and nerves
(b) Incision into the spine
(c) Condition of softening of the meninges
(d) Disease of spinal cord and brain
(e) Instrument to view ventricles

Test 8F

(a) Meningopathy
(b) Cephalometer
(c) Radiculomyelitis
(d) Encephalorrhagia
(e) Neurocytology

The eye

Test 9A

(a) 3   (e) 1   (h) 9
(b) 4   (f) 7   (i) 6
(c) 2   (g) 8   (j) 10
(d) 5

Test 9B

(a) 12   (h) 20   (o) 8
(b) 10   (i) 15   (p) 7
(c) 18   (j) 6   (q) 17
(d) 19   (k) 16   (r) 2
(e) 1   (l) 4/5   (s) 9
(f) 14   (m) 3   (t) 5/4
(g) 13   (n) 11

Test 9C

(a) 17   (h) 10   (o) 3
(b) 14   (i) 4   (p) 11
(c) 9   (j) 2   (q) 5
(d) 18   (k) 20/19 (r) 8
(e) 1   (l) 16/15 (s) 13
(f) 12   (m) 15/16 (t) 7
(g) 19/20 (n) 6

Test 9D

(a) Surgical repair/reconstruction of the eye
(b) Surgical fixation of the retina
(c) Excessive flow of pus from tear ducts
(d) Inflammation of the iris and sclera
(e) Nerve which stimulates movement/action of the eye

Test 9E

(a) Ophthalmoscopy
(b) Blepharitis
(c) Keratopathy
(d) Retinoscope
(e) Iridoplegia

The ear

Test 10A

(a)	8	(e)	3	(h)	1
(b)	5	(f)	4	(i)	6
(c)	7	(g)	10	(j)	2
(d)	9				

Test 10B

(a)	8/9/10	(h)	3	(o)	11
(b)	9/8/10	(i)	15	(p)	13
(c)	14	(j)	17	(q)	2
(d)	10/9/8	(k)	6	(r)	5
(e)	16	(l)	18	(s)	4
(f)	19	(m)	7	(t)	1
(g)	12	(n)	20		

Test 10C

(a)	12	(h)	17	(o)	3
(b)	5/6	(i)	11	(p)	4
(c)	7	(j)	13	(q)	1
(d)	15	(k)	18	(r)	14
(e)	20	(l)	6/5	(s)	8
(f)	2	(m)	16	(t)	9
(g)	10	(n)	19		

Test 10D

(a) Study of the larynx and ear
(b) Hardening within middle ear (around ear ossicles)
(c) Pertaining to the vestibular apparatus and stapes
(d) Pertaining to the malleus and tympanic membrane
(e) Pertaining to the cochlea and vestibular apparatus

Test 10E

(a) Mastoidocentesis
(b) Myringectomy
(c) Otoplasty
(d) Otalgia
(e) Tympanogenic

The skin

Test 11A

(a)	5	(c)	1	(e)	2
(b)	4	(d)	6	(f)	3

Test 11B

(a)	18	(h)	4	(o)	20
(b)	19	(i)	3	(p)	1
(c)	17	(j)	14	(q)	7
(d)	8	(k)	6	(r)	12
(e)	13	(l)	5	(s)	15
(f)	2	(m)	10	(t)	9
(g)	16	(n)	11		

Test 11C

(a)	11	(e)	12	(i)	8
(b)	7	(f)	2	(j)	4/5
(c)	9	(g)	3	(k)	10
(d)	1	(h)	6	(l)	5/4

Test 11D

(a) Abnormal condition of skin plants (fungal infection)
(b) Epidermal cell
(c) Condition of without hair sensation
(d) Tumour of a sweat gland
(e) Abnormal condition of fungi in the epidermis

Test 11E

(a) Dermatitis
(b) Onychosis
(c) Melanonychia
(d) Dermatology
(e) Pachyonychia

The nose and mouth

Test 12A

(a)	4	(d)	5	(g)	3
(b)	8	(e)	2	(h)	1
(c)	6	(f)	7		

Test 12B

(a)	19	(h)	8	(o)	6
(b)	14	(i)	7	(p)	11
(c)	13	(j)	9	(q)	20
(d)	15	(k)	18	(r)	10
(e)	16	(l)	5	(s)	3
(f)	4	(m)	1	(t)	2
(g)	17	(n)	12		

Test 12C

(a)	9	(h)	12	(o)	8
(b)	13	(i)	16/15	(p)	20/19

(c)	15/16	(j)	5	(q)	3
(d)	17	(k)	4	(r)	11
(e)	18	(l)	2	(s)	10
(f)	1	(m)	14	(t)	6
(g)	7	(n)	19/20		

Test 12D

(a) Instrument to measure power/force of the tongue
(b) Measurement of saliva
(c) Inflammation of the tongue and mouth
(d) Splitting of the palate and jaw
(e) Pertaining to formation of/originating in teeth

Test 12E

(a) Sialadenotomy
(b) Palatorrhaphy
(c) Rhinomycosis
(d) Labial
(e) Palatoplasty

The muscular system

Test 13A

(a)	18	(h)	17/16	(o)	7
(b)	15	(i)	3	(p)	10
(c)	8	(j)	19	(q)	20
(d)	13	(k)	1	(r)	11
(e)	9	(l)	5	(s)	12
(f)	2	(m)	4	(t)	14
(g)	16/17	(n)	6		

Test 13B

(a) Instrument which measures electrical activity of muscle
(b) Study of movement
(c) Incision into a tendon and muscle
(d) Without nourishment of muscle (muscle wasting)
(e) Pertaining to an aponeurosis and muscle

Test 13C

(a) Myomalacia
(b) Myogenic
(c) Myopathy
(d) Tenorrhaphy
(e) Tenotomy

The skeletal system

Test 14A

| (a) | 4 | (c) | 2 | (e) | 6 |
| (b) | 3 | (d) | 1 | (f) | 5 |

Test 14B

| (a) | 14/15 | (h) | 13 | (o) | 3 |

(b)	4	(i)	15/14	(p)	2
(c)	18	(j)	20	(q)	6
(d)	12	(k)	11	(r)	16
(e)	7	(l)	8	(s)	5
(f)	19	(m)	9	(t)	10
(g)	17	(n)	1		

Test 14C

(a)	5	(h)	15	(o)	19
(b)	7	(i)	16	(p)	18
(c)	9	(j)	11	(q)	4
(d)	12	(k)	10	(r)	13
(e)	17	(l)	2	(s)	6
(f)	20	(m)	1	(t)	3
(g)	14	(n)	8		

Test 14D

(a) Inflammation of cartilage of a joint
(b) Stone in a bursa
(c) Binding together of vertebrae
(d) Cell which breaks down cartilage
(e) Pertaining to having a hump/hunchback

Test 14E

(a) Arthralgia
(b) Osteosynovitis
(c) Spondylomalacia
(d) Osteoarthropathy
(e) Synovioblast

The male reproductive system

Test 15A

(a)	3	(d)	6	(g)	4
(b)	7	(e)	2	(h)	8
(c)	5	(f)	1		

Test 15B

(a)	16	(h)	13	(o)	14
(b)	18	(i)	20	(p)	19
(c)	3	(j)	12/11	(q)	2
(d)	9	(k)	1	(r)	5
(e)	15	(l)	7	(s)	6
(f)	17	(m)	10	(t)	4
(g)	11/12	(n)	8		

Test 15C

(a)	4	(f)	15	(k)	13
(b)	14	(g)	2	(l)	7
(c)	8	(h)	3	(m)	9
(d)	1	(i)	6	(n)	10
(e)	12	(j)	5	(o)	11

Test 15D

(a) Removal of the epididymes and testes
(b) Flow from the penis (abnormal)

(c)   Removal of the vas deferens and epididymis
(d)   Tying off of the vas deferens
(e)   Condition of sperm in the urine

Test 15E

(a)   Orchidorrhaphy/orchiorrhaphy
(b)   Prostatalgia
(c)   Epididymovasostomy
(d)   Scrotitis
(e)   Prostatorrhoea (Am. prostatorrhea)

The female reproductive system

Test 16A

(a)	3	(d)	6	(g)	8
(b)	4	(e)	2	(h)	7
(c)	1	(f)	5		

Test 16B

(a)	5	(h)	17	(o)	18
(b)	10/11	(i)	7	(p)	8
(c)	12	(j)	15	(q)	16
(d)	19	(k)	3	(r)	1
(e)	20	(l)	13	(s)	14
(f)	2	(m)	6	(t)	9
(g)	4	(n)	11/10		

Test 16C

(a)	22	(j)	4	(r)	9
(b)	17/18	(k)	13/12/14	(s)	7
(c)	16	(l)	5	(t)	23
(d)	8	(m)	10	(u)	15
(e)	1	(n)	19	(v)	14/12/13
(f)	12/13/14	(o)	20/21	(w)	17/18
(g)	24	(p)	21/20	(x)	25
(h)	2/3	(q)	11	(y)	6
(i)	3/2				

Test 16D

(a)   Instrument which measures labour (uterine contractions)
(b)   Removal of the uterus and ovaries
(c)   Surgical fixation of the breasts
(d)   Rupture of the uterus
(e)   Disease of the uterus

Test 16E

(a)   Culdoplasty
(b)   Salpingostomy
(c)   Amniorrhexis
(d)   Colpoptosis
(e)   Colpocytology

The endocrine system

Test 17A

(a)	4	(d)	2	(g)	1

(b)	3	(e)	5	(h)	8
(c)	7	(f)	6		

Test 17B

(a)	16	(h)	10	(o)	9
(b)	11	(i)	15	(p)	4
(c)	20	(j)	2	(q)	5
(d)	1	(k)	7	(r)	12
(e)	19	(l)	3	(s)	14
(f)	8	(m)	17	(t)	13
(g)	18	(n)	6		

Test 17C

(a)   Removal of the parathyroid and thyroid gland
(b)   Pituitary cell
(c)   Enlargement of the adrenal
(d)   Pertaining to acting on/affinity for sugar
(e)   Condition of above normal level of ketones in the blood

Test 17D

(a)   Hyperinsulinism
(b)   Hyponatraemia (Am. hyponatremia)
(c)   Thyrotrophic
(d)   Adrenotropic
(e)   Hypoparathyroidism

Radiology and nuclear medicine

Test 18A

(a)	11	(h)	19	(o)	10
(b)	13	(i)	9	(p)	7
(c)	15	(j)	3	(q)	4
(d)	20	(k)	1	(r)	8
(e)	17	(l)	2	(s)	6
(f)	14	(m)	18	(t)	5
(g)	12	(n)	16		

Test 18B

(a)   Treatment with X-rays
(b)   Specialist who studies sound (ultrasound images)
(c)   Treatment with X-rays and heat
(d)   Instrument which produces a moving X-ray picture
(e)   Technique of making a recording/picture of a slice through the body using ultrasound

Test 18C

(a)   Ultrasonotherapy
(b)   Fluoroscopic
(c)   Scintiangiography
(d)   Thermograph
(e)   Echoencephalography

Oncology

Test 19A

(a)	9	(h)	16	(o)	11

(b)	20	(i)	17	(p)	6	(c)	17	(j)	3	(q)	11
(c)	10	(j)	18	(q)	5	(d)	20	(k)	19	(r)	4
(d)	14	(k)	4	(r)	15	(e)	1	(l)	5/6	(s)	15
(e)	12	(l)	2	(s)	7	(f)	14	(m)	7	(t)	6/5
(f)	3	(m)	19	(t)	8	(g)	2	(n)	16		
(g)	1	(n)	13								

Test 19B

(a) Malignant tumour of fibrous tissue
(b) Malignant glandular tumour of stomach
(c) Malignant tumour of liver cells
(d) Malignant, disordered tumour of the thyroid (refers to appearance of backward growth, i.e. becoming disordered)
(e) Malignant tumour originating in the bronchus

Test 19C

(a) Lymphosarcoma
(b) Chondroma
(c) Osteosarcoma
(d) Neoplasia
(e) Oncotherapy

Anatomical position

Test 20A

(a)	13	(h)	8/9	(o)	10
(b)	18	(i)	12	(p)	9/8

Test 20B

(a)	9	(h)	15	(o)	8/7
(b)	12	(i)	19	(p)	13
(c)	7/8	(j)	5	(q)	10
(d)	14	(k)	18	(r)	3
(e)	1/2	(l)	6	(s)	17
(f)	20	(m)	11	(t)	4
(g)	16	(n)	2/1		

Test 20C

(a) Pertaining to between the phalanges (fingers and toes)
(b) A turning to the right
(c) Pertaining to behind/back of cheek
(d) Pertaining to above the ribs
(e) Pertaining to within cells

Test 20D

(a) Lateral
(b) Laevoversion (Am. levoversion)
(c) Postganglionic
(d) Infrahepatic
(e) Transdermal

Abbreviations

The abbreviations listed here are used in medical records in hospitals and general practice. Students should be aware that whilst certain abbreviations are standard terms others are not and may vary from one hospital or practice to another. Some abbreviations have several different meanings. Those given here are widely used and many are related to the body systems discussed in this book.

A	anaemia (Am. anemia)
AAA	abdominal aortic aneurysm
A&E	accident and emergency
AAFB	acid- and alcohol-fast bacilli
AB1	one abortion
Ab, ab	antibody/abortion
ABC	airway, breathing, circulation
Abdo	abdomen
ABG	arterial blood gases
abor	abortion
ABX	antibiotics
AC	air conduction
ac	ante cibum (before meals/food)
Accom	accommodation of eye
ACE	angiotensin-converting enzyme
ACTH	adrenocorticotrophic hormone
ACU	acute care unit
AD or ad	auris dextra (right ear)
ADA	adenosine deaminase
ADD	attention deficit disorder
ADH	antidiuretic hormone
ADL/ALs	aids to daily living or activities of living
ADR	adverse drug reaction
AEM	ambulatory electrocardiogram monitoring
AF	atrial fibrillation/amniotic fluid
AFB	acid-fast bacilli
AFP	alpha-fetoprotein
A/G	albumin/globulin ratio
Ag	antigen
AGA	appropriate for gestational age
AI	artificial insemination/aortic insufficiency/incompetence
AID	artificial insemination by donor
AIDS	acquired immunodeficiency syndrome
AIH	artificial insemination by husband
A/K	above knee (amputation)
ALL	acute lymphocytic leukaemia (Am. leukemia)
ALS	amyotrophic lateral sclerosis

ALT	alanine transaminase
amb	ambulant/ambulatory
AMI	acute myocardial infarction
AML	acute myeloid leukaemia (Am. leukemia)
ANF	antinuclear factor
ANS	autonomic nervous system
ANT or ant	anterior
APH	antepartum haemorrhage (Am. hemorrhage)
APSAC	acylated plasminogen streptokinase activator complex (anistreplase)
APTT	activated partial thromboplastin time
A-R	apical-radial (pulse)
ARC	aids-related complex
ARDS	adult respiratory distress syndrome
ARF	acute renal failure
AS	auris sinistra (left ear)/alimentary system
ASC	altered state of consciousness
ASCVD	arteriosclerotic cardiovascular disease
ASD	atrial septal defect
ASHD	arteriosclerotic heart disease
ASO	antistreptolysin O
ASOM	acute suppurative otitis media
AST	aspartate transaminase
Astigm	astigmatism of eye
ASX	asymptomatic
ATN	acute tubular necrosis
ATP	adenosine triphosphate
ATS	antitetanus serum
aud	audiology
aur dextr	to the right ear
AV	atrioventricular (1) node (2) bundle/arteriovenous
AVM	arteriovenous malformation
AVP	vasopressin
A&W	alive and well
AXR	abdominal X-ray
AZT	azidothymidine
Ba	barium
BaE	barium enema
BAL	blood alcohol level
BBA	born before arrival
BBB	bundle branch block/blood–brain barrier
BBT	basal body temperature
BC	bone conduction/birth control
BCC	basal cell carcinoma
BCG	bacille Calmette–Guérin
BD or b.d.	bis diurnal (twice a day)

BE	barium enema/bacterial endocarditis
BI	bone injury
BID	brought in dead
b.i.d.	bis in die (twice daily)
B/K	below knee (amputation)
BMR	basal metabolic rate
BM (T)	bone marrow (trephine)/bowel movement
BMT	bone marrow transplant
BNO	bowels not open
BNF	British National Formulary
BOR	bowels open regularly
BP	blood pressure/British Pharmacopoeia
BPH	benign prostatic hypertrophy
BRO	bronchoscopy
BS	blood sugar/bowel sounds/breath sounds
BSE	breast self-examination/bovine spongiform encephalopathy
BSS	blood sugar series
BT	bone tumour/brain tumour/breast tumour/bedtime
BTS	blood transfusion service
BUN	blood urea nitrogen
BX, Bx or bx.	biopsy
c	with
C 1–7	cervical vertebrae
CA, Ca or ca.	cancer/carcinoma
CABG	coronary artery bypass grafting
CACX	cancer of the cervix
CAD	coronary artery disease
CAH	chronic active hepatitis/congenital adrenal hyperplasia
CAL	computer-assisted learning
CAPD	continuous ambulatory peritoneal dialysis
CAT	computerized axial tomography/computer-assisted tomography
CBC	complete blood count
CBE	clinical breast examination
CBF	cerebral blood flow
CCF	congestive cardiac failure/chronic cardiac failure
CCIE	countercurrent immunoelectrophoresis
CCU	coronary care unit
CD	Crohn's disease/curriculum development
CDH	congenital dislocation of the hip joint
CEA	carcinoembryonic antigen
CF	cancer free/cystic fibrosis
CFT	complement fixation test
CFTR	cystic fibrosis transmembrane regulator
CH	cholesterol
CHD	coronary heart disease
CHF	congestive heart failure

CHI	creatinine height index
CHR	chronic
CIBD	chronic inflammatory bowel disease
CIN	cervical intraepithelial neoplasia
CJD	Creutzfeldt–Jakob disease
CL	clubbing
CLL	chronic lymphocytic leukaemia (Am. leukemia)
CMF	cyclophosphamide, methotrexate, 5-fluorouracil
CML	chronic myeloid leukaemia (Am. leukemia)
CMV	cytomegalovirus
CN	cranial nerve
CNS	central nervous system
CO	complains of/cardiac output/carbon monoxide
COAD	chronic obstructive airways disease
COLD	chronic obstructive lung disease
COPD	chronic obstructive pulmonary disease
COP	colloid osmotic pressure
CP	cor pulmonale/cerebral palsy
CPAR	continuous positive airway pressure
CPK	creatinine phosphokinase
CPR	cardiopulmonary resuscitation
CRF	chronic renal failure
CRH	corticotrophin-releasing hormone
C+S	culture and sensitivity (test)
C-sect, or c/sect	caesarean section (Am. cesarean)
CSF	cerebrospinal fluid
CSOM	chronic suppurative otitis media
CSU	catheter specimen of urine
CT	coronary thrombosis/computerized tomography/cerebral tumour/continue treatment
CVA	cerebrovascular accident/costovertebral angle
CVD	cardiovascular disease
CVP	central venous pressure
CVS	cardiovascular system/chorionic villus sampling
Cx	cervix
CXR	chest X-ray
CY	cyanosis
Cysto	cystoscopy
D	diagnosis
DBP	diastolic blood pressure
D & C	dilatation and curettage
DC or d/c	direct current/discharge/discontinue/decrease
DCCT	Diabetes Control and Complications Trial
DD	differential diagnosis
DDA	Dangerous Drugs Act
DDAVP	desmopressin (synthetic vasopressin)
ddC/DDC	dideooxycytidine/zalcitabine
ddI/DDI	didanosine/dideoxyinosine

D & E	dilatation and evacuation	ENG	electronystagmogram
Derm, derm	dermatology	ENT	ear, nose and throat
DES	diethylstilboestrol (Am. diethylstilbestrol)	EOG	electrooculogram
		EOM	extraocular movement
d4T	stavudine	EP	ectopic pregnancy
DIC	disseminated intravascular coagulation	ESR	erythrocyte sedimentation rate
		ERCP	endoscopic retrograde cholangiopancreatography
DIDMOAD	diabetes insipidus, diabetes mellitus, optic atrophy and deafness	ERV	expiratory reserve volume
		ESV	end-systolic volume
Diff	differential blood count (of cell types)	ESWL	extracorporeal shock wave lithotripsy
DIMS	disorders of initiating and maintaining sleep	ET	endotracheal/embryo transfer
		ETF	Eustachian tube function
DIP	distal interphalangeal	EUA	examination under anaesthesia (Am. anesthesia)
DKA	diabetics ketoacidosis		
DM	diabetes mellitus	EXP	expansion
DMD	Duchenne muscular dystrophy	Ez	eczema
dmft	decayed missing and filled teeth (deciduous)		
		FA	folic acid
DMFT	decayed missing and filled teeth (permanent)	FAS	fetal alcohol syndrome
		FB	foreign body/finger breadth/fasting blood sugar
D/N	day/night (frequency of urine)		
DNA	deoxyribose nucleic acid/did not attend	FBC	full blood count
		FBE	full blood examination
DOA	dead on arrival	FBS	fasting blood sugar
DOE	dyspnoea on exertion (Am. dyspnea)	FDIU	fetal death in utero
DOES	disorders of excessive somnolence	FET	forced expiratory technique
DS	Down's syndrome	FEV_1	forced expiratory volume in 1 second
DSA	digital subtraction angiography	FFA	free fatty acids
DTR	deep tendon reflex	FFP	fresh frozen plasma
DTs	delirium tremens	FH	family history
DU	duodenal ulcer	FLP	fasting lipid profile
DUB	dysfunctional uterine bleeding	FNAB	fine needle aspiration biopsy
D+V	diarrhoea (Am. diarrhea) and vomiting	FOBT	fecal occult blood testing
		FP	false positive
DVT	deep venous thrombosis	FRC	functional residual capacity
Dx	diagnosis	FROM	full range of movement
DXT	deep X-ray therapy	FSH	follicle-stimulating hormone
DXRT	deep X-ray radiotherapy	FSHRH	follicle-stimulating hormone releasing hormone
EBM	expressed breast milk		
EBV	Epstein–Barr virus	FTND	full term, normal delivery
ECF	extracellular fluid	FUO	fever of unknown origin
ECG	electrocardiogram	FVC	forced vital capacity
ECSL	extracorporeal shock wave lithotripsy	FX, Fx or fx.	fracture
ECT	electroconvulsive therapy	g	gauge
EDC	expected date of confinement	GA	general anaesthesia (Am. anesthesia)
EDD	expected date of delivery	GABA	gamma-aminobutyric acid
EDV	end-diastolic volume	G&S/XM	group and save/cross-match
EEG	electroencephalography/gram	GB	gall bladder
EENT	eyes, ears, nose and throat	GC	gonococci
EFM	electronic fetal monitoring	GCSF	granulocyte colony stimulating factor
ELISA	enzyme-linked immunosorbent assay	GFR	glomerular filtration rate
Em	emmetropia (good vision)	GGTP	gamma-glutamyl transpeptidase
EMI	elderly mentally infirm	γGT	gamma-glutamyl transferase
EMD	electromechanical dissociation	GH	growth hormone
EMG	electromyogram/electromyography	GHIH	growth hormone-inhibiting hormone
EMU	early morning urine	GHRH	growth hormone-releasing hormone

GHRIH	growth hormone release-inhibiting hormone	HRM	human resource management
GI and GII	gravida I and gravida II (first and second pregnancy)	HRT	hormone replacement therapy
		HSA	human serum albumin
GI	gastrointestinal	HSV	herpes simplex virus
GIFT	gamete intrafallopian transfer	HTLV	human T-cell leukaemia-lymphoma virus (Am. leukemia)
ging	gingiva (gum)		
GIS	gastrointestinal system	HTVD	hypertensive vascular disease
GIT	gastrointestinal tract		
GKI	glucose/potassium/insulin	IABP	intra-aortic balloon pump
GN	glomerulonephritis	IBD	inflammatory bowel disease
GnRH	gonadotrophin-releasing hormone	IBS	irritable bowel syndrome
GR1	one pregnancy	ICF	intracellular fluid
grav	gravid (pregnant)	ICM	intracostal margin
GS	genital system	ICP	intracranial pressure
GTN	glyceryl trinitrate	ICS	intercostal space
gtt	guttae (drops)	ICSH	interstitial cell-stimulating hormone
GTT	glucose tolerance test	ICU	intensive care unit
GU	gastric ulcer/genitourinary	ID or id	intradermal/identity
GUS	genitourinary system	I & D	incision and drainage
GVHD	graft-versus-host disease	IDDM	insulin-dependent diabetes mellitus
Gyn	gynaecology (Am. gynecology)	Ig	immunoglobulin (e.g. IgA, IgG)
		IGT	impaired glucose tolerance
H	hypodermic	IHD	ischaemic heart disease (Am. ischemic)
HAV	hepatitis A virus		
HB or Hb	haemoglobin (Am. hemoglobin)	i.m.	intramuscular
HBGM	home blood glucose monitoring	IM	infectious mononucleosis/ intramuscular
HBsAg	hepatitis B surface antigen		
HBV	hepatitis B virus	IMHP	intramuscular high potency
HC	head circumference	IMP	impression
HCG (hCG)	human chorionic gonadotrophin	IMV	intermittent mandatory ventilation
H/ct or/H.ct	haematocrit (Am. hematocrit)	inf	inferior
HCV	hepatitis C virus	INR	international normalized ratio
HCVD	hypertensive cardiovascular disease	int	inter/between
HD	haemodialysis (Am. hemodialysis)/ Huntington's disease/Hodgkin's disease	IOFB	intraocular foreign body
		IOL	intraocular lens
		IOP	intraocular pressure
		in utero	within uterus
HDLs	high density lipoproteins	i.p.	intraperitoneal
HDV	hepatitis delta virus	IPA	immunosuppressive acid protein
HEENT	head, eyes, ears, nose and throat	IPPB	intermittent positive pressure breathing
HF	heart failure		
HGH or hGH	human growth hormone	IPPV	intermittent positive pressure ventilation
HGP	human genome project		
HHNK	hyperglycaemic (Am. hyperglycemic) hyperosmolar nonketonic	IQ	intelligence quotient
		IRV	inspiratory reserve volume
Hist.	histology (lab)	ISQ	idem status quo (i.e. unchanged)
HIV	human immunodeficiency virus	ITCP	idiopathic thrombocytopenic purpura
HIVD	herniated intervertebral disc	ITP	idiopathic thrombocytopenic purpura
HLA	human leucocyte antigen	ITU	intensive therapy unit
HMG (hMG)	human menopausal gonadotrophin	IU	international units
HOCM	hypertrophic obstructive cardiomyopathy	IUC	idiopathic ulcerative colitis
		IUCD	intrauterine contraceptive device
HO	house officer	IUD	intrauterine death
H & P	history and physical	IUFB	intrauterine foreign body
HPC	history of present condition	IUGR	intrauterine growth retardation
hpf	high power field	IV or i.v.	intravenous
HPI	history of present illness	IVC	inferior vena cava/intravenous cholecystogram
HR	heart rate		

IVF	in vitro fertilization/in vivo fertilization
IVHP	intravenous high potency
IVI	intravenous infusion
IVP	intravenous pyelogram
IVT	intravenous transfusion
IVU	intravenous urography
J	jaundice
JVP	jugular vein pressure/jugular venous pressure
KCCT	kaolin cephalin clotting time
KCO	transfer factor for carbon monoxide
KJ	knee jerk
KO	keep open
KS	Karposi's sarcoma
KUB	kidney, ureter and bladder
KVO	keep vein open
L	lymphadenopathy
(L)	left
L 1–5	lumbar vertebrae
LA	local anaesthetic/left atrium (Am. anesthetic)
La	labial (lips)
LAD	left axis deviation
LaG	labia and gingiva (lips and gums)
LAS	lymphadenopathy syndrome
LAT or lat	lateral
LBBB	left bundle branch block
LCCS	low cervical caesarean section (Am. cesarean)
LD	lethal dose
LDH	lactic dehydrogenase
LDLs	low density lipoproteins
LE	lupus erythematosus
LFTs	liver function tests
LGA	large for gestational age
LH	luteinizing hormone
LHRH	luteinizing hormone-releasing hormone
LIF	left iliac fossa
LIH	left inguinal hernia
LKKS	liver, kidney, kidney, spleen
LLETZ	large loop excision of the transformation zone
LLL	left lower lobe (lung)/left lower lid (eye)
LLQ	left lower quadrant
LMP	last menstrual period
LOC	level of consciousness
LP	lumbar puncture
LSB	long stay bed (geriatric)
LSD	lysergic acid diethylamide
LUQ	left upper quadrant
LV	left ventricle
LVEDP	left ventricular end-diastolic pressure
LVF	left ventricular failure

LVH	left ventricular hypertrophy
Lymphos	lymphocytes
M	murmur
MAb	monoclonal antibody
MAC	mid-arm circumference/*Mycobacterium avium* complex
MAMC	mid-arm muscle circumference
mane	in the morning
MAOI	monoamine oxidase inhibitor
MAP	muscle action potential
MCH	mean corpuscular (red cell) haemoglobin (Am. hemoglobin)
MCHC	mean corpuscular haemoglobin concentration (Am. hemoglobin)
MCL	mid-clavicular line
MCV	mean corpuscular volume
MD	muscular dystrophy
ME	myalgic encephalopathy
med	medial
MEN	multiple endocrine neoplasia
meQ	milliequivalent
mEq/1	milliequivalent per litre
Metas	metastasis
MF	myocardial fibrosis/mycoses fungoides
MFT	muscle function test
MG	myasthenia gravis
MHC	major histocompatibility complex
MHz	megahertz (megacycles per second)
MI	myocardial infarction/mitral incompetence/insufficiency
MIBG	meta-iodobenzyl guanidine
MIC	minimum inhibitory concentration
mmHg	millimetres of mercury
MMM	mitozantrone, methotrexate, mitomycin C
mmol	millimole
MNJ	myoneural junction
MODY	maturity-onset diabetes of the young
MPQ	McGill Pain Questionnaire
MRI	magnetic resonance imaging
mRNA	messenger ribonucleic acid
MRSA	multiple-resistant or methicillin-resistant *Staphylococcus aureus*
MS	mitral stenosis/muscle shortening/muscle strength/musculoskeletal/musculoskeletal system/multiple sclerosis
MSAFP	maternal serum alpha-fetoprotein
MSH	melanocyte-stimulating hormone
MSSU	midstream specimen of urine
MSU	midstream urine
MTA	mid-thigh amputation
My, my	myopia
N	normal
NAD	nothing abnormal discovered/no acute distress

N & V	nausea and vomiting	oto	otology
NANB	non A, non B viruses	OU	oculus unitas (both eyes
NG	nasogastric		together)/oculus uterque
NGU	non-gonococcal urethritis		(for each eye)/oculus utro
NAP	neutrophil alkaline phosphatase		(in each eye)
NAS, nas	nasal/no added salt		
NBM	nil (nothing) by mouth	PA	pulmonary artery/pernicious
NCVs	nerve conduction velocities		anaemia/posterior–anterior
NEC	necrotizing enterocolitis	PABA	para-aminobenzoic acid
NFTD	normal full-term delivery	PAP	primary atypical pneumonia
NIDDM	non-insulin-dependent diabetes	Pap.	Papanicolaou smear test
	mellitus	PAS	p-aminosalycilic acid
NK	natural killer (cells)	PAT	paroxysmal atrial tachycardia
NMR	nuclear magnetic resonance	PAWP	pulmonary artery wedge pressure
#NOF	fractured neck of femur	PBC	primary biliary cirrhosis
NP	nasopharynx	PBI	protein-bound iodine
NPN	non-protein nitrogen	pc	post cibum (after meals/food)
NPO, npo	non per os/nothing by mouth	PCA	patient-controlled analgesia
NREM	non-rapid eye movement (sleep)	PCN	penicillin
NRS	numerical rating scale	PCNL	percutaneous nephrolithotomy
NS	nervous system	pCO_2	partial pressure of carbon dioxide
NSAIDs	non-steroidal anti-inflammatory	PCP	*Pneumocystis carinii* pneumonia
	drugs	PCT	prothrombin clotting time
NSR	normal sinus rhythm	PCV	packed cell volume
NST	non-shivering thermogenesis	PCWP	pulmonary capillary wedge pressure
		PD	Parkinson's disease
OA	osteoarthritis/on admission	PDA	patent ductus arteriosus
OB	occult blood	PE	pulmonary embolism/physical
Ob-Gyn	obstetrics and gynaecology		examination
	(Am. gynecology)	PEC	pneumoencephalogram
Obst-Gyn	obstetrics and gynaecology	PED	paediatrics (Am. pediatrics)
	(Am. gynecology)	PEEP	positive end-expiratory pressure
OC	oral cholecystogram/oral	PEFR	peak expiratory flow rate
	contraceptive	PEM	protein–energy malnutrition
OCP	oral contraceptive pill	PERLAC	pupils equal, react to light,
OD	oculus dexter (right eye)/oculo		accommodation consensual
	dextro (in the right eye)/overdose	PERRLA	pupils equal, round, react to light,
od	every day		accommodation consensual
Odont	odontology	PET	positron emission tomography/
ODQ	on direct questioning		pre-eclamptic toxaemia (Am. toxemia)
OE	otitis externa/on examination	PF	peak flow
OGTT	oral glucose tolerance test	PFTs	pulmonary function tests
OM	otitis media/olim mane	PGL	persistent generalized
	(once daily in the morning)		lymphadenopathy
OOB	out of bed	PID	prolapsed intervertebral disc/pelvic
OPA	outpatient appointment		inflammatory disease
Ophth	ophthalmology	PIH	prolactin inhibiting hormone
OPT	orthopantomogram	PIP	proximal interphalangeal
OR	operating room	PKU	phenylketonuria
Ortho	orthopaedics (Am. orthopedics)	PM	postmortem
Orthop	orthopnoea (Am. orthopnea)	PMB	postmenopausal bleeding
OS	oculus sinister (left eye)/oculo	PMH	past medical history
	sinistro (in left eye)	PMI	point of maximum impulse
Os	mouth	PML	progressive multifocal
osteo	osteomyelitis		leukoencephalopathy
OT	old tuberculin/occupational	PMN	polymorphonuclear leucocytes
	therapy/oxytocin	PMS	premenstrual syndrome
OTC	over the counter (remedies)	PMT	premenstrual tension

PN	percussion note	RAST	radioallergosorbent test
PND	paroxysmal nocturnal dyspnoea (Am. dyspnea)/post-nasal drip	rDNA	recombinant deoxyribose nucleic acid
PNS	peripheral nervous system	RBBB	right bundle branch block
PO or p.o.	per os/by mouth	RBC	red blood count/red blood cell
pO_2	partial pressure of oxygen	RBS	random blood sugar
POAG	primary open angle glaucoma	RCC	red cell count/red cell concentrate
POLY	polymorphonuclear leucocytes	RDA	recommended dietary allowance
POP	plaster of paris	RDS	respiratory distress syndrome
pos	position	RE	rectal examination
post	posterior	REM	rapid eye movement (in sleep)
PPAM	pneumatic post-amputation mobility	RES	reticuloendothelial system
PPD	purified protein derivative (of tuberculin)/packs per day	RF	rheumatoid factor/rheumatic fever
		RFLA	rheumatoid-factor-like activity
PPE	personal protective equipment	RFTs	respiratory function tests
PPH	postpartum haemorrhage (Am. hemorrhage)	Rh	rhesus
		RHD	rheumatic heart disease
PPS	plasma protein solution	RIF	right iliac fossa
PPT	partial prothrombin time	RLE	right lower extremity
p.r. or PR	per rectum/plantar reflex	RLL	right lower lobe
PRH	prolactin-releasing hormone	RLQ	right lower quadrant
PRN or p.r.n.	pro re nata (as required)	RM	radical mastectomy
PRL	prolactin	RNA	ribose nucleic acid
PROG	progesterone	R/O	rule out
PRV	polycythaemia rubra vera (Am. polycythemia)	ROM	range of movement (exercises)
		ROS	review of symptoms
pros	prostate	RPE	retinal pigment epithelial (cells, layer)
prox	proximal		
PSA	prostate-specific antigen	RQ	respiratory quotient
PSCT	pain and symptom control team	RR	recovery room/respiratory rate
PSD	personal and social development	RS	respiratory system
pt or PT	patient/prothrombin time/physical therapy	RSI	repetitive strain injury
		RSV	respiratory syncytial virus
PTA	prior to admission	RT	radiotherapy
PTC	percutaneous transhepatic cholangiogram/graphy	RTA	road traffic accident/renal tubular acidosis
PTCA	percutaneous transluminal coronary angioplasty	RUQ	right upper quadrant
		RV	residual volume/right ventricle
PTH	parathyroid hormone/parathormone	RVF	right ventricular failure
PTR	prothrombin ratio	RVH	right ventricular hypertrophy
PTT	partial thromboplastin time		
PTX	pneumothorax	s	without
PU	peptic ulcer	S1	first heart sound
PUO	pyrexia of unknown origin	S2	second heart sound
PUVA	psoralen + ultraviolet light A	SA	sarcoma/sinus arrhythmia/sinoatrial (node)
PV	per vagina		
PVC	premature ventricular contraction	SACD	subacute combined degeneration
PVD	peripheral vascular disease	SAD	seasonal affective disorder
		SAH	subarachnoid haemorrhage (Am. hemorrhage)
QDS or q.d.s.	quater diurnale summensum (four times a day)		
		SB	seen by
(R)	right	SBE	subacute bacterial endocarditis
RA	rheumatoid arthritis/right auricle/atrium	SBP	systolic blood pressure
		s.c.	subcutaneous/subclavian
Ra	radium	SCC	squamous cell carcinoma
RAD	right axis deviation	SCD	sequential pneumatic compression device/sudden cardiac death
rad	radical		
RAS	reticular activating system	SCID	severe combined immunodeficiency syndrome

SDH	subdural haematoma (Am. hematoma)		THR	total hip replacement
SED	skin erythema dose		TI	thymus-independent cells
SG	skin graft		TIA	transient ischaemic attack (Am. ischemic)
SGA	small for gestational age		TIBC	total iron-binding capacity
SGOT	serum glutamic oxaloacetic transaminase, now serum aspartate transferase		t.i.d.	ter in die (three times daily)
			TIP	terminal interphalangeal
			TIPS	transjugular intrahepatic portosystemic shunting
SCPT	serum glutamic pyruvic transaminase		TJ	triceps jerk
SH	social history		TKVO	to keep vein open
SIADH	syndrome of inappropriate antidiuretic hormone		TLC	total lung capacity/tender loving care
SIDS	sudden infant death syndrome		TLD	thoracic lymph duct
SIG	sigmoidoscopy		TM	tympanic membrane
s.l.	sublingual		TNF	tumour necrosis factor
SLE	systemic lupus erythematosus		TNM	tumour, node, metastases
SLS	social and life skills		TOP	termination of pregnancy
SMD	senile macular degeneration		tPA	recombinant tissue-type plasminogen activator
SOA	swelling of ankles			
SOB	short of breath/stools for occult blood		TPHI	*Treponema pallidum* haemagglutination inhibition (Am. hemagglutination)
SOBOE	short of breath on exertion			
SOS	swelling of sacrum		TPI	*Treponema pallidum* immobilization
SPF	sun protection factor		TPN	total parenteral nutrition
SPP	suprapubic prostatectomy		TPR	temperature, pulse, respiration
SR	sedimentation rate		TRH	thyrotrophin-releasing hormone
SS	saline solution		TSA	tumour-specific antigen
ST	skin test/sinus tachycardia		TSH	thyroid-stimulating hormone
STD	skin test dose/sexually transmitted disease		TSS	toxic shock syndrome
			TT	tetanus toxoid/thrombin clotting time
STU	skin test unit		TTO	to take out (to home)
Subcu	subcutaneous		TUR	transurethral resection (of prostate)
subling	sublingual/under the tongue		TURP	transurethral resection of the prostate
sup	superior			
SV	stroke volume		TURT	transurethral resection of tumour
SVC	superior vena cava		TV	tidal volume
SVT	supraventricular tachycardia		Tx	treatment/therapy
SWS	slow wave sleep			
Sx	symptoms		U	unit
syph.	syphilis		UA	uric acid/urinalysis
			U & E	urea and electrolytes
T	tumour/temperature		UG	urogenital
t	terminal		UGH	uveitis + glaucoma + hyphaema syndrome (Am. hyphema)
T1–12	thoracic vertebrae			
T_3, T_4	triiodothyronine, tetraiodothyronine (thyroid hormones)		UGI	upper gastrointestinal
			ung	ointment (unguentum)
T & A	tonsils and adenoids or tonsillectomy/adenoidectomy		URI	upper respiratory (tract) infection
			URT	upper respiratory tract
TAH	total abdominal hysterectomy		URTI	upper respiratory tract infection
Tb or TB	tuberculosis (tubercle bacillus)		US	ultrasonography/ultrasound/urinary system
TBG	thyroid-binding globulin			
TBW	total body water		USS	ultrasound scan
TCP	thrombocytopenia		UVA	ultraviolet light A
TD	thymus-dependent cells		UVB	ultraviolet light B
TDS	ter diurnale summensum (three times a day)		UVC	ultraviolet light C
			UTI	urinary tract infection
TED	thromboembolic deterrent (stockings)			
TENS	transcutaneous electrical nerve stimulation		VA	visual acuity

VAC	vincristine, adriamycin, cyclophosphamide
VAS	visual analogue scale
VD	venereal disease
VDRL	venereal disease research laboratory (test)
VE	vaginal examination
VF	visual field/ventricular fibrillation
VMA	vanillyl-mandelic acid
VP	venous pressure
VRS	verbal rating scale
VS	vital signs
VSD	ventricular septal defect
VT	ventricular tachycardia
VWF	von Willebrand factor
VV	varicose veins/vulva and vagina
WBC	white blood (cell) count/white blood cell
WCC	white cell count
WNL	within normal limits
WPW	Wolff–Parkinson–White
WR	Wasserman reaction (test for syphilis)
X-match	cross-match
XR	X-ray
XRT	X-ray therapy
ZN	Ziehl–Neelsen stain

Symbols

♂	male
♀	female
*	birth
α	alpha
β	beta
γ	gamma
Δ	delta/diagnosis
ΔΔ	differential diagnosis
#	fracture
†	dead

Glossary

Here is a reference list of prefixes, suffixes and combining forms frequently used in medical words. Use this list to decipher the meaning of unfamiliar words. Note, a dash is added to indicate whether the component usually precedes or follows the other elements of a compound word, e.g. ante- precedes a word root as in **ante**natal whilst -algia follows the root as in neur**algia**. The combining vowels of roots are used or dropped by the application of rules described in the introduction to this book.

a-	without, not (n is added before words beginning with a vowel)
ab-	away from
abdomin/o	abdomen
ac-	to/toward/near/pertaining to
acanth/o	spiny
acar/i/o	mites of the order Acarina
acarin/o	mites of the order Acarina
acetabul/o	acetabulum
acet/o	vinegar
aceton-	ketones/acetone
achill/o	Achilles tendon
acid/o	acid
acin/i	sac-like dilatation
acou-	hear/hearing
-acousia	condition of hearing
acoust/o	hear/hearing/sound
acro-	extremities, point
acromi/o	acromion
act-	do, drive, act
actin/o	rays, e.g. of sun/ultraviolet radiation
acu-	hear/hearing/severe/sudden
ad-	to/toward/in the direction of
adamant/o	dental enamel
aden/o	gland
adenoid/o	adenoid
adip/o	adipose tissue/fat
adren/o	adrenal gland
adrenocortic/o	adrenal cortex
-aem-	blood
-aemia	condition of blood
aer/o	air/gas
aesthesi/o	sensation/sensitivity
aeti/o	cause
af-	to/towards/near
ag-	to/towards/near
agglutin/o	sticking/clumping together
-agogic	pertaining to inducing/stimulating
-agogue	inducing/promoting

agora-	market place/open space
-agra	seizure/sudden pain
-al	pertaining to
alb/o	white
albin/o	white
album-	white
albumin/o	albumin/albumen
alg/o	pain
algesi/o	sense of pain
-algia	condition of pain
all/o	other/different from normal
alve/o	trough/channel/cavity
alveol/o	alveoli (of lungs)
ambi-	on both sides
ambyl/o	dull/dim
ameb/o (Am.)	ameba, a type of protozoan
amel/o	dental enamel
-amine	nitrogen-containing compound
amni/o	amnion/fetal membrane
amoeb/o	amoeba, a type of protozoan (Am. ameb/o)
amph/i	both/doubly
amyl/o	starch
an-	without/not
ana-	backward/apart/up/again
an/o	anus
andr/o	male
aneurysm/o	aneurysm
angi/o	vessel
aniso-	unequal/dissimilar
ankyl/o	crooked/stiffening/fusing/bent
-ant	having the characteristic of
ante-	before in time or place/in front
anter/o	front/in front of
anthrac/o	coal dust
anthrop/o	man/human
ant/i	against
antr/o	antrum/maxillary sinus
aort/o	aorta
ap-	to/toward/near
-apheresis	removal
ap/o	away from/detached/derived from
aponeur/o	aponeurosis (flat tendon)
append/ic/o	appendix
aqua-	water
-ar	pertaining to
arachn/o	spider
-arch/e-	beginning
arrhen/o	male/masculine
arteri/o	artery
arteriol/o	arteriole

arthr/o	joint	cac/o	bad/ill/abnormal
articul/o	joint	caec/o	caecum (Am. cecum)
-ary	pertaining to/connected with	calcane/o	calcaneus/heel bone
as-	to/towards/near	calc/i	calcium/lime/heel
-ase	an enzyme	calcin/o	calcium
-asia	state or condition	cali/o	calyx/cup-shaped organ or cavity (Am. calix) .
-asis	state or condition		
asthen/o	weakness	calor/i	heat
at-	to/towards/near	cancer/o	cancer (general term)
atel-	imperfect/incomplete	canth/o	canthus
ather/o	porridge-like plaque lining blood vessel	capit-	head
		-capnia	condition relating to carbon (dioxide)
-ation	action/condition		
atri/o	atrium	caps-	container
audi/o	hearing	carb/o	carbon/bicarbonate
-aural	pertaining to the ear	carcin/o	cancerous/malignant
aur/i	ear	-cardia	condition of heart
auricul/o	ear/pinna	cardi/o	heart
auto-	self	carp/o	carpal/wrist bones
aux/i	increase	cary/o	nucleus
-auxis	increase	cat/a	down/negative
aux/o	increase	caud-	tail
axill/o	armpit	caudad	towards the tail
ax/o	axis	cav-	hollow
axi/o	axis	cec/o (Am.)	cecum
axon/o	axis	-cele	swelling/protrusion/hernia
azot/o	urea/nitrogen	celi/o	abdomen
		cel/o (Am.)	hollow
ba-	go/walk/stand	cell-	cell
bacill/o	bacillus (a bacterium)	cen/o	new/empty/common
bacter/i/o	rod	-centesis	surgical puncture to remove fluid
balan/o	glans penis	centi-	hundred/one-hundredth
ball-	throw/movement	centr/i/o	centre/central location
bar/o	weight/pressure	cephalad-	towards the head
bartholin/o	Bartholin's glands of vagina	cephal/o	head
basi-	base/basic/alkaline	cerat/o	horny/epidermis/cornea (syn. kerat/o)
baso-	basic/alkaline		
bathy-	deep	cerebell/o	cerebellum
bi-	two/twice/life	cerebr/o	cerebrum/brain
bili-	bile	cer/o	wax
bin-	two each/double	cerumin/o	cerumen/ear wax
bio-	life/living	cervic/o	cervix
blast/o	early/growth/germ/development	-chalasis	slackening/loosening
-blast	germ cell/embryonic/immature/ growing thing	cheil/o	lip
		cheir/o	hand
blenn/o	mucus	chem/o	chemical
blephar/o	eyelid	chir/o	hand
bol-	ball	chlor/o	green/chlorine
brachi/o	arm	chol/e	bile
brachy-	short	cholecyst/o	gall bladder
brady-	slow	choledoch/o	common bile duct
bromidr/o	stench/smell of sweat	cholester/o	cholesterol
bronchi/o	bronchus/bronchial tube	chondr/o	cartilage
bronchiol/o	bronchiole	chord/o	string/cord
bronch/o	bronchus/windpipe	chori/o	chorion/outer fetal membrane
bucca-	cheek	choroid/o	choroid layer of eye
bucc/o	cheek	chromat/o	colour
burs/o	bursa (fluid-filled sac)	chrom/o	colour

-chromia	haemoglobin (Am. hemoglobin)/ pertaining to colour
chron/o	time
chrys/o	gold
chyl/o	chyle, lymphatic fluid formed by lacteals in intestine
chym/o	chyme, creamy material produced by digestion of food
-cide	something that kills/killing
cili/o	cilia/ciliary body of eye/eyelash
cinemat/o	movement/motion (picture)
cine/o	movement/motion
circum-	around
cirrh/o	yellow
cirs/o	varicose vein/varix
-cis-	cut/kill
cistern/o	cistern/enclosed space (subarachnoid space)
-clasis	breaking
-clast	a cell which breaks
claustr/o	barrier
clavicul/o	clavicle
cleid/o	clavicle
clin/o	bend/incline
clitor/i/o	clitoris
-clysis	infusion/injection/irrigation
co-	with/together
-coccus	bacterium (berry-like structure)
coccyg/o	coccyx
cochle/o	cochlea
coel/o	hollow
col-	with/together
col/o	colon
colon/o	colon
colp/o	vagina
com-	with/together
con-	with/together
coni/o	dust
conjunctiv/o	conjunctiva
contra-	against/opposite
-conus	cone-like protrusion
copr/o	faeces (Am. feces)
cor-	with/together
cord/o	a cord
corne/o	cornea/horny (consisting of keratin)
cor/o	pupil
core/o	pupil
coron/o-	crown-like projection/encircling
corpor/o	body
cortex-	outer part/bark
cortic/o	cortex
cost/o	rib
crani/o	skull
cren/o	crenated
-crine	secrete
crin/o	secrete
-crit	separate/device for measuring cells

crur/o	leg
cry/o	relating to cold
crypt/o	hidden
culd/o	cul-de-sac/rectouterine pouch
cut-	skin
cutane/o	skin
cyan/o	blue
cycl/o	ciliary body
-cyesis	pregnancy
cyst/o	bladder
-cyte	cell
cyt/o	cell
-cytosis	abnormal increase/condition of cells
dacry/o	tear/lacrimal apparatus
dacryocyst/o	lacrimal sac
dactyl/o	digits/fingers or toes
de-	down/away from/loss of/ reversing
deca-	ten
deci-	one-tenth
dendr/o	tree/tree-like
dentin/o	dentine of tooth (Am. dentin)
dent/o	tooth
derm/a	skin
dermat/o	skin
derm/o	skin
descemet/o	Descemet's membrane (of cornea)
-desis	fixation/to bind together by surgery/sticking together
desm/o	band/ligament
dextro-	right
di-	two/double
dia-	through/apart/across/between
-dialysis	separate
diaphor/o	sweating (excessive)
didym-	twin
digit/o	finger/toe
dipl/o-	double
dips/o	thirst
dis-	reversal/separation/duplication
disc/o	intervertebral disc (Am. disk/o)
disk/o (Am.)	intervertebral disc
dist/o	far from point of origin
diverticul/o	diverticulum
doch/o	duct/to receive
dolor/i/o	pain (dol – unit of pain)
-dorsal	pertaining to back (of body)
dors/i	back (of body)
dorso-	back (of body)
-drome	a course/conduction/flowing
drom/o	a course/conduction/flowing
duoden/o	duodenum
dur/o	dura mater/hard
dynam/o	force/power
-dynia	condition of pain
dys-	difficult/painful/bad

e-	out/outside
-eal	pertaining to
ec-	out/outside/away from
ech/o	reflected sound/echo
ect-	out/outside/outer part
ecto-	out/outside/outer part
-ectasis	dilatation, stretching
-ectomy	removal, excision
-edema (Am.)	swelling due to fluid
ef-	out/away from
eikon/o	icon
electro-	electrical
ellipto-	shaped like an ellipse
em-	in
-ema	swelling/distension
embol/o	embolus/plug/blockage
-emesis	vomiting
-emia (Am.)	condition of blood
emmetr/o	in due measure
-emphraxis	blocking/stopping up
en-	within/in
encephal/o	brain
end/o	within, inside
endometri/o	endometrium of uterus (lining)
enter/o	intestine
ento-	within, inside
eosin/o	red/dawn-coloured/like eosin, a red acid dye
ep-	above/upon/on
epi-	above/upon/on
epididym/o	epididymis
epiglott/o	epiglottis
epilept/i/o	epilepsy
episi/o	vulva
-er	one who
erg/o/n/o	work
-erysis	drag/draw/suck out
erythr/o	red
-esis	state/condition
es/o (Am.)	within
esophag/o (Am.)	esophagus/gullet
esthesi/o (Am.)	sensation/sensitivity
estr/o (Am.)	estrogen/female/estrus
ethm/o	ethmoid bone
eti-	causation
eu-	good/normal/easily
eury-	wide/broad
ex-	out/out of/away from
exo-	out/away from/outside
-externa	external
extra-	outside of
faci/o	face
falc/i	falx/sickle-shaped structure
fasci/o	fascia/fibrous tissue, e.g. covering muscles
febr/o	fever
fec/o (Am.)	feces
femor/o	femur/thigh

fer/o	to carry/to bear
ferr/o	iron
fet/o	fetus
fibr/o	fibre
fibrin/o	fibrinogen
fibul/o	fibula
fil/o	thread
flagell/o	flagellum/whip
flav/o	yellow
fluor/o	fluorescent/luminous/flow
foet/o	foetus
follicul/o	small sac/follicle
fore-	before/in front of
-form	having form of
front-	front/forehead
-fuge	agent that suppresses/gets rid of
furc/o	branching
galact/o	milk
gangli/o	ganglion/swelling/plexus
gastr/o	stomach
-gen-	cause/produce/originate
-gen	agent that produces/precursor, e.g. pepsinogen
-genesis	capable of causing/pertaining to formation
-genic	pertaining to formation/originating in
ger-	old age/the aged
ger/o	old age/the aged
geront/o	old age/the aged
gingiv/o	gum
gli/o	glue-like (pertains to neuroglial cells of CNS)
-globin	protein
-globulin	protein
glomerul/o	glomerulus of kidney
gloss/o	tongue
gluc/o	sugar/sweet
glyc/o	sugar/sweet
glycogen/o	glycogen, a polysaccharide
glycos	sugar (obsolete variant of glucose)
gnath/o	jaw
-gno-	to know/known or knowledge/judgment
-gnos-	to know/known or knowledge/judgment
-gnosis	to know/known or knowledge/judgment
gon/o	seed/semen/knee
gonad/o	gonads (ovaries or testes)
gonecyst/o	seminal vesicle
goni/o	angle/corner
gony/o	knee
-grade	to go
-gram	X-ray/tracing/recording/one-thousandth of a kilogram (g)

granul/o	granule/granular		condition resulting from
-graph	usually recording instrument/a recording/X-ray/mathematical curve representing data	-iatr/o	medical treatment/doctor
		-ic	pertaining to
		ichthy/o	dry/scaly/fish-like
-graphy	technique of recording/making X-ray	-ician	person associated with
		-ics	art or science of
-gravida	pregnancy/pregnant woman	icter/o	jaundice
gyn-	woman	-ide	binary chemical compound, e.g. glycoside
gynaec/o	woman (Am. gynec/o)		
gyne-	woman	idi/o	self/one's own/peculiar to an organism
gyn/o	woman		
gynec/o (Am.)	woman	il-	in/none
-gyric	pertaining to circular motion	ile/o	ileum
		ili/o	ilium/flank
haem/a	blood (Am. hem/a)	im-	in/none/not
haem/o	blood (Am. hem/o)	immun/o	immune
haemat/o	blood (Am. hemat/o)	in-	in/none/not
haemoglobin/o	haemoglobin (Am. hemoglobin)	-in	used as suffix for various chemicals, e.g. glycerin
hallux	great toe		
hapt-	touch	incud/o	anvil/incus (ear ossicle)
hecto-	one hundred	-ine	used as suffix for chemicals derived or thought to be derived from ammonia, e.g. amine
helc/o	ulcer		
heli/o	sun		
helic/o	helix/spiral form	infer/o	inferior
helmint/h/o	worms	infra-	below/inferior to
hem/a (Am.)	blood	inguin/o	groin
hem/o (Am.)	blood	insulin/o	insulin
hemat/o (Am.)	blood	inter-	between
hemi-	half/on one side	-interna	internal
hepat/o	liver	intestin/o	intestine
hepatic/o	hepatic bile duct	intra-	within/inside
hept/a	seven	intro-	into/within
herni/o	hernia	intus-	in/into
heter/o	other/another/different	-ion	action/condition resulting from action
hex-	six/hold/being		
hidr/o	sweat/perspiration	-ior	pertaining to
histi/o	type of macrophage (histiocyte)	ipsi-	the same/self
hist/o	tissue	ir-	in/none/not
hol/o	entire/whole	ir/o	iris
homeo-	alike/resembling/unchanging/constant	irid/o	iris
		isch/o	condition of holding back/reducing/suppress
homo-	the same		
humer/o	humerus	ischi/o	ischium
hyal/o	glass-like	-ism	process/state or condition
hydatid/i/o	hydatid cyst	is/o-	same/equal
hydr/o	water	-ist	specialist
hygr/o	moisture	-ite	end product, e.g. metabolite
hymen/o	hymen	-itis	inflammation
hy/o	hyoid bone	-ium	structure/anatomical part
hyper-	above normal/excessive/over	-ive	pertaining to
hypn/o	sleep		
hypo-	below normal/under	jejun/o	jejunum
hyster/o	uterus/womb	juxta-	adjoining/near
-ia	condition of	kal/i	potassium
-iac	pertaining to	kary/o	nucleus
-ian	pertaining to	kerat/o	horny/epidermis/cornea
-iasis	abnormal condition/process or	ket/o/n	ketones/carbonyl group

kine-	movement	-lytic	pertaining to breakdown/ disintegration
kinesi/o	movement		
-kinesis	a movement		
kinet/o	movement	macro-	large
kilo-	one-thousand	macul/o	spot/blotch
kolp/o (Am.)	vagina	mal-	bad/diseased or impaired
-kymia	condition of involuntary twitching of muscle/a wave of contraction in a muscle	-malacia	condition of softening
		malle/o	hammer/malleus (ear ossicle)
		mamm/o	breast/mammary gland
kyph/o	crooked/hump	man/o	pressure/hand
		mandibul/o	mandible
labi/o	lip	mast/o	breast/mammary gland
labyrinth/o	labyrinth of ear	mastoid/o	nipple-shaped/mastoid process
lacrim/o	tear/tear ducts/lacrimal apparatus	maxill/o	maxilla
lact/i/o	milk	medi-	middle
laevo-	left (Am. levo-)	-media	middle
-lalia	condition of talking	-medulla	inner part
lamell/a	thin leaf or plate	mega-	abnormally large
lamin/o	lamina/thin plate/part of vertebral arch	megal/o	abnormally large
		-megaly	enlargement
lapar/o	abdomen/flank	melan/o	melanin/dark pigment
-lapaxy	empty/wash out/evacuate	mening/o	membranes (of CNS)
laryng/o	larynx	menisc/o	meniscus
later/o	side	men/o	menses/menstruation/monthly flow
lei/o	smooth		
leiomy/o	smooth muscle	ment/o	chin/mind
lent/i	lens	meso-	middle/intermediate
lept/o	thin/fine/slender	meta-	change in form/position/after
leuc/o	white	metacarp/o	metacarpal
leuk/o	white	metatars/o	metatarsal
levo- (Am.)	left	-meter	measuring instrument
-lexia	condition of speech/words	-metrist	person who measures
lien/o	spleen	metr/o	uterus/womb/a measure
-ligation	tying off of a vessel with a suture	-metry	process of measuring
lingu/a/o	tongue	micro-	small/one-millionth
lip/o	fat/fatty tissue	-mileusis	to carve
lith/o	stone	milli-	one-thousandth
-lith-	stone	mi/o	make smaller/less
-lithiasis	abnormal condition of stones	mito-	thread-like
lob/o	lobe	mono-	one/single
lochi/o	vaginal discharge (lochia)	morph/o	shape/form
-logist	specialist who studies	mort/o	death
log/o	words/speech/study	motor	moving/action/set in motion
-logy	study of	muc/o	mucus
lord/o	bend forward	multi-	many
lumb/o	loin/lower back	muscul/o	muscle
lute/o	yellow/corpus luteum of ovary	my- (from myein)	to close/squint
lymph/o	lymph	myc/o	fungus
lymphaden/o	lymph gland	mycet/o	fungus
lymphangi/o	lymph vessel	myel/o	bone marrow/spinal cord
-lyo-	breakdown/disintegration/ dissolve	my/o	muscle
		myocardi/o	myocardium (heart muscle)
-lys-	breakdown/disintegration/ dissolve	myom/a	muscle tumour
		myring/o	ear drum/tympanic membrane
-lysis	breakdown/disintegration/ dissolve	myx/o	mucus
-lyt-	breakdown/disintegration/ dissolve	nano-	one billionth (10^{-9})
		narc/o	stupor/numbness

nas/o	nose	orch/i/o	testis
-natal	pertaining to birth	orchid/o	testis
nat/o	birth	organ/o	organ
natr/i	sodium	orth/o-	straight
necr/o	death/dead tissue	-ory	pertaining to
neo-	new	os-	body/oral cavity/bone
nephr/o	kidney	-ose	carbohydrate/sugars/starches/
neur/o	nerve (rarely tendon)		full of/pertaining to
neutr/o	neutral	-osis	abnormal condition/disease
noc/i	harm		of/abnormal increase
noct/i	night/darkness	osm/o	odour/smell/osmosis
nom/o	distribute	oss-	bone
non-	without	ossicul/o	ear ossicles/bones
normo-	normal	ost/e/o	bone
nos/o	disease	ot/o	ear
not/o	back	-ous	pertaining to
nucle/o	nucleus	ov-	egg/ovum
nulli-	none	ovari/o	ovary
nyct/o	night/darkness	-oxia	condition of oxygen
-nyxis	perforation/pricking/puncture	ox/o	oxygen
		oxy-	oxygen
obstetric-	pertaining to midwifery		
occipt/o	occiput, posterior region of the	pachy-	thick
	skull	paed/o	child (Am. ped/o)
octa-	eight	palat/o	palate
ocul/o	eye	palm/o	palm
odont/o	tooth/teeth	palpebr/a	eyelid
-oedema	swelling due to fluid (Am. edema)	pan-	all
oes/o	within	pancreat/o	pancreas
oesophag/o	oesophagus/gullet	pancreatic/o	pancreatic duct
oestr/o	oestrogen/female/oestrus	pannicul/o	fatty layer, e.g. of abdomen
-oid	resembling	papill/o	nipple-like/optic disc
olecran/o	elbow/olecranon (bony projection	para-	beside/near
	of ulna)	-para(re)	to bear/bring forth offspring
ole/o	oil		(woman who has borne viable
olig/o	deficiency/few/little		young)
-olithesis	slipping	parathyr/o	parathyroid gland
-oma	tumour/swelling	parathyroid/o	parathyroid gland
oment/o	omentum (peritoneal fold of	-paresis	slight paralysis
	stomach)	-parous	pertaining to production of live
om/o	shoulder		young
omphal/o	umbilicus	-partum	birth
onc/o	tumour/mass	patell/o	patella/knee cap
onych/o	nail	-pathia	condition of disease
oo-	egg	pathic	pertaining to disease
oophor/o	ovary	path/o	disease
-op-	seeing/looking at	-pathy	disease/emotion
ophthalm/o	eye	-pause	stopping
-ophthalmos	eye	pect-	chest/breast/thorax
-opia	condition of vision/defective	ped/o (Am.)	foot/(child
	vision	pelv/i/o	pelvis
opistho-	backward	-penia	lack of/condition of deficiency
-opsia	condition of vision/defective	peps-	digestion/pepsin
	vision	pept-	digestion/pepsin
optic/o	vision/eye/optic nerve	per-	throughout/completely
opt/o	vision/eye	peri-	around
orbit/o	orbit (bony cavity) of eye	pericardi/o	pericardium
or/o	mouth	perine/o	perineum

peritone/o	peritoneum	-pnoea	breathing (Am. -pnea)
petr/o	stone/rock	pod/o	foot
-pexy	surgical fixation/fix in place	pogon/o	beard
phac/o	lens	-poiesis	formation
phag/o	eating/consuming	poikil/o	varied/irregular
-phagia	condition of eating/swallowing	polio-	grey matter (of CNS)
-phagy	eating or swallowing	pollex	thumb
phak/o	lens	poly-	many/much
phalang/o	phalange/finger/toe	polyp/o	polyp/small growth
phall/o	penis	pont/o	pons (part of metencephalon of brain)
pharm-	pharmacy		
pharmac/o	drug/medicine	por/o	passage/pore
pharyng/o	pharynx	port/o	portal vein
-phasia	condition of speaking/speech	post-	after/behind
phe/o	dusky/dark	poster/o	back of body/behind/posterior
-phil	loving/affinity for	posth/o	prepuce/foreskin
phleb/o	vein	-prandial	meal
-phobia	condition of fear	-praxia	condition of purposeful movement/conduct
phon/o	sound/voice		
-phonia	condition of having voice	pre-	before/in front of
-phoresis	carrying	preputi/o	prepuce/foreskin
-phoria	condition of mental state/feeling	presby/o	old man/old age
phot/o	light	primi-	first
phren/o	diaphragm/mind/phrenic nerve	pro-	before/favouring
phthisis	wasting away	proct/o	rectum/anus
-phyma	tumour/boil	progest/o	progesterone
phys/i/o-	nature/physical things	prostat/o	prostate gland
-physis	growth	prosth/o	adding (replacement part)
-phyt/e/o	plant/fungus	proto-	first
pil/o	hair	proxim/o	near
pineal/o	pineal gland	pseudo-	false
pituitar-	pituitary gland	psych/o	mind
placent/o	placenta	-ptosis	falling/displacement/prolapse
-plakia	condition of broad/flat (patch)	-ptotic	pertaining to falling/displacement/prolapse
-plania	condition of wandering, e.g. a cell moving position		
		ptyal/o	saliva
plan/o	flat	-ptysis	spitting/cough up
plant/i	sole of foot	pub/o	pubis
-plasia	condition of growth/formation (increase in number of cells)	pulm/o	lung
		pulmon/o	lung
-plasm	formative substance	pupill/o	pupil
plasma-	plasma cell	pyel/o	pelvis/trough of kidney
plasm/o	anything moulded, shaped or formed/formative substance/growth	pyle/o	portal vein
		pylor/o	pylorus
		py/o	pus
-plasty	surgical repair/reconstruction	pyr/o	heat/fire/burning
platy-	flat		
-plegia	condition of paralysis	quadr/i/u-	four
pleo-	more	quinqu-	five
plethysm/o	volume	quint-	five
pleur/o	pleural membranes/rib/side		
plex/o	network of nerves, blood or lymph vessels	rachi/o	spine
		radic/o	nerve root
-plexy	strike/paralyse	radicul/o	nerve root
-pnea (Am.)	breathing	radi/o	radiation/X-ray/radius
pneum/a/o	gas/air also lung/breath	re-	back/contrary/again
pneumat/o	gas/air/breath	rect/o	rectum
pneumon/o	lung/air	ren/o	kidney

reticul/o	net-like/reticulum	sex-	six
retin/o	retina	sial/o	saliva/salivary glands
retro-	backwards/behind	sialaden/o	salivary glands
rhabd/o	striated/striped	sider/o	iron
rhabdomy/o	striated muscle	sigmoid/o	sigmoid colon
rhe/o	electric current/flow	sinistr/o	left/left side
rheumat/o	rheumatism	sin/o	sinus
rhin/o	nose	sinus/o	sinus
rhiz/o	root/nerve root	sinus-	sinus
rhod/o	red	-sis	condition/state of
roentgen/o	X-ray/Roentgen rays	sit/o	food
-rostral-	superior/pertaining to or resembling a rostrum/beak	somat/o	body
		somn/i/o	sleep
-rrhage	bursting forth of blood/bleeding	son/o	sound
-rrhagia	condition of bursting forth of blood/bleeding	-spadia	condition of drawing out
		-spasm	involuntary contraction of muscle
-rrhaphy	suture/suturing/stitching	sperm/i/o	sperm
-rrhea (Am.)	excessive discharge/flow	spermat/o	sperm
-rrhexis	breaking/rupturing	sphen/o	sphenoid bone/wedge-shaped
-rrhoea	excessive discharge/flow (Am. -rrhea)	spher/o	sphere-shaped/round
		sphincter/o	sphincter/ring-like muscle
rubr-	red	sphygm/o	pulse
		-sphyx-	pulsing
sacchar/o	sugar/sweet	spir/o	to breathe
sacr/o	sacrum	splanchn/o	viscera/splanchnic nerve
salping/o	Eustachian tube/Fallopian tube	splen/o	spleen
sangui-	blood	spondyl/o	vertebra/vertebrae/spinal column
sapr/o	decay/decayed matter	spongi/o	sponge-like
sarc/o	fleshy/connective tissue	spor/o	spore
sarcomat/o	sarcoma (malignant tumour, e.g. of connective tissues)	stapedi/o	stirrup/stapes (ear ossicle)
		staphyl/o	resembling bunch of grapes/clusters
scapul/o	scapula		
scat/o	faeces/faecal matter (Am. feces)	-stasis	stopping/controlling/cessation of movement
-schisis	cleaving/splitting/parting		
schiz/o	split/cleft/divided	-static	pertaining to stopping/controlling/standing
scint/i	spark/flash of light		
scirrh/o	hard	-staxis	dripping/a dropping, e.g. of blood
scler/o	hard/sclera (white of eye)	stear/o	fat
-sclerosis	abnormal condition of hardening	steat/o	fat
scoli/o	crooked/twisted	sten/o	narrow/constricted
-scope	instrument to view	-stenosis	abnormal condition of narrowing
-scopist	specialist who uses viewing instrument	sterc/o	faeces (Am. feces)
		ster/e/o	solid/three-dimensional
-scopy	visual examination	stern/o	sternum
scot/o	darkness	steth/o	chest/breast
scotom/o	scotoma/blind spot	-sthenia	strength
scrot/o	scrotum	stomat/o	mouth
seb/o	sebum	stom/o	mouth
-sect (ion)	cut	-stomy	to form a new opening or outlet/communication/an opening
secundi-	second		
semi-	half/partly	strept/o	twisted chain
semin/i	semen	styl/o	stake/styloid process (of temporal bone)
sens/o	sense		
sensor/i	sense/sensation	sub-	under
seps/o	infection	sud/o	sweat/perspiration
septic/o	sepsis/infection/putrefaction	super/o	superior/above/excess
sept/o	septum, e.g. nasal septum	supra-	above/over
ser/o	serum	sy-	with/together

syl-	with/together	-trauma	injury/wound
sym-	with/together	-tresia	condition of an opening
sympathic/o	sympathetic nervous system/nerves	tri-	three
		trich/o	hair
symphisi/o	symphysis pubis	trichin/o	*Trichinella spiralis* (parasitic nematode worm)
syn-	together/in association		
syndesm/o	ligament/connective tissue	trigon/o	trigone
-synechia	condition of adhering together	-tripsy	act of crushing
synovi/o	synovial fluid/membranes	-triptor	instrument designed to crush or fragment
syring/o	tube/cavity		
		-trite	instrument designed to crush or fragment
tachy-	fast		
tact-	touch	-trophic	pertaining to nourishment
tars/o	tarsus/ankle	-trophy	nourishment/development/ increase in cell size
tax/o	ordered movement		
-taxia	condition of ordered movement	-tropia	condition of turning
tele-	far away/operating at a distance	-tropic	pertaining to affinity for/ stimulating/changing in response to a stimulus
telo-	end		
ten/o	tendon		
tend/o	tendon	-tubal	pertaining to a tube
tendin/o	tendon	tympan/o	tympanic membrane/middle ear
tenont/o	tendon	typhl/o	caecum (Am. cecum)
ter-	three		
terat/o	monster/deformed fetus	uln/o	ulna
testicul/o	testicle/testis	ul/o	scar/gingiva (gums)
tetra-	four	ultra-	beyond
thalam/o	thalamus (part of cerebral cortex)	-um	thing/structure
thanat/o	death	un-	not/opposite of/release from
thec/o	sheath	ungu/o	nail
thel/e/o	nipple	uni-	one
-therapy	treatment	-ur-	urine
-thermia	condition of heat	uran/o	palate
therm/o	heat	-uresis	excrete in urine/urinate
-thermy	heat	ureter/o	ureter
thorac/o	thorax	urethr/o	urethra
thromb/o	thrombus/clot	-uria	condition of urine/urination
thrombocyt/o	platelet	urin/a/o	urine
thym/o	thymus gland	ur/o	urine/urinary tract
thymic/o	thymus gland	-us	thing/structure/anatomical part
thyr/o	thyroid gland	uter/o	uterus
thyroid/o	thyroid gland	uve/o	uvea (pigmented parts of eye)
tibi/o	tibia	uvul/o	uvula
-tic	pertaining to		
toc/o	labour/birth	vagin/o	vagina
-tome	cutting instrument	valv/o	valve
tom/o	slice/section	valvul/o	valve
-tomy	incision into	varic/o	dilated veins/varicose vein
-tonia	condition of tension/tone	vas/o	vessel
ton/o	stretching/tension/tone	vascul/o	vessel
tonsill/o	tonsil	ven/o	vein
top/o	place/particular area	venacav/o	vena cava/great vein
tox/o	poison	ventricul/o	ventricle of heart or brain
tox/i	poison	ventro-	belly side of body
toxic/o	poison	-version	turning
-toxic	pertaining to poisoning	vertebr/o	vertebra
trache/o	trachea	vesic/o	bladder/blister
trachel/o	neck	vesicul/o	seminal vesicle
trans-	across	vestibul/o	vestibule of inner ear

viscer/o	viscera/internal organs (esp. abdomen)	xer/o	dry
		xiph/i/o	xiphoid process
viv/i	life		
vit/o	life	-y	process/condition
vitre/o	glass		
vol/o	palm	zo/o	animal
vulv/o	vulva	zyg/o	joined
xanth/o	yellow		
xen/o	strange/foreign		